Child Public Health

Child Public Health

SECOND EDITION

Mitch Blair
Sarah Stewart-Brown
Tony Waterston
Rachel Crowther

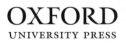

OXFORD
UNIVERSITY PRESS

OXFORD
UNIVERSITY PRESS

Great Clarendon Street, Oxford OX2 6DP

Oxford University Press is a department of the University of Oxford.
It furthers the University's objective of excellence in research, scholarship,
and education by publishing worldwide in

Oxford New York

Auckland Cape Town Dar es Salaam Hong Kong Karachi
Kuala Lumpur Madrid Melbourne Mexico City Nairobi
New Delhi Shanghai Taipei Toronto

With offices in

Argentina Austria Brazil Chile Czech Republic France Greece
Guatemala Hungary Italy Japan Poland Portugal Singapore
South Korea Switzerland Thailand Turkey Ukraine Vietnam

Oxford is a registered trade mark of Oxford University Press
in the UK and in certain other countries

Published in the United States
by Oxford University Press Inc., New York

© Oxford University Press, 2010

The moral rights of the author have been asserted
Database right Oxford University Press (maker)

First edition published 2003
Reprinted 2004
Second edition published 2010

British Library Cataloguing in Publication Data
Data available

Library of Congress Cataloging in Publication Data
Data available

Typeset in Minion by Glyph International Bangalore, India
Printed in Great Britain
on acid-free paper by
Clays Ltd, St Ives

ISBN 978-0-19-954750-0

10 9 8 7 6 5 4 3 2 1

Oxford University Press makes no representation, express or implied, that the drug
dosages in this book are correct. Readers must therefore always check the product
information and clinical procedures with the most up-to-date published product
information and data sheets provided by the manufacturers and the most recent codes of
conduct and safety regulations. The authors and the publishers do not accept responsibility
or legal liability for any errors in the text or for the misuse or misapplication of material in
this work. Except where otherwise stated, drug dosages and recommendations are for the
non-pregnant adult who is not breastfeeding.

To our children and our parents and to all those who have, or have had, the power and will to transform the health and wellbeing of children.

Foreword

A plaque on the wall of a community child health clinic in one of the most deprived parts of south London reads: 'The health of the people is the highest law.' As a junior doctor, whenever I cycled past this building I was inspired again and again by these wise words of Cicero's. I wanted my future to be more about promoting and protecting health and preventing disease among the people at large, than treading the traditional path through one-on-one medical care.

That simple aspiration is the essence of public health – together with the inherent drive to eliminate inequity and reduce inequalities. And nowhere in the broad field of public health are these challenges more up-front and pivotal than in the world of children and young people.

What makes child public health so exciting? Is it because the health and wellbeing of children and young people are crucial in terms of the rest of their lives? Is it because the inequalities brought to bear in childhood can have such profound effects? Is it because of the kaleidoscopic complexity of factors influencing a child's health? Or is it because things happen so fast with children, you have to get it right first time?

To my mind it is all of these things and more. The stuff of child public health has such potency and immediacy, such breadth and depth, so many facets and nuances, and carries such huge responsibilities. It is a great melting pot of influences – genes, family, peers, school, behaviour, environment, culture, practice, health systems, macroeconomics, climate. Child public health is where nature and nurture come together with explosive life-changing force. It is at the core of all public health.

And to address this enormity, the scope of this book is truly immense. The authors have taken a commendably broad, all-embracing approach – examining the changing patterns of child health and disease in the UK and internationally, analysing the key determinants, drawing upon important lessons from the past, and then moving on to look at child public health in practice, illustrated by a series of scenarios dealing with common child public health challenges in today's world.

But to my mind one of this book's most compelling themes is the way it conveys the new energy and dynamism in child public health. There is a real sense of moving to a different level. Working in new ways, making new connections across many disciplines and sectors, winning new hearts and minds. The book in effect spearheads a whole new movement embracing the concepts of human rights and social justice.

So much so that I now have the barely controllable urge to go back to that plaque on the clinic wall in south London and scrawl an addendum: 'But the health of children is the heart of humanity.'

Professor Alan Maryon-Davis FRCP, FFPH,
President, UK Faculty of Public Health
London

Foreword

It gives me great pleasure to write the foreword for the second edition of *Child Public Health*. In my experience as a Medical School Dean, when medical students set off on their journey through medical school, public health is rarely top of their list of ambitions compared to the more dramatic and exciting specialties of surgery, intensive care and neonatology. However, for me, an introduction to public health as an undergraduate was an epiphany. In my naivety, as a young student, I had not appreciated until then how much of health is determined by our environment and social background. After graduation, having chosen to specialise in paediatrics, it became even more apparent to me that the inequalities of one generation are visited on the next generation. It became clear that poor nutrition, passive smoking and poverty in pregnancy and childhood stored up long-term consequences for the health of adults. With most common paediatric problems such as cot death, asthma, gastroenteritis, child abuse, childhood accidents and teenage pregnancy there is a very steep social gradient. In improving the health of children globally, measures to improve water sanitation and hygiene have had infinitely more impact than new tests and treatments. To improve the health of children in developed countries, the quickest wins would result from bringing the health of children from the poorest sections of society up to the current standard of health of those from the most affluent sections.

This second edition gives a fascinating overview of the whole field of public health as it pertains to children, with a broad introduction on the need for public health and then chapters on epidemiology, determinants, prevention and transition to adult health. Interspersed with these chapters on the core body of knowledge which underpins public health are helpful sections on definitions, approaches to research and public health for the practitioner with 'real world' scenarios.

I warmly commend this book to you and congratulate the authors on their very important contribution.

Professor Terence Stephenson
President, Royal College of Paediatrics and Child Health

Contents

Authors' biographies

Mitch Blair MSc, FRCPCH, FFPH
Mitch Blair is Reader in Paediatrics and Child Public Health at Imperial College London, Consultant Paediatrician at Northwick Park Hospital Harrow and Hon Professor at Thames Valley University. He has held posts in London and Nottingham. He has a long standing interest in undergraduate and postgraduate teaching, and research interests in child health promotion programmes, international child health indicators and complementary medicines use in children. He is married and has two adult children.

Sarah Stewart-Brown BM BCh, PhD, FFPH, FRCPCH, FRCP
Sarah Stewart-Brown is Professor of Public Health and Director of the Health Sciences Research Institute at Warwick Medical School in the University of Warwick, England. During her career she has worked in both NHS and academic public health and paediatrics. She has a long standing interest in the public health issues of childhood as they relate to children and parents, and as they relate to future adults. In recent years she has focused on emotional and social development as the bedrock on which future health and wellbeing is founded. She has two children and one grandchild.

Tony Waterston MD FRCPCH
Tony Waterston is a retired consultant paediatrician living in Newcastle upon Tyne. He worked for over twenty years as a community paediatrician in an inner city area where families face a high level of deprivation, following spells as a clinician and teacher in Zambia and Zimbabwe. His main interests are the health consequences of poverttitten extensively. He has lead the advocacy work of the Royal College of Paediatrics and Child Health and established their paediatric teaching programme in the occupied Palestinian territories. He has three children and three grandchildren.

Rachel Crowther MB BChir, MSc, FFPH
Rachel Crowther is a consultant in public health medicine working at the South East Public Health Observatory in Oxford. Her special interests are in child public health and health intelligence, and she has contributed to several books in the fields of public health and paediatrics. She is also interested in teaching, especially the integration of public health teaching into other curricula, medical and otherwise. She has five children aged between four and eighteen and currently lives in a boarding house in a secondary school in which she plays an active pastoral role. She also writes fiction and has had a number of short stories published.

Why child public health?

Who is this book for?

For well over a century, policy makers and medical professionals alike have understood the importance of child health for society. Healthy children have a much greater chance of growing up into strong, healthy, fulfilled, and productive adults, able themselves to nurture the next generation and carry society forwards—but that is not all. Ensuring that our children are healthy and happy is an important end in itself. The right of children to enjoy childhood to the fullest extent possible is enshrined in the United Nations Convention on the Rights of the Child as well as in the legal framework of many countries. Children make up around 20% of the UK population, and as much as 50% in some other countries. They are a vulnerable group, politically disempowered as non-voters with no formal civic representation. They need others to advocate for them and to ensure that their rights—including the right to health—are protected.

Child public health involves promoting the health and wellbeing of young people in the widest sense. It requires the commitment and co-operation of a wide range of individuals and organizations: not only those working in health, social care, and education (including professionals, managers, commissioners, and policy makers) but also local and national government (including departments of transport, housing, and leisure); the voluntary sector, at local, national, and international levels; the police force, legal, and criminal justice systems; and of course children and young people themselves, and their parents, families, friends, and carers. This book is for all these people. It aims to support all health care professionals interested in the health of children and young people, especially those working or training in the fields of public health, primary care, and paediatrics. It also provides an introduction to the principles and practice of child public health for everyone with an interest in the subject—from doctors, nurses, and public health practitioners to social workers and teachers, managers and commissioners, and from parents and voluntary workers to probation officers.

For those working in child health in both community and hospital settings, this book aims to explore the preventive aspects of clinical practice, demonstrating the importance of public health principles both in everyday practice and in the planning of future services. For the public health professional with a wide portfolio to address, it seeks to highlight some common public health issues specific to children that are amenable to the approaches described in later chapters. Primary health care teams are being given an increasingly important role in the modern NHS with regard to health needs assessment and the commissioning of services. This text will appeal to primary care professionals with an interest in children's health and will help them with these responsibilities. Mental health is a key issue for child health today, and this book will also be of value to professionals working in child and adolescent mental health services, who have an interest in prevention.

Some of the material will be familiar to some readers, but the aim is to bridge a number of divides—between branches of the medical profession, between different professions and disciplines, between the statutory and voluntary sectors, and between the professional and lay perspective. We hope that there will be something here to interest and inform every reader.

Whilst the book has been written by people working in the UK and uses mainly UK examples, the global perspective is well recognized, and the principles and approaches espoused are relevant to those practising or intending to practice child public health throughout the developed world.

What is child public health?

Definitions of health and of public health are dealt with in some detail in Chapter 4. Suffice it to say here that child public health is neither a single nor a simple entity, and that it involves a range of ideals, activities, and academic disciplines. It covers the study of patterns of health and illness in children and young people, investigation of the factors which affect their health, and the ways in which we—as individuals, organizations, professions, and societies—can modify these factors in order to improve the health and wellbeing of all young people. We define child public health as

> The art and science of promoting and protecting health and wellbeing and preventing disease in infants, children, and young people, through the skills and organized efforts of professionals, practitioners, their teams, wider organizations, and society as a whole.

We have chosen not to define precisely what we mean by a child, nor to divide this book into sections according to the various age groups that make up childhood and adolescence. This is partly because we perceive the process of growing up as a continuous one, which different individuals undertake at different paces. Although the patterns of ill health and the factors influencing health shift as a child gets older, many of the important determinants of child health, and resulting health problems, affect children and young people at several different stages of development. This book is structured on a thematic basis, recognizing the need for action across a range of ages, sectors, and professional boundaries. Its inclusive approach covers children from conception through to the teenage years, and the transition to adulthood.

Although children and young people themselves are of central importance, it is essential to see them in context—within their families, communities, environments, and wider social and political setting. All these constitute layers of influence on the individual child and the child population, and spheres of activity for child public health practice. We cannot hope to improve the lot of children and young people, now or in the future, without addressing social policy, family relationships, environmental concerns, and community structures (see Chapter 4).

Why is child public health important?

Child public health is emerging—or perhaps re-emerging—as a subspecialty of both public health and paediatrics, and as a broadly based interdisciplinary movement. We have already hinted at some of the reasons why this is a welcome and an important development and why, therefore, we feel the need to devote a whole book to public health with a child focus.

Defining a common interest

As a secondary interest of many professionals and practitioners but the particular focus of few, child public health has tended until recently to fall between several different stools. Most current public health literature and action addresses the proportionately (and literally!) larger adult population. Very few public health practitioners have a predominantly child health focus, perhaps with the exception of health visitors and school nurses.

Many of those working in paediatrics and general practice tend to focus on personal health services and interventions at the level of the individual, and are not used to considering problems or solutions at community or population level. Most have, however, noticed considerable changes in their case loads and the problems presenting to them over the last few decades. These changes often reflect social, economic, and political factors as well as medical ones, and need to be tackled at population level as well as through individual consultations.

The public health and clinical approaches are often presented in contrast to one another, as qualitatively different ways of responding to health and disease. The former is seen to focus on populations and the latter on individuals—or the one 'upstream', concerned with the causes of ill health, and the other 'downstream', dealing with the consequences. In practice, many child health workers combine individual and population perspectives in their day-to-day work and share a similar aim—that of optimizing the health and wellbeing of all children and young people. Defining common ground, and understanding what those with different backgrounds can contribute to the common cause, is an important objective of child public health.

But the need for common understanding and co-operation goes much wider than the health sector. Many teachers, social workers, educational psychologists, and others working with children in a variety of disciplines are becoming increasingly aware that health and behaviour problems impinge on, and are affected by, factors within their own spheres of operation. Many, however, feel they lack the means—or indeed the time—to address them.

There is a need to draw together all these perspectives into a coherent movement that tackles the health and health-related problems of children. Those working with and for children across different disciplines need to act together on the broader determinants of child health. This means acquiring new knowledge and skills and working in new ways, and this book aims to provide some of the necessary information and tools.

Understanding and responding to changes in child health

A key objective of child public health is to explore and elucidate changes in health and disease in children, to provide professionals with the tools needed to assess the health needs of their child population, and to provide guidance on appropriate ways of meeting them.

There has been a major shift in the patterns of morbidity and mortality (ill health and death) over the past century in developed countries, and it is important to understand the reasons for these changes and to respond to them.

As the burden of perinatal and infant mortality, infectious disease, and malnutrition has declined, there has been an increase in multifactorial disorders and conditions which require a more complex preventive approach. These include mental, emotional, and behavioural problems, physical and neurodevelopmental disabilities, and problems like obesity and asthma, which are attributable to changes in how we live and the environment we create for ourselves. These are often referred to as 'millennial' morbidities, and they require an eclectic approach and set of skills in order to tackle them.

Child health as an end in itself and as a major determinant of adult health

Children deserve the best possible health and protection from harmful influences. The United Nations Convention on the Rights of the Child enshrines many important principles of child public health, including the right of children to health, safety, identity, to be heard and listened to, and to participate in their health care. As a society, we have a responsibility to ensure that children have as good a start in life as we can give them, and can enjoy their early years as free as they can be from disease, disability, and distress, with their wishes and needs understood and respected.

In particular, we have a responsibility towards less advantaged children in this and other countries—children whose rights are more likely to be infringed and whose health, development, and self-expression is more likely to be compromised. Inequalities in health are common, as we shall see: those from the lowest social class have twice the chance of dying before their first birthday as those from the highest social class, and almost all illnesses and causes of death are more common in poorer and socially excluded children. The collective endeavour that is child public health has a crucial role in safeguarding children's rights, tackling health inequalities in children, and ensuring that children's health is kept at the forefront of social policy, health care planning, and our national (and international) conscience.

Recent research has illuminated the contribution which exposure to physical and emotional factors in infancy and childhood makes to adult health and disease. This has added additional impetus to research on child health and to the development of disease prevention and health promotion initiatives among children as future adults.

Pioneers in child public health

A number of pioneering individuals from different parts of the world and different professional backgrounds have brought a public health perspective to bear on child health problems over the last couple of centuries, making significant contributions to the health and wellbeing of children and setting examples of the wide sphere of influence of child public health interventions. Some of their work is described below.

United Kingdom

One of the earliest pioneers of child public health, Edward Jenner (1749–1823), a Gloucestershire country physician, made the important observation that milkmaids who had contracted cowpox seemed to be immune from catching smallpox. Jenner inoculated a small boy, James Phepps, with cowpox material by scratching it onto his arm, and then proceeded to test his hypothesis by inoculating him with smallpox. The discovery that James was indeed protected from smallpox heralded the era of vaccination and the later development of what remains one of the most successful preventive measures available to the medical profession.

John Snow (1813–1858) is also remembered for his historic contribution to tackling cholera. During the London cholera epidemic of 1854, over five hundred people died in ten days within a radius of 250 yards of Broad Street. Snow's meticulous geographical plotting of the cases, and exploration of their water supply, led to the conclusion that the Broad Street water pump was the source of the disease and to the removal of the pump handle to prevent further cases. Cholera is associated with a high mortality rate in infants and children and can devastate the lives of those who do not die by leaving them as orphans. Snow's work had an indirect as well as a direct effect on child health; the famous episode of the Broad Street pump contributed significantly to the evidence for infectious agents as specific causes of disease, opening the door to the

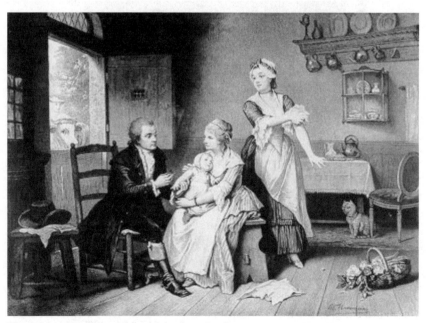

Fig. 1 Edward Jenner and the birth of vaccination.

treatment and prevention of the infectious diseases that constituted a major cause of mortality and morbidity in children at the time.

Edwin Chadwick (1800–1890) was Secretary to the Poor Law Commissioners. Together with Anthony Cooper, the Seventh Earl of Shaftesbury, he was instrumental in protecting the wellbeing of children by limiting the age at which they could be legally employed in the factories and mills of the time. The Factory Act of 1833 excluded children under the age of nine from working in factories, limited work by children under fourteen to 48 hours per week, and made provision for them to attend school for at least two hours a day. Opponents to the Act were concerned that the country's industrial welfare would be severely threatened by the loss of two hours labour per day of up to 30,000 girl workers, fearing that 'our manufacturing supremacy would depart from us'. Chadwick also authored a major review of the sanitary condition of the labouring classes in England and Wales, published in 1842. Amongst his recommendations were the development of water and sanitation supplies to major towns—a public health measure to help prevent the cholera epidemics like that from the Broad Street pump. At this time, four out of five houses in Birmingham and eleven out of twelve in Newcastle had no water supply. Chadwick was said to be a harsh, domineering man, but he had the qualities of persistence and tenacity often required to make fundamental changes in social policy.

Charles Dickens (1812–1870) was another influential child public health figure. His novels and serials, in particular *Oliver Twist* and *David Copperfield*, described the effects of the Industrial Revolution and the immense social changes of the nineteenth century and gave a vivid picture of the plight of children living in poor social

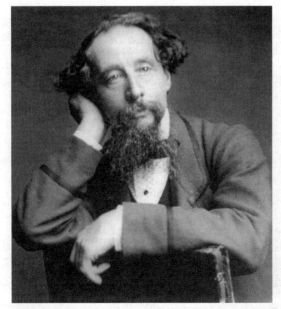

Fig. 2 Charles Dickens.
From Ackroyd P. Dickens Public Life and Private Passion. BBC Books 2002.
Source: © Getty Images, with permission.

circumstances. His attention to detail often caused shock and disbelief at his public readings. His work as an advocate for children was recognized in his invitation to speak at the opening of the Hospital for Sick Children in Great Ormond Street, London.

James Spence (1892–1954) was the first Professor of Child Health (as opposed to clinical paediatrics) in England and set up the first babies' hospital where mothers could 'room in' (stay in the hospital with their children). His survey of the causes of infant mortality in the North East, undertaken with the co-operation of the city councils, was one of the first population-based (as opposed to hospital-based) investigations carried out by a paediatrician. He took a similar 'community approach' with the establishment of the 'Thousand Families' project, which followed up all babies born in May and June of 1947. This was one of the first studies to show clearly the association between poverty and ill health. It was also one of the first studies to show that the ill effects of poverty could be traced from one generation to another in intergenerational cycles of disadvantage.

Donald Court (1912–1994) succeeded James Spence on his death, and was influential for his recognition of the importance of community paediatric services, and for his calls to strengthen the study of social determinants of health and disease in the child and family. Court ensured that these factors were included in the education of health

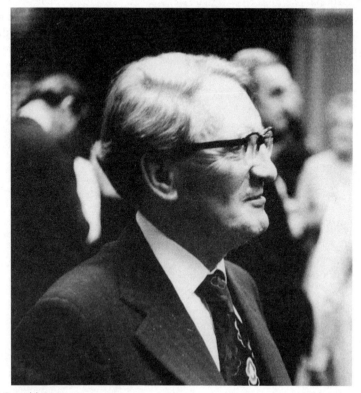

Fig. 3 Donald Court.
Source: Used with kind permission of the Court family.

professionals. He chaired the UK Commission of Enquiry into the Child Health Services, 'Fit for the Future', which reported in 1976 and recommended the establishment of multidisciplinary teams, integrated community and hospital paediatric services, and primary paediatric care delivered by GPs. Court always maintained that preventive medicine should be given the same status as curative medicine:

> Without continuing enquiry, there is no progression. My plea is that we should apply the same critical energy to the study of social as we do to cellular behaviour.

Whilst working in Nigeria in the 1950s, the paediatrician Professor David Morley (1923–2009) revolutionized child health care. He set up under-fives clinics, training local women to immunize children, chart their growth, and educate the local population about family health. He was probably the originator of the parent-held child health record, a concept which, like charting children's growth, spread to the developed world. He developed low cost alternatives to inhalers (plastic bottles), and measures for preparing oral rehydration fluids (the two ended spoon), and set up a charity which provided low cost educational aids. His prime philosophy was of empowerment of local people. His writing has been profoundly influential for child health workers in the Third World.

Europe

Lennart Kohler (1933) trained as a paediatrician and became the head of child health services in Sweden. He was professor, first in social and preventive medicine, then in social paediatrics at the Nordic School of Public Health in Goteborg. He was also Dean

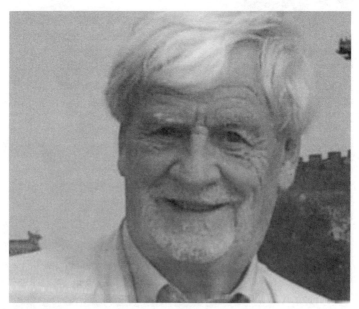

Fig. 4 Lennart Kohler.
Source: Used with kind permission of Lennart Kohler.

of the Nordic School för many years. He developed the concept of social paediatrics, and in 1977, founded the European Society of Social Paediatrics (ESSOP) – an organization which is still bringing together not only Europeans, but also like-minded Australians and Americans. Social paediatrics is defined as a global, holistic, and multidisciplinary approach to child health; it considers the health of children within the context of their society, environment, school, and family. It thus integrates the physical, mental, and social dimensions of child health and development as well as care, prevention, and promotion of health and quality of life. Social paediatrics acts in three areas – child health problems with social causes, child health problems with social consequences, and child health care in society. The concept was gradually widened into child public health and, in many ways, Lennart Kohler can be seen as the father of child public health. He developed research in the field as well as developing numerous courses, which attracted public health researchers, health planners, physicians, psychologists, social workers, and nurses from all of the Nordic countries and also from further afield.

United States of America

Abraham Jacobi (1830–1919) was a radical socialist paediatrician, the first Professor in the Diseases of Children in the US and President of the American Medical Association. On the basis of careful studies of the causes of infant mortality, he called for the development of high-quality maternity services and midwifery schools. He was a great advocate of breast-feeding, especially amongst the poor of New York, and was one of the first to speak out against artificial milk manufacturers. He recognized the need for doctors to:

> … enlighten and direct public opinion in regard to the broad problems of hygiene, and of representing to the world the practical accomplishments of scientific medicine.

During the 1870s, Jacobi set up summer corps of doctors to work in the tenements of New York – a case of positive discrimination in health service provision towards those most in need. In later decades, he was heavily involved in the formation of the Society for the Prevention of Cruelty to Children and other welfare organizations.

James P. Grant (1922–1995) led UNICEF as its third executive director from 1980. Over the period of the next 15 years, he was responsible for a worldwide campaign, 'child survival revolution', which saved the lives of at least 25 million children by mobilizing international, national, and local initiatives to improve immunization, oral rehydration therapy, and breastfeeding. The campaign was helped enormously by the then Director General of the WHO, Dr Halfdan Mahler, who was the architect of the Alma Ata declaration on primary health care in 1978. Between 1981 and 1990, the worldwide vaccination rate for children increased from 20% to 80%. Grant also helped to bring about the adoption by the UN General Assembly, in 1989, of the Convention on the Rights of the Child. This led ultimately to the World Summit for Children, when heads of state and government gathered to create a global plan of action and to establish concrete goals for children's health, education, wellbeing, and protection.

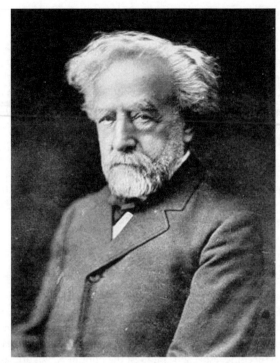

Fig. 5 Abraham Jacobi.

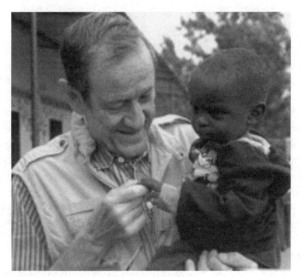

Fig. 6 James Grant.
Source: UNICEF/NYHQ1994–0481/press, with permission.

Australia

Professor Fiona Stanley worked as a doctor with aboriginal communities in Western Australia, drawing attention to the profound effect of the environment on child health. She developed a unique population database (Western Australian Maternal and Child Health Research Database) to predict trends in maternal and child health and the effects of preventive programmes. She and her colleagues made the connection between the lack of folic acid in mothers' diets and spina bifida in babies. In 1990, Stanley became the founding director of the Telethon Institute for Child Health Research in Perth, a multidisciplinary research facility that investigates the causes and prevention of major childhood diseases and disabilities. She was instrumental in launching the Australian Research Alliance for Children and Youth, which aims to progress collaboration and evidence-based action to improve the wellbeing of young Australians. She often uses the phrase 'modernity's paradox' (coined by Professor Clyde Hertzman) to describe the way that the boon of increasing wealth and opportunity has also resulted in increased social differences and more problems for children and young people.

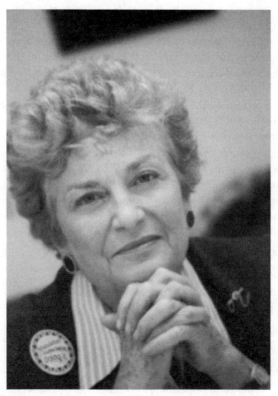

Fig. 7 Fiona Stanley.
Source: With kind permission of Fiona Stanley.

The structure of this book

The rest of this book is divided into eight chapters. The first describes the landscape of child health in the UK and Europe. The second highlights the very different child health problems facing developing countries, many related to poverty, and outlines the significant connection and interdependence that exists between the developed and developing worlds. This chapter aims to provide a global perspective for child health in the UK and suggests that international child health should be a matter of concern for us all. Chapter 3 describes the major determinants of child health, reflecting on major changes in recent decades and setting out the key challenges for child public health today.

Chapter 4 provides an historical review of child public health. It explains how the cause of child health has fared through the centuries, highlighting key milestones and identifying lessons for practice today. These are particularly important to draw on as the agenda for child health is redefined at the start of the twenty-first century. Chapter 5 covers some essential concepts and definitions in child public health practice. It explores the nature of health and disease, the epidemiological notions of causality and risk, and some of the key activities of public health including health promotion and disease prevention. This chapter aims to provide a brief overview for those exploring these topics for the first time, and should also be a useful refresher for those trained in public health, offering a child health perspective on familiar concepts.

One of the most exciting areas of research in recent years has been the unravelling of how early human growth and development affects later adult health. Chapter 6 provides a critical review of current knowledge about these links, exploring the implications this has for child public health.

The last two chapters move the reader from theoretical to practical matters. Chapter 7 addresses techniques and resources for assessing health needs, comparing the clinical and public health process of making a 'diagnosis', and describes the sources of information available to support public health practice. It also considers approaches to evaluation and the generation of evidence in public health, and shows how these differ from approaches appropriate to clinical care. The final chapter contains an overview of the community diagnosis process in practice through ten child public health scenarios, each of which considers a different issue. The aim is to illustrate a range of 'real' problems in child public health and possible approaches to tackling them. The topics covered are:

- walking the patch–developing a public health approach to a locality
- promoting infant mental health
- reducing unintentional injury due to motor vehicles
- promoting breast-feeding
- child health surveillance programmes–delay in diagnoses
- mitigating the impact of social deprivation
- investigating declining vaccine uptake
- investigating systems for responding to child deaths from abuse

◆ responding to the epidemic of youth obesity

◆ a whole country approach to tackling child malnutrition

Each scenario aims to 'bring to life' the approaches and techniques described in earlier chapters, applying them to key child public health issues with down-to-earth descriptions of child public health in practice. It is hoped that they will help practitioners from a range of disciplines to get started on addressing the problems they face in their own practice.

Chapter 1

Child health in the UK and Europe

A time traveller from a previous century would probably conclude that most children in Europe today are extremely healthy and that most of their needs are met. There have been great advances in living conditions and technology which have led to increased survival over the last 150 years. Child mortality and morbidity have fallen dramatically, children are growing taller, they are participating more in society, disease and disability are better treated, and there are better and more focused services for preschool children. Improvements have been achieved in the treatment of childhood cancer, in mortality and morbidity from accidents, and of course in the prevention and treatment of infectious diseases. There is no doubt that we have much to be proud of and that children in the UK and Europe are healthier than at almost any time in the past. This is due largely to improved nutrition and housing, smaller families, water and sewage treatment, and also to the beneficial effects of immunization and a highly successful 'Back to Sleep' campaign in the 1990s to reduce Sudden Infant Death syndrome (SIDS) (Fig. 1.1).

Yet the last 50 years have witnessed profound changes to the lives of children in Europe and in other parts of the developed world—in family structure, socioeconomic environment, transport, communications technology, lifestyle and the type of food we eat—and the perceptive time traveller would also notice a new set of child health problems, some of which may not be manifest until later in life. Emotional, behavioural and mental health problems are increasingly pervasive. Teachers in inner-city schools report difficulties in controlling children's behaviour even in the Reception Year, and many older children are beyond the control of their parents. Truancy rates are increasing, and newspapers carry stories about crimes committed by children as young as 10 or 11. Obesity in childhood has risen sharply; more young people are committing suicide; smoking and binge drinking are at epidemic proportions in teenagers. Children watch more and more television, and the use of mobile phones is increasing dramatically. These phenomena significantly affect children's patterns of social interaction and have consequences for their health.

Certain groups of children—including children of asylum seekers, those with disabilities, and the socially excluded—fail to benefit from the opportunities available to others in society. Up to 20% of UK children are considered to be vulnerable or in need (see box).

Vulnerable children—children who would benefit from extra help from public agencies to optimize their life chances and for the risk of social exclusion to be averted. They include:

+ Children in public care
+ Children with disabilities
+ Pupils with behaviour and attendance problems
+ Children in need of protection
+ Children in need of family support
+ Young offenders
+ Young carers
+ Children and adolescents with mental health problems
+ Young drug misusers
+ Teenage parents
+ Children of asylum seekers

Children in need—a subset of vulnerable children who are in need of protection or family support, or in public care.

These children often have a very different experience of life—and of health—from their peers.

Although many of these new child health problems present to health professionals, including GPs, paediatricians, health visitors, school nurses, and child psychiatrists, these are problems which cannot be solved by health services alone. As Chapter 3 will illustrate, their causes lie in a wide range of social, economic, and environmental factors, and in order to tackle them action is needed across just as broad a spectrum. Professionals in other voluntary and statutory agencies (including education, social services, probation, and the police) encounter the same problems, and have a shared

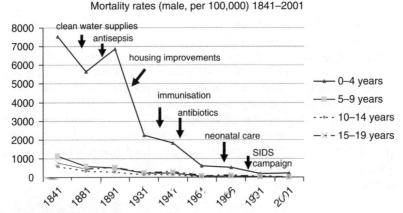

Fig. 1.1 Changing mortality and ameliorative measures.

interest in addressing them. The child public health approach—assessing and grappling with the determinants of health through joint working with a wide range of agencies and the involvement of communities—is essential if we are to tackle these issues. Many of these problems are examined in more detail throughout the course of this book, and the final chapter will explore the application of the public health perspective to their solution.

Key messages

- Changing pattern of children's health
- Food availability high and fewer infectious diseases
- High levels of mental health problems, teenage pregnancy, obesity, drug taking, and smoking
- Child public health approach essential for tackling these problems

---

Measuring health and disease

As we discuss in Chapter 5, health is a positive concept, more than just the absence of disease. Those concerned with children's health in policy making, practice and research are beginning to focus on the positive end of the spectrum and there is a welcome trend to collect data on children's subjective experiences of their health and wellbeing, e.g. the WHO Health Behaviours of School Children Survey (HBSC) or the TellUs survey in England). However it is diseases and health problems that are generally measured when statistics are collected. Much of the information in this section thus relates not to health but to the absence of health.

Causes of death in childhood

The most commonly presented statistics of child health and indeed of the health of whole communities are those which count deaths. Whilst a far cry from a measurement of health, mortality statistics have for centuries acted as a remarkably reliable indicator of health in general. With regard to the UK and the rest of Europe, what they tell us reflects what we have said in the introduction – that child health has improved dramatically over the course of the last century.

The charts below in Figs 1.2 and 1.3 indicate how child mortality rates from all causes vary across Europe and between the English regions, and how causes of death vary with age.

Post infancy, accidents are now the most important cause of death. Together with self harm and other injury, accidents make up nearly 50% of all deaths at age 15–19, with an especially high rate among boys. Cancers are a significant cause of death for the 'middle years'—the 1–4, 5–9, and 10–14 age groups – even though childhood cancer survival has improved dramatically over the last 20 years. There are important variations in mortality across geographical, socio-economic, and ethnic boundaries which are explained elsewhere in this book.

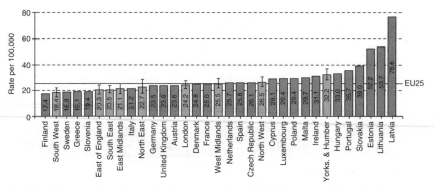

Fig. 1.2 All causes directly standardized mortality rate by European nation/English region 2001–03 (ages 1–19 years).
Source: Reproduced from Indications of Public Health in the English Regions 5: Child Health, Association of Public Health Observatories, 2006, with permission.

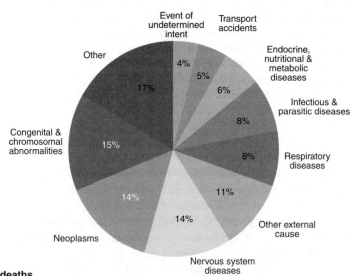

N=1596 deaths

Fig. 1.3a Deaths by cause category England 2002–04 (ages 1–4 years).
Source: Reproduced from Indications of Public Health in the English Regions 5: Child Health, Association of Public Health Observatories, 2006, with permission.

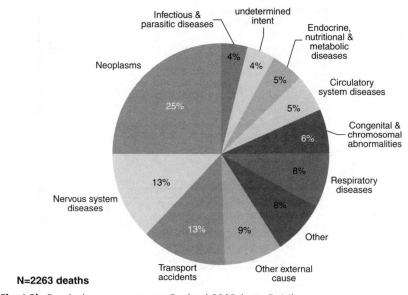

Fig. 1.3b Deaths by cause category England 2002 (ages 5–14).
Source: Reproduced from Indications of Public Health in the English Regions 5: Child Health, Association of Public Health Observatories, 2006, with permission.

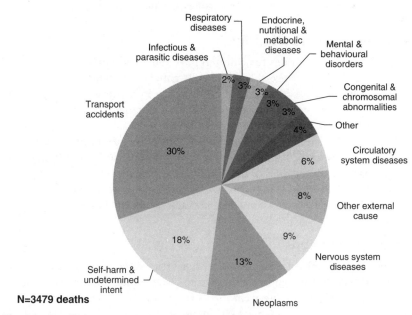

Fig. 1.3c Deaths by cause category England ages (15–19).
Source: Reproduced from Indications of Public Health in the English Regions 5: Child Health, Association of Public Health Observatories, 2006, with permission.

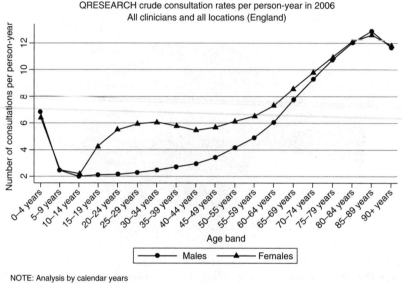

QRESEARCH crude consultation rates per person-year in 2006
All clinicians and all locations (England)

NOTE: Analysis by calendar years
copyright QRESEARCH 2003–2007 (Database version 13)

Fig. 1.4 Graph of GP consultation rates by age.

Source: Reproduced from *Trends in Consultation Rates in General Practice 1995 to 2006: Analysis of the QRESEARCH database*. Final Report to the Information Centre and Department of Health July 2007 Copyright © 2009, Re-used with the permission of The Health and Social Care Information Centre. All rights reserved.

Health service consultations

While GP consultation rates for children have remained fairly steady over the last three decades, attendance at a hospital out-patient or accident and emergency department has increased substantially—doubling in the case of 0–4 year-olds. Children aged 0–4 have an average of six GP consultations per year; those aged 5–15 have between two (boys) and three (girls) Fig. 1.4.

Telephone consultation has increased from 3% in 1995 to 10% in 2006 as a proportion of all primary care consultations. The proportion of nurse consultations has also risen, making up one third of the total in 2006, in contrast to 20% in 1995. It is estimated that NHS Direct, the telephone consultation service for the UK National Health Service, is now the largest provider of health services in Europe.

Hospital admissions

Children under 1 year have the highest admission rate, largely accounted for by emergencies (240.5 per 1,000 population per annum). The number of emergency admissions decreases with age; the rate of emergency admissions is 96.0 per 1,000 population in the 1–4 age group and 39.5 per 1,000 population in the 10–14 age group. (ISD Scotland 2008 data)

The main conditions for which children are admitted to hospital are shown below in Fig. 1.5.

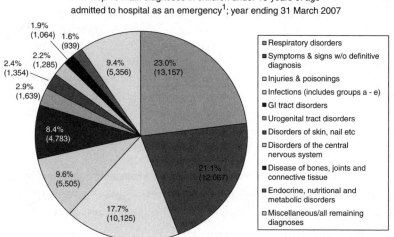

Top 10 main diagnoses in children under 15 years of age
admitted to hospital as an emergency[1]; year ending 31 March 2007

- Respiratory disorders
- Symptoms & signs w/o definitive diagnosis
- Injuries & poisonings
- Infections (includes groups a - e)
- GI tract disorders
- Urogenital tract disorders
- Disorders of skin, nail etc
- Disorders of the central nervous system
- Disease of bones, joints and connective tissue
- Endocrine, nutritional and metabolic disorders
- Miscellaneous/all remaining diagnoses

Fig. 1.5 Causes (ICD10) of hospital admission children.
Source: Data from ISD Scotland Child Health Statistics website, extracted February 2008.

There has been an increase in admissions to hospital over the last few years, particularly for infants see (Fig. 1.6).

For the 0–19 age group, the number of emergency admissions via the A&E department:

- increased by 4% between 1996/97 and 2002/03 (359,000 to 373,000)
- increased by 30% between 2002/03 and 2006/07 (373,000 to 484,000)

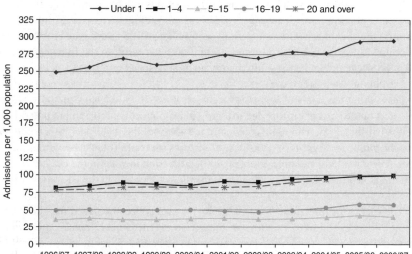

Fig. 1.6 Graph of emergency admission trends.
Source: Trends in Children and Young People's Care: Emergency Admission Statistics,
1996/97–2006/07, England DH 2008, with permission.

Factors contributing to this rise include increased expectations among both parents and professionals of children being healthy; parental anxieties about children's illness in general; and the availability of a wider range of medical interventions for both illness and disability (e.g. cancer, short stature, cystic fibrosis). Contractual changes may also have caused a shift from GP consultation to A&E. However, several studies suggest that there has also been a genuine increase in some common childhood health problems.

Important child health problems

Children's health problems can be grouped as follows:

- **Acute illnesses** such as otitis media, meningitis, bronchiolitis, and anaphylaxis
- **Chronic illnesses** such as asthma, epilepsy, diabetes, cancer, HIV, and AIDS
- **Disabilities** including physical and learning disabilities, and sensory impairments
- **Injury**—accidental and non-accidental
- **Disorders of eating and nutrition** including failure to thrive, obesity, anorexia nervosa, and bulimia
- **Mental health disorders** such as attention deficit hyperactivity disorder (ADHD), challenging behaviour, poor sleeping, depression, anxiety, autism, and psychoses

Acute illnesses

Many acute illnesses are becoming less common and less serious as a result of immunization, better social conditions, and improved primary care. There are fewer admissions for vaccine-preventable diseases; indeed one of the successes of recent years has been the introduction of vaccines against Haemophilus influenzae, meningococcus C, and pneumococcus, which are causes of serious morbidities such as epiglottitis, pneumonia, and meningitis. Other infections such as hepatitis B and C and TB have risen recently, however, and poor immunization intake can result in the re-emergence of vaccine-preventable diseases, often with surprising speed and spread as is demonstrated in the Table 1.1 below.

Fears about the safety of pertussis vaccine in the 1970s and 1980s, and of MMR at the start of the current century, led to a drop in immunization rates and to potentially serious outbreaks of whooping cough and measles (see Fig. 1.7). There is a tendency for the public to forget the seriousness of diseases successfully tackled by immunization (there were, for example, over 250,000 deaths from measles in the UK during the twentieth century). In 2002–4, the rate of measles vaccination in the UK was amongst the lowest in Europe (Fig. 1.8).

The spectre of infectious diseases has by no means been banished for good, and minor illnesses still have a significant impact on parents and children. Expectations have changed: parents do not expect children to be ill these days and have less experience in managing illness at home, so common infectious diseases such as respiratory infections can be very worrying, and the level of help sought from health professionals high. Partly as a result of the assumption that specific treatment is now available for all

Table 1.1 Numbers of notifiable diseases 1994–2007 England

Disease	1994	1995	1996	1997	1998	1999	2000	2001	2002	2003	2004	2005	2006	2007
Acute poliomyelitis	–	1	1	2	2	–	–	–	–	–	–	–	–	–
Cholera	30	32	32	33	48	29	30	28	17	26	31	34	37	41
Diphtheria ‡	9	12	11	22	23	23	19	13	20	13	10	9	10	9
Dysentery	6,956	4,651	2,312	2,274	1,813	1,538	1,494	1,388	1,087	1,047	1,203	1,237	1,122	1217
Food poisoning	81,833	82,041	83,233	93,901	93,932	86,316	86,528	85,468	72,649	70,895	70,311	70,407	70,603	72,382
Malaria	1,139	1,300	1,659	1,476	1,110	1,005	1,128	1,081	847	791	609	679	613	426
Measles ‡	16,375	7,447	5,614	3,962	3,728	2,438	2,378	2,250	3,187	2,488	2,356	2,089	3,705	3670
Meningitis	1,800	2,285	2,686	2,345	2,072	2,094	2,432	2,623	1,545	1,472	1,267	1,381	1,494	1251
meningococcal	*938*	*1,146*	*1,164*	*1,220*	*1,152*	*1,145*	*1,164*	*1,020*	*706*	*646*	*554*	*579*	*618*	*557*
Meningococcal septicaemia	430	707	1,129	1,440	1,509	1,822	1,614	1,238	842	732	691	721	657	673
Mumps ‡	2,494	1,936	1,747	1,914	1,587	1,691	2,168	2,741	1,997	4,204	16,367	56,256	12,841	7196
Rubella ‡	6,326	6,196	9,081	3,260	3,208	1,954	1,653	1,483	1,660	1,361	1,287	1,155	1,221	1082
Scarlet fever	6,193	5,296	4,873	3,569	3,339	2,086	1,933	1,756	2,159	2,553	2,201	1,678	2,166	1948
Tuberculosis	5,591	5,608	5,654	5,859	6,087	6,144	6,572	6,714	6,753	6,518	6,723	7,628	7,621	6989
hepatitis A	*2,715*	*2,120*	*1,339*	*1,837*	*1,515*	*1,676*	*1,271*	*1,138*	*1,381*	*1,194*	*784*	*513*	*433*	*333*
hepatitis B	*528*	*623*	*613*	*730*	*886*	*864*	*1,035*	*1,028*	*1,073*	*1,151*	*1,215*	*1,325*	*1,165*	*1265*
hepatitis C	*n/a*	*n/a*	*n/a*	*n/a*	*n/a*	*743*	*1,042*	*1,061*	*1,340*	*1,574*	*1,851*	*2,120*	*2,194*	*2040*
Whooping cough	3,964	1,869	2,387	2,989	1,577	1,139	712	888	883	409	504	594	550	1089

Source: Data from Report: Statutory Notifications of Infectious Diseases (NOIDs) – Annual Totals 1994 to 2008 – England and Wales, Health Protection Agency.

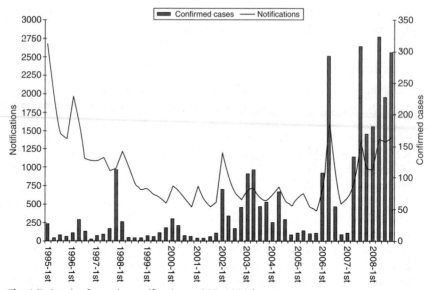

Fig. 1.7 Graph of measles notifications 1995–2009 by qtr.
Source: Reproduced from Health Protection Agency UK, http://www.hpa.org.uk/web/
HPAweb&HPAwebStandard/HPAweb_C/1195733808276, with permission.

illnesses, antibiotics may be inappropriately used for some conditions, leading to increasing antibiotic resistance among common pathogens and the potential for untreatable 'super bugs' in the future.

In addition, the emergence of new infectious diseases (most notably HIV, but also a range of others including the viral haemorrhagic fevers such as Lassa and Ebola) poses a threat worldwide.

Whilst infectious diseases have generally declined in incidence and severity, the incidence of other acute conditions such as allergy and anaphylaxis has increased.

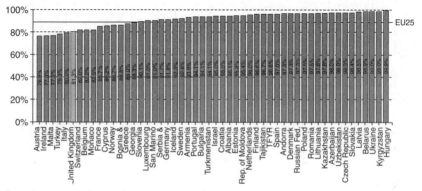

Fig. 1.8 European immunization rate measles.
Source: Reproduced from Indications of Public Health in the English Regions 5: Child Health, Association of Public Health Observatories, 2006, with permission.

Between 2001 and 2005, the incidence of multiple allergic disorders rose by nearly one third and their prevalence by nearly 50%.

Chronic illnesses

As childhood mortality rates have fallen, there has been a proportional increase in chronic diseases. This paradox reflects increasing expectations of health, greater recognition and diagnosis of certain diseases (e.g. asthma, eczema), and better survival rates of children with conditions such as cerebral palsy or cystic fibrosis. The appearance of HIV and AIDS in the UK and Europe has posed particular challenges.

Although increased recognition and diagnosis has played a part in inflating the apparent rise in asthma, there is evidence that there has also been a real increase. This is believed to be due in part to air pollution from motor vehicles and other sources as well as possible immunoadaptive (T cell subclass differentiation) and lifestyle changes (see Further reading). There is an association between TV viewing in the early years and the risk of developing asthma in later childhood. In one study, children who watched television for 2 hours a day were almost twice as likely to develop asthma by 11.5 years of age as those watching for 1–2 hours a day (adjusted odds ratio 1.8; 95% confidence intervals 1.2 to 2.6).

The prevalence of diabetes mellitus is also increasing, and more and more children are presenting with Type II diabetes (traditionally 'maturity onset' diabetes associated with obesity, sometimes known as 'diabesity') as well as the traditional childhood Type I, or insulin-dependent, diabetes.

Chronic illnesses are of great significance because of their impact on daily life. A child with chronic illness may find it difficult to participate fully in the usual pursuits of his or her age group. One of the parents (usually the mother) often has to devote a considerable amount of time to caring for the child, and her own needs may become subservient. Employment and family income may suffer, and marital relationships are often strained. Children with chronic illnesses—and those with disabilities—may require intensive services from both health and other agencies, although they and their parents usually become expert in the management of their condition.

The challenge facing those managing chronic illnesses in childhood is to balance the short term and the long term, and to take account of the child's perspective and values. Meticulous blood glucose control may carry huge benefits for the future, but if the diabetic child's life is entirely dominated by his or her condition then those benefits may be obtained at the cost of compromising the experience of childhood. Adolescents with cancer may find the side-effects of chemotherapy such an intolerable insult to their body image that they may say they would prefer not to be treated. The adults responsible for their care need to be aware of these concerns in deciding jointly what is best for the child. These patients are often amongst the most challenging for clinicians in terms of balancing the rights of children and their carers.

Disabilities

It is estimated that approximately 1 in 20 children have a significant disability, although definitions vary a great deal. Spencer et al. have analyzed routine sources such as the

Family Resources Survey of 16,000 households, providing useful data on the functional impact of disability in children (Table 1.2).

Analyses such as these focus on physical and sensory disability. A previous survey carried out in the UK by what was then the Office for Populations Censuses and Surveys (Fig. 1.9) is the only study to have addressed equivalence in levels of disability in functioning across mental and physical domains. This survey showed what those working in the field of child health know from day to day experience, that mental health problems are by far the most important cause of disability in childhood. Manifested as emotional and behavioural problems, mental illness in childhood devastates families and causes profound disruption in schools. Because special surveys are required to pick up data on mental health, and these problems are a rare cause of hospital admission, GP consultation, or mortality, they often get downplayed in analyses of child health.

As for chronic illnesses, quality of life is a major consideration for children with disabilities and their parents (see Chapter 5). Expectations of the services and treatment available, both from health services and other agencies such as education and social services, are higher than they used to be. The demands on professionals are great, especially in the context of limited resources, and the inability to deliver the support needed by a family can be a major source of frustration.

Therapeutic improvements have affected the incidence of some conditions. The incidence of bilateral spastic cerebral palsy has declined considerably in very low

Table 1.2 Chronic illness and disability

Difficulty/problem experienced	% of population		% of children with DDA defined disability			
	All		Male		Female	
	n	%	n	%	n	%
Mobility	193,950	1.5	119,282	20.5	74,668	20.2
Lifting and carrying	84,759	0.7	50,482	8.7	34,277	9.3
Manual dexterity	107,798	0.8	76,293	13.1	31,505	8.5
Continence	88,748	0.7	54,264	9.3	34,484	9.3
Communication	255,534	2.0	170,783	29.3	84,751	22.9
Memory, concentration, learning	288,203	2.2	211,743	36.3	76,460	20.7
Recognising physical danger	171,352	1.3	126,622	21.7	44,730	12.1
Physical coordination	167,585	1.3	116,841	30.0	50,744	13.7
Other	268,427	2.1	166,668	28.6	101,759	27.5

Chronic ILLNESS Family Resources Services Disabilty Discrmination Act definition: Any longstanding illness, disability or infirmity which has troubled child over a period of time or likely to affect him/her over a period of time and which limits child in some way with 1 or more substantial difficulties with daily activities.
Source: Spencer N and Blackburn C.
www2.warwick.ac.uk/fac/cross_fac/healthatwarwick/research/currentfundedres/disabled children/, with permission.

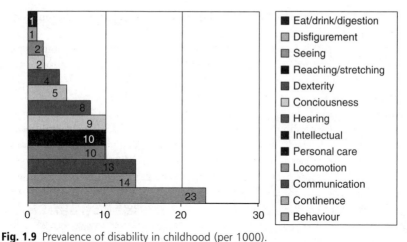

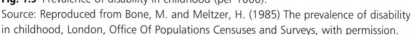

Fig. 1.9 Prevalence of disability in childhood (per 1000).
Source: Reproduced from Bone, M. and Meltzer, H. (1985) The prevalence of disability in childhood, London, Office Of Populations Censuses and Surveys, with permission.

birthweight infants (1000–1500gms) as a result of improvements in neonatal intensive care. However, the rate has remained stable in extremely low birthweight infants (below 1000g). These babies are increasingly surviving to later ages, often with disability.

There has been an increase in notifications of all congenital anomalies in Europe over the last 20 years, although the incidence of some anomalies has fallen dramatically with improvements in antenatal care. These include screening and termination for Down's syndrome and neural tube disorders (spina bifida and anencephaly), immunization against rubella (both post-partum and in childhood), greater awareness of the teratogenic potential of certain drugs, and the promotion of folic acid intake in pregnancy, which has reduced the incidence of neural tube disorders. Figure 1.10 illustrates the incidence of anencephaly in two cities and shows considerable differences between them. Some of the variation may be due to differences in ascertainment and case definition.

Accidental injury

After infancy, accidental injury continues to be the main cause of death. Although absolute rates have fallen over the last few decades, they have not declined as much as other causes, so that injuries represent a growing proportion of deaths among children and young people. Transport-related deaths account for 1 in 20 deaths in under fives, 1 in 9 between 5 and 14 years and nearly 1 in 3 in the later teens.

UK death and injury rates for child pedestrians have improved recently and are now amongst the lowest in Europe (Fig. 1.11).

However, socio-economic inequalities in accidental death and injury rates are particularly marked. The children of parents who have never worked or are long-term unemployed are 13 times more likely to die from unintentional injury and 37 times

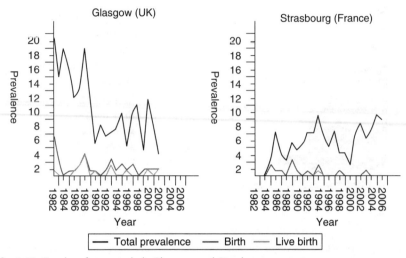

Fig. 1.10 Graphs of anencephaly Glasgow and Strasbourg.
Source: Reproduced from EUROCAT Website Database: http://www.eurocat.ulster.ac.uk/
pubdata/tables.html (data uploaded 31/03/2009), with permission.

more likely to die from exposure to smoke, fire, or flames than those whose parents
are in higher managerial or professional occupations (see Chapter 3).

Although transport accidents account for a large proportion of *deaths* from injury,
the morbidity from other forms of injury is greater (Fig. 1.12). Many hospital emergency attendances are for injuries sustained at home or school.

Data gathered in the National Child Development Study cohort show that injury is
now also the most common cause of physical disability in young adults.

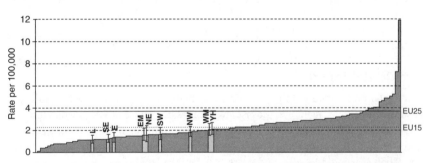
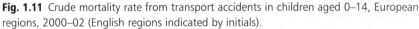

Fig. 1.11 Crude mortality rate from transport accidents in children aged 0–14, European
regions, 2000–02 (English regions indicated by initials).
Legend: *Transport accident crude mortality rate by European region 2000–02 (ages
0–14 years) English Regions initials.*
Source: Reproduced from Indications of Public Health in the English Regions 5: Child
Health, Association of Public Health Observatories, 2006, with permission.

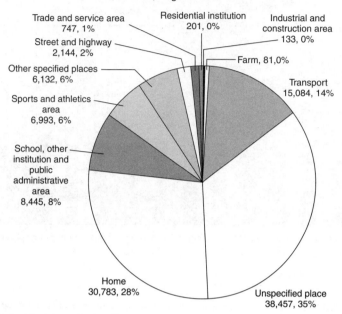

Emergency hospital admissions aged 0–17 years resulting from transport accidents and place of occurrence of non-transport accidents, England 2006-07

Trade and service area
747, 1%

Street and highway
2,144, 2%

Other specified places
6,132, 6%

Sports and athletics
area
6,993, 6%

School, other
institution and
public
administrative
area
8,445, 8%

Residential institution
201, 0%

Industrial and
construction area
133, 0%

Farm, 81,0%

Transport
15,084, 14%

Home
30,783, 28%

Unspecified place
38,457, 35%

Fig. 1.12 Accident types by location.
Source: Reproduced from Accident Prevention Amongst Children and Young People A Priority Review Feb 2009 DH, DCSF, Dept Transport, with permission.

Disorders of eating and nutrition

In the UK, eating disorders relate mainly to inappropriate or excessive dietary intake, although certain problems of undernutrition —anorexia nervosa among adolescents and failure to thrive in infants—remain important causes of ill health in childhood.

The number of overweight and obese children continues to rise, amounting to what is now described as an obesity epidemic. The International Obesity Task Force has established age- and gender-specific cut-offs that correspond to a BMI of 25 at age 25 years. Figure 1.13 below shows the increase in rates of overweight and obesity among children in the UK over the last decade.

It is significant that over the period covered by these charts, obesity has risen more sharply than overweight, indicating a shift of the BMI distribution upwards. Childhood obesity has significant implications for health in later life as well as impacting adversely on children's peer relationships and self-esteem (see Chapter 8, scenario I).

Even among children of normal weight there are concerns about diet, with many children consuming excessive amounts of saturated fat and sugar, and too little fresh fruit and vegetables and essential fatty acids, such as those contained in fish oils. Dietary patterns vary between social classes, with children from more deprived backgrounds having poorer diets. Iron deficiency is prevalent in 15–40% of some child populations, particularly those from poorer backgrounds. This has consequences for child growth

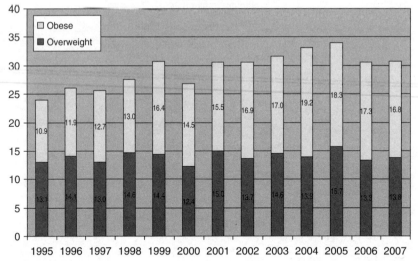

Fig. 1.13 Obesity rates.
Source: Data from General Households Survey.

and brain development. The UK government's 'Five a Day' initiative, which promotes the consumption of at least five portions of fruit and vegetables a day, and schemes to provide free fruit in schools, have had some impact on children's diets. Twenty-one percent of children ate five or more portions in 2007 compared to 11% in 2001.

The rise in food poisoning in recent years is also of concern, especially to younger and immunocompromised children, who are at greater risk of serious illness from infections such as E. coli 0157.

Eating disorders such as anorexia nervosa and bulimia are an increasing problem, especially among adolescent girls. Such girls are highly subject to media images of underweight women appearing as fashion models, and also to peer influences, which can generate 'outbreaks' in schools.

A new area of concern for child health is the rising incidence of allergies to foodstuffs. Peanut allergy is the best known example, leading to acute anaphylaxis in a very small number of children. Much larger numbers of children suffer less dramatic allergies to a wide range of foodstuffs including dairy products, soy, wheat, and eggs. Colonization of the gut by 'friendly' microbes in very early life appears to play a part in the development of the normal and abnormal immune response, and widespread use of broad spectrum antibiotics in the neonatal period is therefore a potential cause of this increase (see Chapter 6).

The improvement in children's dental health owes a great deal to the addition of fluoride to toothpaste and drinking water, but there are now marked socio-economic and regional variations related to the inequitable geographic distribution of water fluoridation as well as to high sugar consumption. Although dental care is available free on the NHS to children, in some areas NHS dentists are hard to find. Regional variations in England and across Europe are shown in Fig. 1.14.

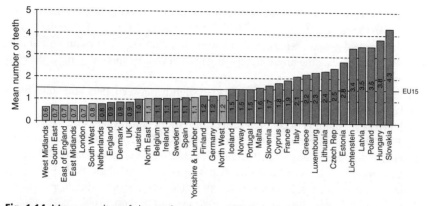

Fig. 1.14 Mean number of decayed, missing or filled teeth in 12-year-old children by European nation and English region 2000–02.
Source: Reproduced from *Indications of Public Health in the English Regions 5: Child Health*, Association of Public Health Observatories, 2006, with permission.

Mental health problems

Mental health problems are increasingly prevalent at all ages and, as noted above, are now the commonest cause of disability in childhood in the developed world. Prevalence figures depend on diagnostic criteria, which may vary from study to study. However, it is estimated that approximately one in ten children over the age of five have a significant mental health disorder. Disorders are commoner in boys at all ages (Fig. 1.15).

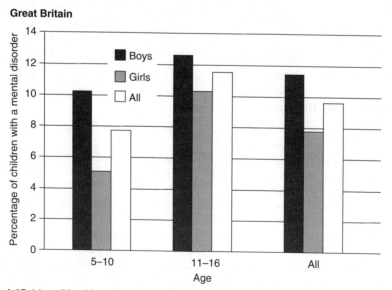

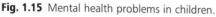

Fig. 1.15 Mental health problems in children.
Source: Reproduced from Mental Health of children and Young People in Great Britain 2004, ONS 2005, with permission.

The commonest are conduct disorders (6%), emotional disorders such as anxiety and depression (3.5%), and hyperkinetic disorders such as ADHD (1.5%). Prevalence varies with age and gender, family size and structure, ethnicity, socioeconomic status, education, and coexisting physical impairments, which are explored in more detail in Chapter 3.

The prevalence of emotional disorders fell slightly between 1999 and 2004, but a similar decrease was not seen for other conditions.

A much larger number of children suffer from emotional and behavioural problems which fall short of diagnostic criteria for mental disorder. These problems are on the increase, and pose challenges to all services for children (health, mental health, social services, and particularly education). Behaviour problems blight children's lives, making it difficult for them to learn at school and to make friends with their peers. As Chapter 6 makes clear, most children do not grow out of these problems. As adolescents they are at high risk of school failure, delinquency, substance misuse, teenage pregnancy, violence, and crime. As adults they are at high risk of personality disorder, depression, anxiety, drug and alcohol abuse, and marital breakdown (see Chapter 6).

The diagnosis of autism and Asperger's syndrome continues to rise steadily, placing great strain on the specialist services needed to provide for these children, especially the early intervention services that offer some hope of better integration in the medium term. There is increasing concern across Europe about suicide attempts, which are a marker of youth distress.

Summary

The reduction in mortality and morbidity from infectious disease has been replaced by the 'morbidities of modern living', which affect the children of most developed countries. Particular areas of concern include a rise in mental ill health and developmental disorders, injury, obesity, and the health effects of poverty. These represent some of the principal challenges facing child public health professionals at the beginning of the twenty-first century.

Further reading

Bone, M. and Meltzer, H. (1985) The prevalence of disability in childhood. Office Of Populations Censuses and Surveys, London.

Sherriff, A., Maitra, A., Ness, A.R., et al. (2009) Association of duration of television viewing in early childhood with the subsequent development of asthma. *Thorax*; **64**: 321–325.

Simpson, C., Newton, J., Hippisley-Cox, J., and Sheikh, A. (2008) Incidence and prevalence of multiple allergic disorders recorded in a national primary care database. *Journal of the Royal Society of Medicine*; **101**: 558–563.

Strachan, D.P. (November 1989) Hay fever, hygiene, and household size. *BMJ*; **299** (6710): 1259–60.

Strachan, D.P. (August 2000) Family size, infection and atopy: the first decade of the "hygiene hypothesis". *Thorax*; **55 Suppl 1**: S2–10.

The Children's Society's Good Childhood Inquiry: http://www.childrenssociety.org.uk/all_about_us/how_we_do_it/the_good_childhood_inquiry/1818.html accessed 17.6.09

Chapter 2

Child health in developing countries/the majority world

Why is international child health important?

> We must move children to the centre of the world's agenda. We must rewrite strategies to reduce poverty so that investments in children are given priority.
>
> *Nelson Mandela*

> Children and mothers are dying because those who have the power to prevent their deaths choose not to act....As health professionals, we should not accept this pervasive disrespect for human life. We have a voice, a platform and a constituency that should be an instrument for radical change.
>
> *Richard Horton, Editor of* The Lancet *2008 371, 1217–19*

It is hardly possible for anyone in the developed world, lay or professional, to be unaware of the many threats to the health and wellbeing of children in the developing world (also known as the majority world). Facts and photographs, crises and appeals populate our newspapers, television screens, and professional journals—especially since the recent growth in global terrorism. Many of us now travel to parts of the world previous generations only read about and see very different societies at first hand. Nevertheless, despite our familiarity with images of life in the developing world, there is a risk that we are all too busy with our own everyday lives to acknowledge our part in the global scheme.

It is salutary to remember that roughly 85% of the world's 1.5 billion children live in developing countries, and that the accident of their country of birth marks them out from the beginning for a very different experience of life and health. A comparison of child health indicators between the top five and bottom five countries in the world, as in Table 2.1, provides a stark illustration of the contrast between them. A child born in Sierra Leone has an almost one in three chance of dying before reaching his or her fifth birthday—almost eighty times higher than for a child born in Sweden, Norway, or Japan. Fewer than 20% of the population in Sierra Leone, Niger, Afghanistan, or

Table 2.1 UNICEF RANKINGS U5M
Comparison of child health indicators in different countries (top five and bottom five under fives mortality)

Country	Under 5s mortality (per 1000 births)	Immunization uptake % (DPT/polio3 by 1 yr)	Exclusive breast-feeding <6 months	% of population with adequate sanitation	Rank for under fives mortality (1=worst)
Sierra Leone	270	64	8	39	1
Angola	260	44	11	31	2
Niger	253	39	14	13	4
Afghanistan	257	77	–	34	3
Mali	217	85	25	46	6
France	4	98	–	–	175
Singapore	3	95	–	100	189
Japan	4	99	–	100	175
Norway	4	93	–	–	175
Sweden	3	99	–	100	189

(– means data unavailable) Source: Data from UNICEF (2008) *State of the World's Children 2008: Child Survival*.

Mali have adequate sanitation, and barely one in two children in these countries receives basic immunizations.

The United Nations developed Millennium Development Goals to be reached by 2015. Goal 4 is to reduce under-fives mortality by two-thirds. In 2008, only 16 of 68 priority countries were on track to reach this goal, and 12 countries were experiencing worse rather than improved under-fives mortality. These set-backs are largely due to failures in policy and commitment by industrialized countries.

The key health problems facing children in different parts of the globe differ significantly. Most child deaths worldwide are due to preventable causes such as perinatal conditions, respiratory infections, and diarrhoeal diseases. Many of these are related to poverty and malnutrition, which are both widespread and increasing—and both of which are significantly affected by the behaviour of more developed countries. Immunization has been a success story, but huge numbers of children still die from vaccine-preventable diseases. Obviously some conditions—such as mental illness, disability, and long term illnesses such as epilepsy—are common to both the developed and developing world. However, their prevalence, their impact on the child and family, and the services available to deal with them differ between industrialized countries and those with a subsistence economy. Similarly, many determinants of health—such as housing conditions and family structure—are relevant to all children worldwide, but their nature, severity, and relative impact on health varies. Table 2.2 highlights some of the contrasts.

So why should we, as individuals concerned with child public health, wish to know more about children growing up in less privileged countries? Do we have responsibilities towards them, and can we do anything to improve their health and wellbeing?

Table 2.2 Comparison of some important determinants of health and key health problems in children in the developed and developing world (see also Chapter 3)

	Developed world	Developing world
Important determinants of health	Inappropriate nutrition e.g. overconsumption of saturated fats and sugar Lack of exercise Risk behaviour e.g. substance misuse Relative poverty/income inequality Family structure and relationships Social attitudes and stigma Time spent watching TV/ playing video games Performance related stress	Malnutrition Absolute poverty Lack of sanitation Availability of education War and violence Famine, drought, and flooding Climate change Availability of health care, especially antenatal, perinatal, and preventive services Family structure and relationships Family planning and family size Child labour Migration Injury risk
Key health problems	Acute illnesses (usually not fatal) Obesity & other lifestyle problems Emotional and behavioural problems Disability (due to increasing survival of preterm infants and injury) Chronic illnesses & malignancy	Respiratory infections Diarrhoeal diseases Vaccine-preventable infectious diseases and other acute illnesses (more often fatal) HIV, TB, and Hepatitis B Disability (related to birth injury, polio, accidents, war and conflict)

Do the choices we make about how we live in the developed world influence the life chances of children in the developing world? Does the situation in far-flung parts of the globe have an impact on our own practice? Could a better understanding of the background to migration and asylum-seeking, for example, help us to plan and provide health services at home? The box below lists some of the reasons why a global health approach is desirable in the countries of the North.

The rationale for a global health approach

♦ Health problems of low-income countries will impact on the North through immigration and population movement

♦ There is wide exchange of health professionals both from North to South and South to North

The rationale for a global health approach (continued)

- ◆ Many of the health problems in the South are the result of policies in the North (e.g. marketing of unhealthy products, the pharmaceutical industry, the exploitation of natural resources)
- ◆ Climate change, which will have a huge impact on children in the South, is the result of excessive and unsustainable energy expenditure in the North

This chapter aims to address the connections between child health in the developed and developing world, offering an international perspective on children in society and their health, exploring the complex links between different parts of the globe, and arguing that there is significant interdependence between them. It discusses the key health problems of children who live in developing countries, where poverty and lack of resources are key mediators, as well as those whose lives have been disrupted by war and infrastructure breakdown. It examines some of the solutions which have been developed through research or innovations in practice—some of which could benefit child public health practice in the developed world too.

This is an enormous subject which is inevitably covered here in summary only, but we hope this chapter offers some insight into what we consider to be a vitally important area of child public health, and that it will be of interest and relevance to readers from all backgrounds.

The global burden of childhood disease

Child health problems in developing countries today are not dissimilar to those seen in Europe in the eighteenth and nineteenth centuries, both in terms of the extent and severity of ill health and of the range of conditions encountered. The diseases of absolute poverty, and common infectious diseases which have largely been conquered in the developed North (though relative poverty has definitely not), are more significant than tropical diseases. The new 'plagues' of the twentieth and twenty-first centuries (especially HIV, mental illness, and injury, including road traffic injury) have added dramatically to the burden of disease, whilst the mitigating effect of socioeconomic, environmental, and technological progress has had little impact in many countries (see Table 2.3).

Children in developing countries today face similar health problems to European children in previous centuries—diseases of poverty and common infectious diseases—but to these are added the new 'plagues' of HIV, mental illness, and road traffic injury.

In Europe and the US, infant mortality is now below 10 per 1,000 births, but in many developing countries it remains above 100 per 1,000 births, and in some cases is as high as 300. The most common causes of infant death in such countries are septicaemia,

Table 2.3 Comparing causes of death in children ages 0–14 years by broad income group

Low and middle income countries				High income countries			
Rank	**Cause**	**Deaths (millions)**	**% Total deaths**	**Rank**	**Cause**	**Deaths (millions)**	**% Total deaths**
1	Perinatal conditions	2.49	20.7	1	Perinatal conditions	0.03	33.9
2	Lower respiratory infections	2.04	17.0	2	Congenital anomalies	0.02	20.0
3	Diarrhoeal diseases	1.61	13.4	3	Road traffic accidents	0.01	5.9
4	Malaria	1.10	9.2	4	Lower respiratory infections	0.00	2.5
5	Measles	0.74	6.2	5	Endocrine disorders	0.00	2.4
6	HIV/AIDS	0.44	3.7	6	Drownings	0.00	2.4
7	Congenital anomalies	0.44	3.7	7	Leukaemia	0.00	1.9
8	Whooping cough	0.3	2.5	8	Violence	0.00	1.8
9	Tetanus	0.22	1.9	9	Fires	0.00	1.2
10	Road traffic accidents	0.18	1.5	10	Meningitis	0.00	1.2

Source: Reproduced with permission from Lopez et al (2006), *Global Burden of Disease and Risk Factors*, © The International Bank for Reconstruction and Development, The World Bank.

tetanus of the newborn, birth injury from unskilled midwifery, low birth weight, and congenital malformations.

Almost 10 million children under five died last year worldwide, most from preventable causes. At least half these deaths took place in sub-Saharan Africa, the majority occurring in just 60 developing countries. Globally, maternal mortality claimed 535,900 lives in 2005 (Maternal Mortality Ratio – the number of maternal deaths per 100,000 live births is 402 globally compared to 11 in US) and, as for child mortality, at least half of these were in sub-Saharan Africa. Malnutrition is implicated in more than half of children's deaths worldwide. The impact of malnutrition is discussed further below, in the section on determinants of health.

> Most child deaths worldwide are due to preventable causes such as perinatal conditions, respiratory infections, and diarrhoeal diseases, many of them related to poverty and malnutrition. Immunization has been a success story, but huge numbers of children still die from vaccine-preventable diseases.

Diseases related to or exacerbated by poverty

The extent and impact of poverty is discussed in detail in the next chapter. Some of the diseases associated with poverty are:

- Malnutrition—which has direct and indirect effects on health (e.g. starvation, vitamin deficiency, and greater susceptibility to disease)
- Diarrhoeal disease
- Acute respiratory infections (measles, pertussis, pneumonia)
- Tuberculosis
- HIV infection
- Skin and eye infections

Common infectious diseases

Many common infectious diseases—most of them now rare causes of death or serious illness in developed countries—remain major killers in poor countries. Measles is a particularly significant example, accounting for 5% of all deaths in children under five in developing countries. Measles is more severe in malnourished children, especially those with vitamin A deficiency, and the risk of serious complications is much higher. Whereas the death rate from measles in developed countries is only 2–3 per 1000 cases, in developing countries it is at least 30–50 per1000 cases, and may be as high as 100–300 per 1000 cases in some areas. This variation is thought to be due to a greater intensity of infecting dose owing to overcrowding. There was no evidence of a reduction of the incidence of measles, mumps, and rubella in Africa between 1990 and 2005.

Over 250,000 children develop tuberculosis every year, and 100,000 children will continue to die each year from TB (WHO data). The vast majority of these live in high prevalence areas (over 40 cases per 100,000 population) such as Africa, South and South East Asia, and South America. The risk of active disease following infection is high in children under three, those with poor nutritional status and living conditions, and particularly in HIV-positive individuals, for whom the risk is increased ten-fold. Effective treatment requires the use of at least three drugs for several months, which may be very difficult to achieve.

Hepatitis B is also a significant problem in many countries, with over 2 billion people infected worldwide and over a million deaths per year. In countries with high prevalence (over 8% of the population) such as Africa, many children are affected, usually by transmission from mother to baby at birth. Children are more likely to become chronic carriers of the virus and to suffer long-term complications such as cirrhosis or cancer of the liver.

Acute respiratory infections, meningitis, and other potentially treatable or preventable diseases are also more common (and often more serious) in developing countries. Lack of availability of what we might consider basic medicines—such as antibiotics—compromise the outcome for children already made more vulnerable to serious disease by poor nutrition and general health.

Immunization was the success story of the twentieth century: smallpox has been eradicated worldwide, and many countries have reduced the burden of measles, polio, and pertussis by effective immunization programmes. Polio could be eradicated, though progress remains slow: in 2008 there were 1652 reported cases of polio worldwide, down from 350,000 in 1988. (See http://www.polioeradication.org/) However, the potential benefits of immunization have not been fully realised. For example, fewer than half of children in certain parts of Africa currently receive measles vaccine. Problems with vaccine delivery and uptake are discussed further in the section on determinants of health.

> 2–3 children die per 1000 cases of measles in developed countries, compared with up to 300 per 1000 cases in some developing countries. TB and Hepatitis B also remain common and potentially serious causes of ill health worldwide.

AIDS and HIV infection

The current global AIDS epidemic is a tragedy for children as well as for their families.

At the end of 2006, 2.3 million children under 15 worldwide were living with HIV. In 2007, 270,000 children died of AIDS, whilst more than 15 million children under 18 had lost one or both parents to the disease. 250,000 children acquire the HIV virus every month. Roughly 10% of all new infections are in children under 15, and 50% are in young people aged 15–24. Almost all children under 15 with HIV acquired the infection through vertical transmission from their mothers, at birth or immediately afterwards. Although studies have shown that vertical transmission can be virtually eliminated with antiretroviral therapy, the expense and lack of availability of these drugs in many countries means that enormous numbers of HIV-positive mothers and their babies fail to benefit from them. Major questions and obstacles remain to be addressed before HIV in children can be successfully prevented and treated.

As well as the direct effects of infection in children, the impact of losing relatives to AIDS is also devastating, with many children being left in charge of families and younger siblings at a young age.

> At the end of 2006, 2.3 million children were living with HIV, and in 2007, 270,000 children under 15 died of AIDS. Most caught it through vertical transmission from their mothers, which can be prevented with antiretroviral therapy.

Injuries

If the global burden of disease is presented in terms of disability adjusted life years (DALYs: see Chapter 7 for definition), then injuries come second only to infectious disease in their impact, accounting, for example, for seven times the burden of disease of nutritional deficiency.

More than 85% of all deaths and 90% of disability adjusted life years lost from road traffic injuries occur in developing countries. Among children aged 0–4 and 5–4 years,

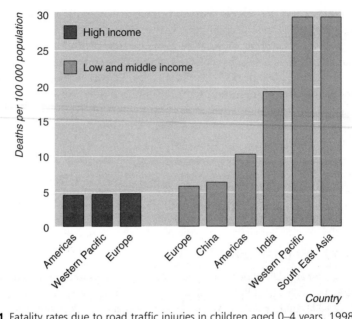

Fig. 2.1 Fatality rates due to road traffic injuries in children aged 0–4 years, 1998.
Source: Reproduced from Nantulya V. M. and Reich M. R. (2002) The neglected
epidemic: road traffic injuries in developing countries, *BMJ* 324: 1139–41, with
permission from the BMJ Publishing Group.

the number of fatalities per 100,000 population in low-income countries is about six
times greater than in high-income countries – including a fourfold greater proportion
of children killed as pedestrians Figs 2.1 and 2.2.

The reasons for this high mortality include the growing numbers of motor vehicles
in developing countries, higher numbers of deaths and injuries per crash, poor

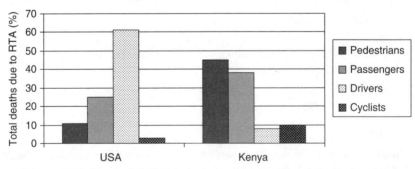

Fig. 2.2 Deaths due to road traffic injuries by road user category in a developed and a
developing country.
Source: Reproduced from Nantulya V. M. and Reich M. R. (2002) The neglected
epidemic: road traffic injuries in developing countries, *BMJ* 324: 1139–41, with
permission from the BMJ Publishing Group.

enforcement of traffic safety regulations, inadequacy of public health service infrastructure, and poor access to health care.

Although road traffic injuries are the single largest cause of death, interpersonal (war) and self-inflicted violence combined contribute an even greater number.

Violence against children

Understand that one person can do something about violence but many people can stop violence
No violence against children is justifiable; all violence against children is preventable
UN Report on Violence against Children, 2006

Violence against children worldwide was highlighted in a 2006 UN report that examined the extent of violence in five settings: home and family, school, care and justice systems, work settings, and the community.

Societal acceptance of violence is posited as an important reason for the epidemic. One hundred and six countries allow corporal punishment in schools and only sixteen countries ban it in the home. It is estimated that that between 80%–98% of children worldwide suffer physical punishment in their homes, with a third or more experiencing severe physical punishment resulting from the use of implements. In developing countries, 20%–65% of school-aged children reported having been verbally or physically bullied in school in the past 30 days.

In care settings, the situation for children can be grim: violence by institutional staff, for the purpose of 'disciplining' children, includes beatings, harassment, torture, isolation, restraint, and rape. Some children with disabilities may be subject to violence under the guise of treatment, such as electro-convulsive treatment (ECT) without the use of muscle relaxants or anaesthesia. Electric shocks may also be used as 'aversion treatment' to control children's behaviour.

Such violence reflects society's lack of protection of children, and our collective failure to promote children's interests and ensure that they have full participation in society – the key tenets of the UN Convention on the Rights of the Child (see p. 43).

Reproductive health

In older children, teenage pregnancy remains a particularly worrying issue. Nearly 15 million girls aged 15–19 years give birth each year, accounting for more than 10% of all babies born worldwide.

In many developing countries, more than one-third of women give birth in their teens. This has a major impact on health, with the risk of death from pregnancy-related causes being four times higher in this age group than among women over 20.

Female genital mutilation still occurs in some parts of the world, although its prevalence is gradually subsiding. The UN document referred to above reported that globally, 100–140 million girls and women have undergone some form of female genital mutilation (FGM) or cutting. In Africa, 3 million girls and women are subjected to genital mutilation or cutting every year. This figure (from UN Violence report p. 62) illustrates the prevalence of FGM in Africa among women and their daughters.

Tropical diseases

As well as the more familiar infectious diseases discussed above, children in many parts of the world are at risk of tropical diseases which can cause death, disability, or severe illness. Some of the more important are listed below:

- Malaria
- Leprosy
- Schistosomiasis
- Trachoma
- Trypanosomiasis
- Yellow fever
- Dengue fever

Malaria is a major cause of illness and death in certain areas where the more severe falciparum malaria remains endemic, including Brazil, South East Asia, and sub-Saharan Africa (where 90% of these deaths occur). It can lead to serious complications and if untreated, the mortality rate in children may reach 40%. The other types of malaria are rarely fatal but can lead to protracted, even lifelong infection, with intermittent relapses.

Leprosy, too, is still a significant problem, affecting over a million people worldwide, including upwards of 5 per 1000 population in some tropical and subtropical countries. Although uncommon in children under three (partly because of its long incubation period), it is seen in older children, and cases do occur even in infancy, probably due to transplacental transmission. Its major impact is the disfigurement and disability that result from chronic infection. As for tuberculosis, treatment is possible but needs to be long-term—at least 12 months of multidrug therapy.

For parasitic infections such as schistosomiasis (bilharzia), the most serious consequences are generally those of chronic infection, which include liver fibrosis, intractable urinary obstruction, and infertility. Trachoma infection in childhood frequently leads to blindness in later life; it is widespread in many parts of the world, including northern and sub-Saharan Africa, parts of Asia, and South America. Trypanosomiasis (sleeping sickness) is confined to tropical Africa, where the tsetse fly is found, and is always fatal without treatment: one form kills within weeks, whereas the other may last for years before finally leading to death.

Yellow fever and dengue fever—both transmitted by mosquitoe—cause acute illness. The fatality rate is generally below 5%, although the more severe form of dengue is more common in children. They have recently been joined by several newer types of viral haemorrhagic fever including Lassa and Ebola.

Disability

The burden of untreated disability in children in developing countries is significant. The causes include the exotic (leprosy and other tropical diseases) and the more familiar (meningitis, polio and other infections, traffic accidents, war, landmines, congenital abnormalities, and birth injuries); many of them are preventable or treatable. The manifestations may be physical (including problems with vision and hearing as well as locomotor impairments) or psychological. Few data are available on mental health problems but these are manifest in association with war, separation and displacement, child exploitation, and child labour. It is likely that they represent a very significant burden which will be recognized as awareness grows.

According to UNICEF, there are 170 million children in the world with disabilities, and one in ten of them have a serious disability. The vast majority have no access to rehabilitative or support services, and many are unable to acquire a formal education. In many cases, disabled children are simply withdrawn from community life; even if they are not actively shunned or maltreated, they are often left without adequate care.

It is estimated that only 2% of disabled children in developing countries have any form of rehabilitation assistance or education.

> The burden of untreated disability in children in developing countries is significant. Lack of surgical facilities, therapists, and adaptive aids and devices means many of those affected do not reach their potential. The impact of their lost labour may be very significant for themselves and their families.

There is a great need for increased emphasis on disability in the training of health workers and the operation of services.

The UN Convention on the Rights of the Child (UNCRC)

One of the reasons why children's health is so poor in the majority world is the relative neglect of children as a focus for government concern. Though this neglect affects children in all countries, it has a greater impact on child mortality and morbidity in countries afflicted by poverty. The UN Convention on the Rights of the Child was introduced for this reason and to ensure that children receive the protection from the state that they deserve.

Promulgated in 1989, this convention is one of the most ratified by states across the world. The CRC is an extremely important means of improving child health and wellbeing and is a vital tool for advocacy by all those concerned with child public health. Whilst only a minority of countries have integrated the convention into their domestic law, the UN carries out a five yearly inspection and issues a report which is of considerable influence. The role of civil society in supporting the upholding of children's rights is very significant. Health care professionals and others concerned with child health and children's rights may join with non-governmental organizations in challenging or supporting the actions taken and the official reports submitted by governments.

The Convention has three main categories: protection (from exploitation, violence and infectious disease), provision (of health and education services) and participation. The last holds children to be rights bearers who should take part in both conception and delivery of services – something that in health is rare. For the clinician, this means listening to the child and ensuring their view is heard; for the public health practitioner, it means including children and young people in the process of consultation and planning. The key principles of the Convention are shown below.

Key principles of the UN Convention on the Rights of the Child

- Best interests of the child to be a primary consideration in legislation
- Relates to all children without discrimination
- Rights to survival and development
- Rights to express their views and freedom of expression
- Access to information of benefit and protection from injurious information
- Protection from violence, abuse, and neglect
- Right to the highest attainable standard of health
- Right to an adequate standard of living
- Protection from economic exploitation

In practical terms, the CRC should be used in health services to ensure that a child-centred view is taken. Children are given choices, are offered confidentiality, provided with information, and their views are sought. Within the country, the convention bears on child labour, children in prison and the armed forces, children affected by violence and sexual exploitation, and children living in poverty. Its comprehensive nature makes it the ideal tool for the child public health professional to work across sectors to improve the present grave situation for children internationally.

Summary

This chapter has highlighted the huge burden of acute and long lasting illness and disability in children living in low income countries. The prospects for improvement are enormous if we in the developed world can muster the political will to place children and their wellbeing ahead of arms and conflict, more consumer goods, and high salaries for the well off in society.

Further reading

A course on teaching children's rights (2009) Royal College of Paediatrics and Child Health and American Academy of Pediatrics. Available on www.essop.org

Children's Rights Alliance for England www.crae.org.uk

Editorial: A renaissance in primary health care (2008) *The Lancet*; 372(9642): 863.

Full text of CRC available at www.unicef.org/crc

Horton, R. (2008) Countdown to 2015: A report card on maternal, neonatal and child survival. *The Lancet*; 371(9620) 1217–1219.

Milennium Development Goals: http://www.un.org/millenniumgoals/bkgd.shtml accessed 17.6.09

The People's Health Movement (2008). *Global Health Watch 2: An alternative world health report*. Zed Books, London. http://www.ghwatch.org/ghw2/ghw2pdf/ghw2.pdf

Waterston, T. and Davies, R. (2006) Series on children's rights *The Lancet*, **367(9511)**: 635.

Waterston, T. and Goldhagen, J. (2007) Why children's rights are central to international child health. *Arch. Dis. Child.*, **92**: 176–180.

WHO Division of Child Health and Development (1997). Integrated management of childhood illness. *Bulletin of the World Health Organisation*; **75 supplement 1**: 119–28.

Chapter 3

Determinants of child health

> It is more important to know what sort of person has a
> disease than to know what sort of disease a person has.
> *Hippocrates, 460 BC–ca. 370 BC*

Over the last ten years, there has been an explosion of knowledge around the determinants of health and disease. A determinant is any factor or characteristic that increases the risk of disease or brings about a change in health, either for the better or for the worse. These factors might be very closely related in time or space to the outcome we are interested in (proximal or 'downstream'), or relatively far away in terms of the causal chain and our understanding of the precise mechanisms through which it acts (distal or 'upstream').

In many respects, we are rediscovering the philosophy of the ancient medical thinkers of Greece, India, China, and Arabia, who described the intimate interface between the physical and social environment, nutrition, emotional wellbeing, and health, and we are attempting to explain the scientific mechanisms underpinning the effects of these different factors. From their writings, it is clear that these early thinkers recognized ways in which different determinants could interact with one another, some potentiating and some reducing risk. With the increasing sophistication of epidemiological and biological methods today, we are beginning to be able to observe and quantify this complex interplay of determinants. Epigenetics – the study of the way in which the expression of disease-related genes is determined by the environment – is a good example.

A number of different conceptual frameworks have been used to describe how the various different determinants of health interrelate. The Mandala diagram is a well-known example that has been used for centuries to describe the wide range of factors that influence our health. Figure 3.1 shows the individual at the centre surrounded by the immediate social environment of the family and the local community; this is encircled by the wider socio-economic, physical, and human-made environment. Health (or, more accurately, sickness) services are represented, along with work and lifestyle, as important determinants of health and wellbeing. The community as a whole is influenced by prevailing culture, and by natural ecology.

We have adapted this framework to describe the determinants of child health and how they interact. Thus parental health and genetic constitution, antenatal and postnatal nutrition, and infection influence early human biological factors such as birthweight. At a family level, support, nurturance, and stimulation influence the development of language, social and emotional health. The family is in turn influenced by resources determined in large part by employment and financial security.

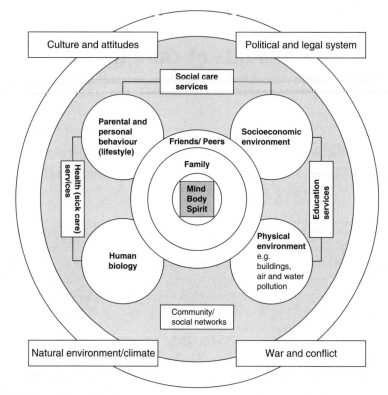

Fig. 3.1 Mandala of Child Health.
Source: Adapted from Hancock, T. (1985), The Mandala diagram of health—a model of the human ecosystem. Family and Community Health 8: 1–10, with permission.

Neighbourhoods and communities play a part in determining what families can and cannot offer their children. Here factors such as safety, social cohesion, and the avoidance of ghettoization of poor and marginalized families are key influences on early childhood development. The way in which we design our cities and their social organization has a major influence at this level. At the widest level of social aggregation, the key factors are sociopolitical organization and programme delivery. Income distribution, patterns of employment and migration, and societal attitudes to children and young people influence the conditions in which children live, learn, and grow up.

We describe each of these levels of influence and give examples of how these determinants effect the child in the centre of the diagram.

Human biology

Genetic predisposition plays a part in determining the personality, temperament, and health of children. For a small number, specific genetic defects lead directly to specific conditions such as cystic fibrosis, Down's syndrome, or haemophilia. Children from certain ethnic backgrounds are at greater risk of particular genetic diseases such as thalassaemia and sickle cell anaemia. Consanguinity increases the risk of certain disabling conditions among groups for whom this is a common cultural practice. It is important that health professionals are aware of these risks and alert to the possibility of rare diseases, so that they can offer appropriate care and counselling. A better understanding of metabolic pathways in rare diseases (such as cystathionine beta synthase deficiency related mental retardation) has led to a greater understanding of possible biological markers for commoner conditions such as heart disease and possible preventive measure with dietary vitamin supplementation.

The rapid rise in understanding of genetic conditions offers the potential for intervention and also for screening, either antenatally or post-natally, or sometimes in later childhood; it also raises complex ethical issues that society needs to address. In the future, genetic manipulation may make it easier for parents to choose to remove defects in their unborn infant. It will be important for health service providers to ensure that information is available to parents of all backgrounds and education.

There is an increasing understanding of the biology of behaviour and emotions, and of the ways in which gene expression affects temperament and the way individuals react to different environments. Twin studies have been helpful in determining the relative influences of genes and environment on different behaviours (see Further reading – Spector, T.D.), and recent epigenetic studies are even more revealing. These have shown that the expression of genes related to conduct disorder and depression is influenced by the quality of parenting (Further reading – Moffitt studies).

The science of epigenetics is giving us insights into how the physical and social environment can interact directly on genetic expression. In one study by Pembrey, paternal (but not maternal) grandsons of Swedish boys who were exposed to famine in the 19th century were less likely to die of cardiovascular disease. Diabetes mortality in the grandchildren increased if food was in plentiful supply, suggesting that this was a transgenerational epigenetic effect which in itself can trigger differential gene expression in different populations.

Parental and personal behaviour

> If we could give every individual the right amount of nourishment and exercise, not too little and not too much, we would have found the safest way to health.
>
> Hippocrates

This advice is clearly as central today as it was in Hippocrates' time. Parental, especially maternal, nutrition is a key determinant of fetal and early infant health. It is of critical importance in the developing world, but also highly relevant in industrialized societies. Other parental lifestyle determinants important in pregnancy and childhood include exercise, alcohol, smoking, and drugs. This section outlines the effects of these factors from both a parental and also a child perspective.

Nutrition

Antenatal

Infants of mothers who are deficient in micronutrients are at a greater risk of death, low birthweight, or congenital anomalies. For example, folate deficiency leads to a greater risk of spina bifida. Table 3.1 below shows the effect of nutrient supplementation (iron and folate and multiple micronutrients) on the risk of infant mortality in a large double blind randomized controlled trial in Indonesia. There was an 18% reduction in early infant mortality in the supplemented mothers.

It is estimated that up to two-thirds of pregnant women in some UK urban environments are Vitamin D deficient. The potential consequences include neonatal convulsions, poor bone health, and increased risk of infections such as TB and HIV. The UK is currently promoting antenatal nutritional health with its Healthy Start campaign. This actively encourages disadvantaged families to have a healthier diet by providing vouchers that are exchangeable in local shops for fruit and vegetables.

Infancy

For the vast majority of mothers, breast-feeding is overwhelmingly the best method of infant feeding. In all countries of the world, both rich and poor, there are significant health benefits from breast-feeding, particularly in the prevention of gastroenteritis and respiratory infections, but also in the reduction of other infections and in enhanced cognitive development. HIV positive mothers are advised not to breast-feed because of the risk of vertical transmission of the HIV virus, but in the developing world, particularly rural areas, the health risks of bottle feeding often outweigh the risks of HIV transmission.

Advantages of breast-feeding

For the baby	For the mother
Lower risk of gastrointestinal infections	Cheap
Lower risk of respiratory infections	Convenient – no sterilizing or bottle preparation
Lower risk of atopic disorders	
Possibly, higher IQ in preterms	No risk of error in composition
Lower risk of sudden infant death	Promotes post-partum weight loss
Lower risk of heart disease in later life	Lower risk of breast cancer
Lower risk of obesity	May promote mother–infant relationship

In the UK breast-feeding rates have improved over the last two or three decades but the increase has been slow in recent years (Fig. 3.2).

The numbers maintaining breast-feeding are low; there is a sharp and continuing decline over the first few weeks and months, so that only 25% of mothers are still breast-feeding at six months (Fig. 3.3). At six months of age, the UK has one of the lowest breast-feeding rates in Europe. The incidence of breast-feeding is higher for first babies than subsequent births, and there are significant differences between social

Table 3.1 Effect of maternal supplementation

	IFA			MMN			Relative risk (95% CI)	p value
	Number of deaths	Number of births*	Events per 1000 births*	Number of deaths	Number of births*	Events per 1000 births		
Early infant mortality[†]	580	13500	43.0	490	13798	35.5	0.82 (0.70–0.95)	0.010
Neonatal mortality	353	13862	25.5	325	14169	22.3	0.90 (0.76–1.06)	0.19
Early neonatal mortality[‡]	267	13971	19.1	247	14287	17.3	0.90 (0.76–1.08)	0.26
Late neonatal mortality[§]	86	13862	6.2	78	14169	5.5	0.88(0.63–1.23)	0.44
Postneonatal mortality[¶]	227	13500	16.8	165	13798	12.0	0.70 (0.55–0.89)	0.0040

Infants with follow-up to the distal timepoint for each outcome were included. IFA= iron and folic acid. MMN=multiple micronutrients. *Refers to livebirths. †From birth to 12 weeks (90 days) after birth. ‡From birth to 7 days after birth. § From 8 days to 28 days after birth. ¶From 29 days to 90 days after birth.

Source: Reprinted from The Lancet, Effect of maternal multiple micronutrient supplementation on fetal loss and infant death in Indonesia: a double-blind cluster-randomised trial The Supplementation with Multiple Micronutrients Intervention Trial (SUMMIT) Study Group* *Lancet* 2008; 371: 215–27.

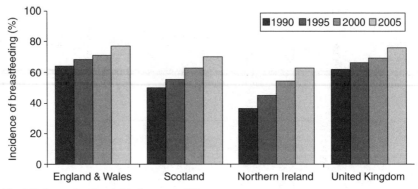

Fig. 3.2 Breast-feeding initiation rates UK.
Source: Reproduced from Infant Feeding Survey 2005, NHS Information Centre 2007.
Copyright © 2009, Re-used with the permission of The Health and Social Care
Information Centre. All rights reserved.

and ethnic groups. The majority of mothers in professional and managerial classes breast-feed, compared to relatively small numbers in routine and manual classes, although figures from 2005 show a narrowing of this gap (Table 3.2).

Breast-feeding rates among mothers from the Asian subcontinent and of African or Caribbean origin are substantially higher than among white mothers (Table 3.3).

There have been improvements in hospital and community support with the development of the UNICEF Baby Friendly Award but these are slow to influence breast-feeding rates.

The risks of bottle feeding are high where access to safe water supplies is limited and advice on appropriate feed composition may not be available. There is a heavy responsibility on health professionals to ensure that they do not advertently or inadvertently offer pro-bottle feeding messages through their advice and their example. Manufacturers of formula milk, seeking to expand their market in the developing world, may promote

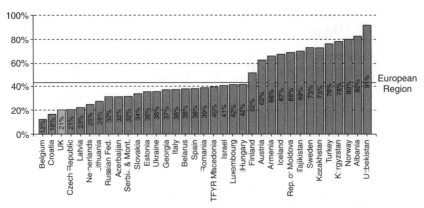

Fig. 3.3 Percentage of women breast-feeding at six months by European nation,
1994–2003 average.
Source: Reproduced from Indications of Public Health in the English Regions 5:
Child Health, Association of Public Health Observatories, 2006, with permission.

Table 3.2 Breast-feeding by socio-economic status

| | England & Wales | |
| | 2000 | 2005 |
% who *breastfed initially*	%	%
Managerial & professional	86	89
Intermediate occupations	75	79
Routine and manual	60	67
Never worked	54	67
Unclassified	68	72
All mothers	**71**	**77**

their products to the detriment of breast-feeding rates. The UNICEF Baby Friendly Hospital and Community awards (see http://www.babyfriendly.org.uk/) ensure that good practice is standard, and there is now evidence that being born or reared in a Baby Friendly environment increases the chances of successful breast-feeding.

Childhood

The food that young children eat is determined primarily by parental choice (a proximal determinant); later the choice of children and young people themselves plays an important part, as well as more distal determinants such as availability, cost, and the influence of marketing.

Unhealthy food is often more convenient for parents and cheaper than healthy options. Several surveys have shown that a 'healthy' food basket (containing fruit, vegetables, and fish, for example) is considerably more expensive than an 'unhealthy' basket (containing food such as pies, chips, and sausages). Attitudes to food may be

Table 3.3 Breast-feeding by ethnicity

| | *Percentage who breastfed initially* | |
| | *2000* | *2005* |
	%	%
White	68	74
Mixed	86	34
Asian or Asian British	87	94
Black or Black British	95	96
Chinese or other ethnic group	85	93
All mothers[†]	**70**	**77**

[†] Includes some mothers for whom ethnicity was not recorded.

heavily influenced by intensive media marketing of high-calorie, high-sugar, and low-fibre foods. It is hard for parents to control food quality as few families grow their own food. Most buy it in the supermarket where the basis for their choice is often marketing (much of it aimed at children) rather than nutritional principles.

The tendency to buy convenient, unhealthy food is greater in inner city estates that lack markets where good-quality vegetables can be purchased cheaply, and in low-income families without a car who are unable to 'shop around' for bargains. When a higher proportion of the household budget goes on food, adults are reluctant to buy food that might be thrown away if the children do not like it. Thus children's preferences, influenced by advertising, may affect the family diet unduly. Families from ethnic minorities, who find it hard to access culturally appropriate ingredients, may well fall back on the most familiar and least healthy options among the 'traditional' UK diet.

Recent research underpinning solutions to childhood obesity has shown that children's preferences are malleable, but that children may need to be exposed to new foods many times before they develop a taste for them. Current advice suggests that parents decide what goes on children's plates (controlling portion size) and that children decide what goes in their mouths. In this way, their tastes can be widened in accordance with their needs, at relatively low cost. The practice of insisting that children finish the food on their plates is inappropriate, interfering with children's developing sense of their own needs.

Nutritional awareness in the community is low and labelling information can be abstruse and confusing, although the 'traffic lights' schemes introduced recently may help. Cooking facilities may be limited, parents increasingly lack culinary skills and knowledge, and many have only ever eaten a very limited range of foods. Food additives are ubiquitous, especially in soft drinks and the convenience foods that are attractively marketed to children; these may cause hyperactivity and migraine and may be addictive. There is also a high 'hidden' salt and sugar content in many products, increasing the risk of coronary heart disease, cancer, obesity, and dental caries.

Currently, about one in five children in the UK eat no fruit. It has been suggested that increasing fruit and vegetable intake to five pieces a day across the population is the second most effective strategy for reducing cancer after curbing smoking, and could reduce deaths from chronic disease overall by 20%. Health education alone cannot change the situation: initiatives such as food co-operatives, farmer's markets in cities, and the government's National School Fruit Scheme can make an important contribution.

The ways in which families eat have changed radically over the last few decades. An increasing and significant proportion of families do not own a table and chairs at which they can eat family meals. Meals are taken 'on the hoof' or in front of the television in a solitary way rather than in a relaxed social atmosphere. These new lifestyles have been shown to increase consumption of calories, particularly the unhealthy calories.

The unintended consequences of food-purchase choices also affect the biosphere/ecology level of the Mandala. Buying food that comes from a long distance – such as vegetables from Africa, fruit from the US, apples from Australia, or bottled water from France (or indeed England) has an environmental cost, increasing our carbon footprint and influencing climate change – which may in turn lead to increased food costs, secondary to harvest failure from flooding. The value to health as well as to the environment of using food which is sourced locally is being increasingly recognized both by individual families and corporate purchasers such as schools and the NHS.

Much of the difference in mortality between the developed and developing world is mediated by malnutrition. Over 50% of the world's malnourished children and low birth weight infants live in south Asia, and one in three of Africa's children are underweight. It is estimated that 226 million children worldwide are stunted by malnutrition which, as we have already seen, has a major impact on their ability to resist and recover from infection. Nutritional deficiencies in minerals and vitamins are estimated to cost some countries the equivalent of more than 5% of their GNP in lost lives, disability, and productivity.

Physical activity among children and young people

The amount of exercise children in the developed world take has dropped precipitously over the last half century. Children are now often driven to school, school playing fields have been sold off, and parents are often too anxious about dangers to let their children 'play out'. Coupled with rapid developments in entertainment technology such as gaming and social websites, this means that children live increasingly sedentary lives. Concerned with the epidemic of childhood obesity, Western countries are now developing policies designed to increase physical activity in schools and create safe routes for children to walk to and from school.

Children are more likely to exercise regularly if their parents do. In one Swedish study, parents' physical activity was strongly associated with that of their children. With two active parents, the odds ratio for children's participation in sport was almost 4 for girls and 9 for boys, compared with having inactive parents (See Eriksson, M. et al.).

The national recommendation is that adults and children should undertake at least 60 minutes of vigorous exercise daily. Physical activity in childhood has an influence on adult health through the prevention of obesity and the promotion of cardiovascular health. Other benefits include protection from depression, anxiety, and insomnia. Regular exercise in childhood also reduces the risk of infectious disease and improves bone health in later adult life. Taking exercise in a team improves social interaction, confidence, and self-esteem. Opportunities for exercise in later childhood and adolescence depend on the availability of play areas and leisure facilities, which are often scarce in socially disadvantaged areas.

Parental alcohol, smoking, drugs

Drinking alcohol during pregnancy has a direct effect on the developing fetus. The fetal brain is particularly sensitive to alcohol: a wide spectrum of conditions, including general cognitive impairment, and mental and behavioural problems, has been shown to be associated with its consumption in pregnancy.

Parental alcohol abuse also acts as an upstream determinant of child health in older children through its effect on emotional and physical development. The quality of parenting is likely to be affected, and there is an increased risk of domestic violence and child abuse, as well as traffic accidents and injury at work. The last may affect the ability of the parent to keep a job, placing the family at socio-economic risk.

Maternal smoking also has a profound effect on the physical growth of the fetus, resulting in low birthweight infants, prematurity, and a high risk of attention deficit hyperactivity disorder (ADHD) in later childhood. There is a strong causal association between parental smoking in the postnatal period and the incidence of glue ear and lower respiratory tract infections in childhood.

It is estimated that in some inner-city areas as many as 15% of pregnant women have taken marijuana or cocaine at some stage during their pregnancy. Cocaine can interfere with endogenous opiate production in the foetal brain, causing irritability in infants during the first few weeks. Many substances can affect the growth and function of the brain many years after the initial fetal exposure.

Risk behaviour and adolescent health

During preadolescence and adolescence, children make choices about health-related lifestyles for themselves. These choices may be heavily influenced by their parents' behaviour and their experiences in the home, but other factors (especially peer influences) also play a part. The lifestyles young people adopt at this stage, although still malleable, affect their health and contribute to the development of the diseases which cause morbidity and premature mortality in adulthood. Diet, nutrition, and exercise are key elements, as are high-risk behaviours such as substance use and misuse (smoking, alcohol, mood altering drugs) and unsafe sex.

As children become more independent financially, they can purchase low-cost, unhealthy food for themselves.

Alcohol, drug, and tobacco abuse increase with age in adolescence, and there are marked gender differences in their use. There is an association with truancy, poor schoolwork, antisocial behaviour, unplanned sexual activity, and involvement with the police. Although the UK has amongst the highest levels of adolescent substance abuse in Europe (40% of 15 year olds report drinking alcohol at least once a week, and a substantial proportion report drunkenness (Fig. 3.4)), there are signs of a reduction in the past few years. Smoking rates are higher in Eastern European countries and high alcohol consumption is more prevalent in other northern European countries, reflecting different environmental and cultural influences. About a quarter of English and nearly a third of Welsh 15-year olds report trying cannabis; approximately 1 in 10 have taken cannabis in the past 30 days.

Many adolescents who experiment with drugs, alcohol, and smoking revert to a healthier lifestyle in young adulthood. However, long term smokers almost invariably started smoking at a young age, and postponing the age of experimentation is therefore considered a worthwhile preventive intervention (Fig. 3.5) Many health education programmes have been developed to discourage experimentation with different substances. Most schools offer children classes on these topics which aim to increase children's knowledge and understanding. Controlled trials have been unable to demonstrate

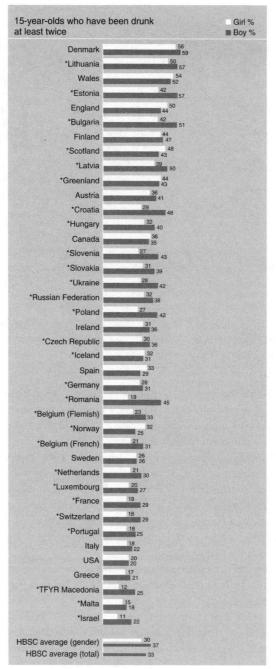

15-year-olds who have been drunk at least twice

Girl %
Boy %

Country	Girl %	Boy %
Denmark	56	59
*Lithuania	50	57
Wales	54	52
*Estonia	42	57
England	50	44
*Bulgaria	42	51
Finland	44	47
*Scotland	48	43
*Latvia	39	50
*Greenland	44	43
Austria	36	41
*Croatia	29	48
*Hungary	32	40
Canada	36	35
*Slovenia	27	43
*Slovakia	31	39
*Ukraine	28	42
*Russian Federation	32	38
*Poland	27	42
Ireland	31	36
*Czech Republic	30	36
*Iceland	32	31
Spain	33	29
*Germany	28	31
*Romania	19	45
*Belgium (Flemish)	23	33
*Norway	32	25
*Belgium (French)	21	31
Sweden	26	26
*Netherlands	21	30
*Luxembourg	20	27
*France	18	29
*Switzerland	18	29
*Portugal	18	25
Italy	18	22
USA	20	20
Greece	17	21
*TFYR Macedonia	12	25
*Malta	15	18
*Israel	11	22
HBSC average (gender)	30	37
HBSC average (total)		33

* indicates a significant gender difference (at p<0.05). No data available for Turkey

Fig. 3.4 Drunkenness.
Source: Reproduced from Currie C et al., eds. *Inequalities in young people's health. HBSC international report from the 2005/2006 survey*. Copenhagen, WHO Regional Office for Europe, 2008: 133, with permission.

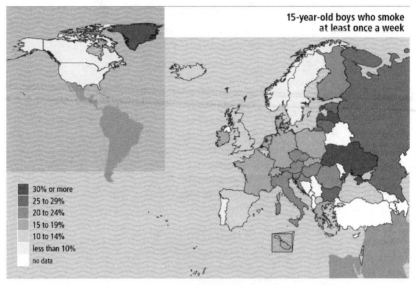

Fig. 3.5 Smoking.
Source: Reproduced from Currie C et al., eds. *Inequalities in young people's health. HBSC international report from the 2005/2006 survey.* Copenhagen, WHO Regional Office for Europe, 2008:122, with permission.

sustained effects on behaviour. There is some evidence that it is possible to delay the onset of smoking but very little that it is possible to influence drug or alcohol misuse. Programmes to improve nutrition and exercise are more effective. The programmes that work best are whole school approaches that aim to change the school ethos and environment and also involve parents and the wider community. These approaches are part of what defines the Health Promoting School approach which is now widespread throughout Europe and has informed the UK's Healthy Schools Programme.

Over the last few years in England, there has been a decline in smoking rates among children. The decline in alcohol consumption has been less marked, partly due to the marketing of beverages such as alcopops, designed to appeal to teenagers, and the relative reduction in the cost of alcohol.

There is concern that sexual activity among adolescents is rising, with a consequent increase in sexually transmitted diseases and unintended teen pregnancies. There are enormous variations within Europe: nearly two thirds of 15-year olds in Greenland have had sexual intercourse compared to only 12% in Slovakia. The figure is around 27% for England, where around 80% report using a condom when last having intercourse, and around 20% report using the contraceptive pill. There were approximately 40,000 pregnancies in 15–17 year olds in England and Wales in 2007, of which half were aborted. There has been a 10% fall in our teenage pregnancy rate since 1997, a slower reduction than in many other countries. This reflects differences in attitudes and policies relating to sexual activity, and access to health education, advice, and practical support. School-based programmes to promote sexual health are worthwhile because they help children develop knowledge and understanding of this topic. However, controlled trials have been unable to show that, on their own, they are effective in reducing sexual activity in the young or increasing safe sex. There is some evidence that those that involve peers may be more worthwhile than those that don't.

Family influences and parenting

Families are a potent influence both on a child's genetic constitution and, as we have seen in the last section, on their health related behaviour. The family also constitutes a child's immediate social network and has a vital influence on the development of socio-emotional health and wellbeing.

Family size and structure

Until fairly recently, epidemiological studies of the influence of families on children's growth and development have concentrated on easily measurable determinants such as family size and structure. In industrialized countries, both of these factors have changed dramatically over the last century, and these changes have had a major influence on the way children are looked after.

Large family size is a distinctive feature in most low-income countries and has been the focus of much aid and education by industrialized countries. These efforts have often been ineffective, and there is now a much better understanding of how reproductive decisions are taken. The key factors in reducing family size in developing countries are increasing income (so that children are not seen as an economic necessity), educating women, and making contraceptive advice available throughout the health service. Countries such as Kerala (a state of Southern India) and Sri Lanka, which have focused on these factors, have had remarkable success in reducing fertility. Family size and short birth interval are important predictors of nutritional status, but far more of the earth's resources are used by the small families of the industrialized countries rather than the large families of the poor world.

The average family size is the UK is now 1.9 children, meaning that only children are now common and large siblingships rare (Fig. 3.6). However, the latter are a risk factor for poverty in the developed as well as developing world (Fig. 3.7).

Partly as a result of changing gender attitudes and expectations (Table 3.4), which have given women greater financial independence, marital breakdown is now very common. Forty per cent of first marriages end in divorce, and in England and Wales in 2007, nearly one in four children (a total of 2,672,000 dependent children) lived in lone-parent families, over 90% of which are headed by the mother (Table 3.5). More than one in ten dependent children (1,284,000) live in a step-family (ONS). The latter are more prone to break down than first time marriages, so many children move in and out of different family structures throughout their childhood. While these changes create problems for many children, (see below) for some they may be a source of resilience. Becoming a single parent is almost invariably associated with a drop in family income, and marital breakdown is therefore an important cause of childhood poverty.

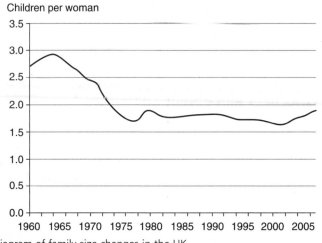

Fig. 3.6 Diagram of family size changes in the UK.
Source: National Statistics website: www.statistics.gov.uk, with permission.

Family break-up and conflict

It is not unusual for children's health and wellbeing to suffer from family breakdown. Emotional and behavioural problems and educational failure are more common, and children in these circumstances are also more likely to be abused. Some have suggested that it is not the single-parent family status or the family breakdown themselves

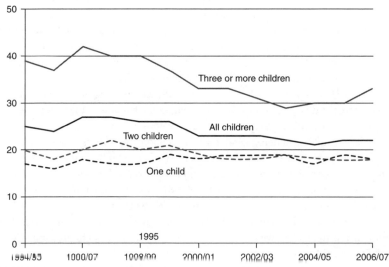

Fig. 3.7 Poverty related to family size. Proportion of children living in households below 60 per cent of median household disposable income: by number of children in family *UK*.
Source: Reproduced from National Statistics website: www.statistics.gov.uk, with permission.

Table 3.4 Attitudes to marriage[1]

Great Britain	Percentages	
	Agreed with statement 2000	Agreed with statement 2006
Married couples make better parents than unmarried ones	28	29
Even though it might not work out for some people, marriage is still the best kind of relationship	59	56
Marriage gives couples more financial security than living together	49	64
There is no point getting married – it's only a piece of paper	9	9

1 Adults aged 18 and over were asked if they agreed with the above statements. Excludes those who responded 'don't know' or did not answer.

Source: Reproduced from Social Trends no.39, ONS 2009, with permission.

which are the problem, but the poverty which often accompanies these situations. Others have suggested that what damages children is exposure to conflict. Persistent unresolved conflict in the home is detrimental to children's social and emotional development. Children who grow up in homes characterized by marital discord,

Table 3.5 Percentage of dependent children living in different family types

Great Britain	Percentages				
	1972	1981	1992[1]	2001[1]	2003[1]
Couple families					
1 child	16	18	18	17	17
2 children	35	41	39	38	37
3 or more children	41	29	27	25	24
Lone mother families					
1 child	2	3	4	6	6
2 children	2	4	5	7	8
3 or more children	2	3	4	5	6
Lone father families					
1 child	–	1	1	1	2
2 or more children	1	1	1	1	1
All children[2]	100	100	100	100	100

1 At spring. These estimates are not seasonally adjusted and have not been adjusted to take account of the Census 2001 results.

2 Excludes cases where the dependent child is a family unit, for example, a foster child.

Source: Table 2.4, Social trends no. 34, ONS 2009, with permission. http://www.statistics.gov.uk/STATBASE/ssdataset.asp?vlnk=7256

particularly where there is verbal or physical aggression, non-verbal conflict, or the 'silent treatment,' are at increased risk of emotional and behavioural problems. Sometimes children, particularly girls, may respond to conflict by adopting a parental role themselves. All these outcomes put children at increased risk of experiencing mental health problems and difficulty in establishing healthy relationships in later life. Persistent unresolved conflict, including domestic violence, occurs in all social classes. Recent research has demonstrated the protective value of retaining a strong influence from the biological father in both reconstituted and single parent families, but it requires a high level of emotional maturity in parents to achieve this.

Child care

Child care is now often shared between two parents who do not live together.

There are considerable variations in care arrangements, with grandparents remaining a very important influence (Table 3.6). Paid (formal) childcare is particularly important for lone parents, and the quality of that care has important repercussions for children's health and wellbeing. Poor quality day care is very common and now known to be damaging to children's emotional and social development. Good quality day care offers young children continuity of relationship and care in small groups, which simulate families. These approaches enable young children to form the all important attachment relationships that they need for the parts of their brains governing emotional and social development to grow in a way which supports good mental health in later childhood. Up until recently day care has been a poorly paid and poorly respected job. But with the growing body of evidence of its importance, degree courses and professional qualifications are increasing in number and the workforce is becoming more skilled. At the same time, child minders who can provide a substitute family environment for babies and young children are becoming better trained and more respected.

Mothers are tending to have their children later, and babies and very young children are increasingly being placed in day care facilities as a result of their parents' changing work patterns and economic circumstances (Fig. 3.8). The long term impact on adult social and emotional functioning of placing large numbers of babies in day care will take a while to emerge.

Early parent–child relationships

In the last few decades, attention has been focused not just on the 'shape' of families, but on what goes on within them. It is now clear that from the moment of birth, the way mothers and fathers relate to their babies has an important influence on their emotional and social development, and studies in both animals and humans have begun to elucidate the biological mechanisms for this process.

Early studies of family relationships focused on the concept of mother–infant attachment, which can be reliably measured in a laboratory setting. Attachment studies – based on the way a one-year old responds to the mother's departure and return – divide children into those who are securely attached (around 70% of the population) and those who are not. Different categories of 'disordered' attachment have been

Table 3.6 Child care arrangements

Child care arrangements for children with working mothers: by family characteristics, 2006

Great Britain

	Percentages[1]		Informal child care				
	Child care not required	Formal child care[2]	Ex partner/ non-resident parent	Grand-parent	Older sibling/ other relative	Other informal[3]	Total informal
Family type							
Lone parent	47	28	14	31	15	11	46
Couple	39	27	1	32	8	7	39
Family type working status							
Lone parent: 1 to 15 hours	54	14	9	20	11	21	37
Lone parent: 16 hours and above	38	29	15	33	15	10	47
Couple – both: 16 hours and above	43	31	2	34	8	8	40
Couple – one only: 16 hours and above	57	17	0	28	9	8	35
Age of child							
0 to 4	21	54	4	42	9	8	49
5 to 10	34	33	6	39	12	12	51
11 to 16	71	6	3	18	8	5	26

1 Percentages do not sum to 100 per cent as respondents could give more than one answer.

2 Includes nurseries/crèches, nursery schools, playgroups, registered childminders, after school clubs/breakfast clubs, and holiday play schemes.

3 A friend, neighbour or babysitter, who came to the home.

Source: Reproduced from Social Trends no.39, ONS 2009, with permission.

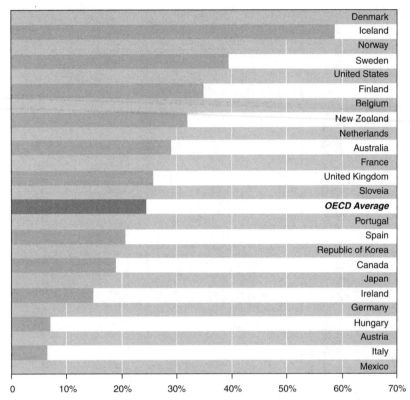

Fig. 3.8 Percentage enrolment of 0–3 year olds in child care. Child care in transition – a league table of early childhood education and care in economically advanced countries. Source: Reproduced from Report Card 8, 2008, UNICEF Innocenti Research Centre, Florence.

described, including avoidant, ambivalent, and the most severely disturbed category – disorganized. Secure early attachment predicts, in later years:

◆ self-confidence

◆ self-efficacy

◆ self-regulation

◆ autonomy

◆ good relationships with peers.

Children who are insecurely attached at one-year of age are likely to be anxious, aggressive, or isolated at school. Adolescents who were securely attached at age one are more competent, more socially orientated and empathetic, able to develop deeper relationships, and more likely to respond to stress by seeking help than those who were insecurely attached infants

There has been an increase, in recent years, in observational research during the first few months of the baby's life, which has refined our understanding of attachment and described differences in parental sensitivity and attunement. Whilst almost all of this research is based on the mother-baby relationship, it is very likely that it also applies to fathers, whose influence on early life is greater than was previously understood. Sensitivity to babies' needs and cues, and appropriate parental responses are critical to socio-emotional development (Fig. 3.9). The babies of mothers who are not able to 'read' their infants and are not in tune with their needs become anxious and withdrawn. In the longer term, these babies fail to develop the self-soothing mechanisms that older children and adults depend on to respond helpfully to stress. Babies who are nurtured in a way that is sensitive to their needs seem better able to weather the adverse consequences of living in poverty and deprivation, emerging unscathed into adulthood. Thus early relationships play an important part in the development of resilience, and insecure attachment creates vulnerability to psychopathology in later life.

The baby's temperament plays a part in this process too. Babies are active players in their early relationships, and some are just much more difficult to soothe than others.

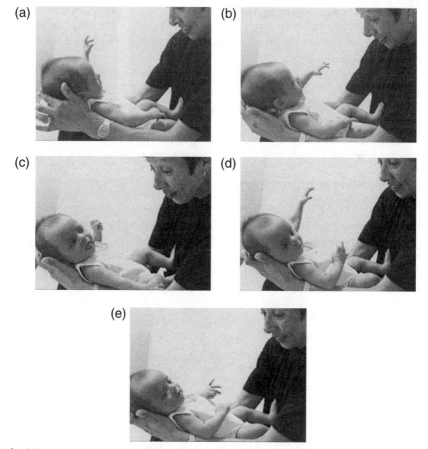

Fig. 3.9 How parents can 'read' their baby. Alexandra shows that she is tiring of the conversation (a,b) by turning her head away (c) and watching her mother from the corner of her eye. She then cuts her gaze completely (d). In (e) she is recharged and shows that she is ready for further conversation.
Source: From The Social Baby. Murray L. and Andrews E. (eds). The Children's Project. www.socialbaby.com

Some research suggests that sensitive, attuned parenting has a greater impact on these babies than on those who have the fortune to be born more robust. Sadly, the most irritable 'difficult' babies are often those of parents who are least well equipped to provide sensitive, attuned care (for example those who have used illegal drugs during pregnancy).

There are strong intergenerational links in attachment styles, and parents tend to parent their children in the way that they themselves were parented, particularly with regard to the more subtle socio-emotional components of the relationship. It can be hard for parents to appreciate that there are alternative ways of parenting, let alone that there are better ones; and it can be equally hard to shift parental relationship patterns that date back to infancy.

Whilst the importance of these very early relationships was being demonstrated, interventions were being developed to support them. These range from video interaction modelling, through cognitive behavioural approaches, to psychotherapeutically-based interventions. Collectively, these interventions aim to promote infant mental health (see Chapter 8 scenarios B). Interventions to support early fathering are now being developed too, but the evidence base to show that these interventions work is not yet well established.

Parental mental illness (see below), most importantly post-natal depression, interrupts attachment. Babies whose mothers have been depressed are more likely to demonstrate difficulties in adjustment to school, difficulties in relating to peers, and emotional and behavioural problems typical of insecurely attached children. Problems with attachment are more common amongst mothers living in social deprivation, and many intervention studies have concentrated on trying to improve attachment in this group.

Parent–child relationships in childhood and adolescence

Sensitive parenting continues to be important throughout childhood, but from the age of two onwards setting and maintaining 'boundaries' becomes an issue of importance for social and emotional development and mental health. Harsh and inconsistent discipline, poor monitoring and supervision, and lack of warmth, affection, and praise are all important determinants of antisocial behaviour and conduct disorder in children, and of delinquency, violence, and criminality in adolescence. Paterson and colleagues at the Oregon Social Learning Centre have shown that these parenting styles account for as much as 40% of the variation in conduct disorder.

A useful classification, which owes its origins to Diana Baumrind, describes parenting styles (Fig. 3.10) as:

authoritative – loving and understanding, with firm, age-appropriate and negotiated boundaries

authoritarian – punitive and unaffectionate, controlling

neglectful – neither loving nor firm

permissive – loving, but failing to exercise any control.

Children of parents who are authoritative do much better at school, have higher self-esteem, and more rewarding peer interactions than those whose parents adopt other styles. Positive approaches to discipline are important (Fig. 3.11).

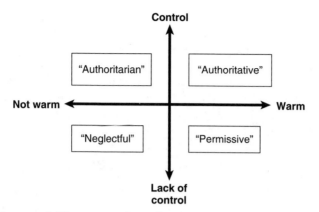

Fig. 3.10 Diagram of different parenting styles.

Another approach to the classification of parenting distinguishes between just two different dimensions of parenting—support and control. This classification emphasizes the positive aspects of parental support and the negative aspects of intrusive parental control. Overcontrolling parenting styles can have a negative impact on the development of autonomy. Children of parents who are controlling and unsupportive are most at risk of unhealthy lifestyles and poor educational outcomes. Good communication with parents (Fig. 3.12), which is unlikely to feature in families where parents are controlling or unsupportive, can protect against the adoption of unhealthy lifestyles.

Recent research with children and adolescents themselves show how perceptive children can be about their parents and parenting. They reveal a remarkable tolerance of different family set ups; the key for children and adolescents is to feel that their parents are interested in them and care about them. They also reveal a quite mature approach to boundaries, supervision and discipline; children recognize this as necessary for their wellbeing and are also clear that positive discipline works better than negative.

A large number of interventions have been developed to help parents of children between 2 and 11 years change the way they parent, and the evidence base for some of these interventions is impressive. These range from books, DVDs, television programmes, and websites through intensive one-to-one programmes delivered in the home or clinic setting. The most common programmes in the UK are group-based (catering for around 10 parents) and offer a two to three hour session once a week for 8–12 weeks. The programmes that are effective are those that can be delivered consistently, where those delivering them receive significant training and supervision, and where they work from a manual. Good quality programmes attend to parents needs by providing crèches and transport if necessary. Good facilitators are respectful and empathetic and take a strengths-based approach. Parents get home work, practise the skills they have learnt through role play, and report back the next week. The best known examples of these sorts of programmes are the Incredible Years Series of programmes from the US and Triple P from Australia. Good quality programmes like Mellow Parenting, Family Links, and Strengthening Families Strengthening Communities have also been developed in the UK.

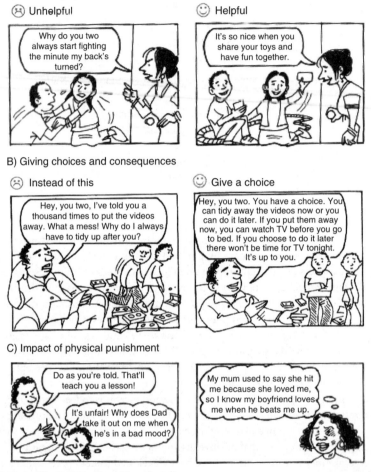

Fig. 3.11 An illustration of positive discipline.
Source: Reproduced from The Parenting Puzzle. Candida Hunt with Annette Mountford. Oxford, Family Links 2003, with permission.

Abuse and neglect

Child abuse and neglect represent the extreme end of the continuum of dysfunctional parenting. Abuse may be physical, emotional, or sexual, or take the form of neglect or failure to thrive. Abuse can occur in families from all social classes, although physical abuse and neglect (but not sexual abuse) are more common in manual class families. It is most common when the parents themselves were abused as children, among parents who abuse alcohol or drugs, or who have mental health problems, and when the child has a disability. Abuse and neglect have profound effects on children's physical and mental health, often leading to failure to thrive, to repeated injuries, to withdrawal, mental illness, and emotional and behavioural problems—and to abusive relationships with partners and children in later life. The most serious cases can be

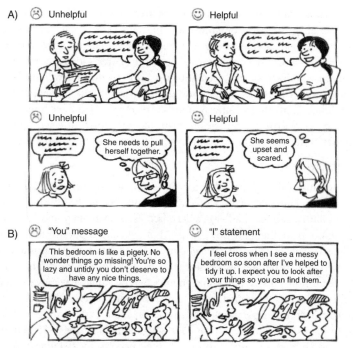

Fig. 3.12 The effect of listening well.
Source: Reproduced from The Parenting Puzzle. Candida Hunt with Annette Mountford.
Oxford, Family Links 2003, with permission.

fatal: one or two children a week die at the hands of their parents or carers in the UK, although the NSPCC believes this to be a significant underestimate.

The boundary between abuse and acceptable punishment is not clearly defined and is changing with time. The acceptability of any form of physical punishment is now questionable. Several studies have shown that, while physical punishment may interrupt problem behaviour and relieve parental frustration, in the longer term it increases rather than reduces antisocial behaviour. Any form of physical punishment is an assault and models the belief that it is acceptable for the powerful to control the powerless by force. It is also in clear breach of the UN Convention on the Rights of the Child. Eighteen European countries now regard physical punishment as abusive and have brought in legislation to protect children from physical discipline; indeed, the UK is now in the minority in permitting a physical assault of a child by a parent, unless a bruise or other injury results.

Risk factors for poor parenting, abuse, and neglect

Risk factors for sub-optimal parenting, abuse, and neglect include poverty and social exclusion. Parenting is more difficult for families who are coping with poverty. However the story here is complex. Whilst there is good evidence that positive parenting is more common among the affluent, variation within social groups is greater than between them. Some studies have suggested that parenting in all its manifestations (psychological, emotional, social and protective) is the mediator through which income inequality influences outcomes for children. There is evidence that children whose parents are able to maintain good parenting in the face of social deprivation are protected from many of the deleterious effects of the latter. Other studies have shown that children who have a caring relationship with an adult outside the immediate home are relatively protected from poor home environments. Social policies which reduce childhood poverty are important for a wide range of child outcomes and create an important backdrop for policies to promote parenting; however the evidence suggests that antipoverty strategies alone will not of themselves improve parenting.

Parental mental health

Mental illness in one or both parents is a strong risk factor for socio-emotional problems and frank mental illness in children. Mediating factors include the severity and length of the parent's illness, and the child's age at its onset. Psychopathology may be passed from one generation to another partly by genetics, but twin and adoption studies show that mental illness is not 'inherited' in a straightforward or specific way. For example, parental bipolar disorder increases the risk of all types of mental illness in the children, including unipolar depression, phobias and schizophrenia. Several studies have suggested that it is not the mere presence of parental mental illness that puts children at risk, but the functional impairment (e.g. in parenting) and impact on family and economic conditions.

While the lifetime risk of mental disorder is high, ranging from 40-75 % in different studies, many children remain unaffected by their parents' mental illness, and studies of resilience and protective factors have played a fruitful part in the development of interventions to prevent transmission. Alongside family income, employment, stable family structure, and social inclusion, they have identified good family relationships and positive parenting as key protective factors.

Families in which one or both parents have a mental illness are often 'hard to reach', partly because of the very real fear such parents have that statutory services will deem them to be a risk to their children and institute child protection proceedings. Adult psychiatrists need to be more attentive to the impact mental illness in their adult patients may have on their children. These children and young people often remain invisible until they come to the attention of school authorities, criminal justice, paediatric, or child and adolescent mental health services (CAMHS). A variety of interventions have been developed recently to help clinicians raise the issue of children and parenting sensitively with their patients, to reduce the isolation, stigma and guilt felt by members of such families, and to support parenting and positive family relationships. Similar intensive interventions are beginning to be developed and trialled in families where parents abuse drugs, a group in which parental mental illness is common.

Community and social network

Peer relationships

As children grow and develop, their lives widen, and relationships with others outside the home, both peers and adults, become increasingly important (Fig. 13.13).

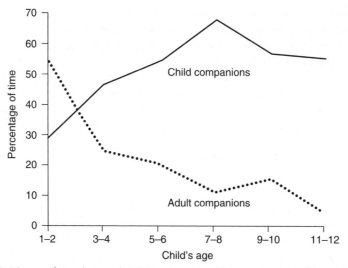

Fig. 3.13 Diagram from the good childhood enquiry. Time spent with adults and other children.
Source: Reproduced from Ellis, Rogoff & Cromer (1981) Age segregation in children's social interactions. Developmental Psychology, 17: 399–406 with permission.

Because of the strong influence of family relationships on the development of the socio-emotional brain and because, by the time they start to make relationships outside the family, children themselves are important players in their relationships, these new relationships have a tendency to echo those experienced within the family. Such children therefore experience 'double jeopardy', finding themselves on the receiving end of dysfunctional relationships both at home and amongst their peers, without the opportunity to experience positive relationships in either setting.

School ethos

While children's socio-emotional environment is affected by the quality of their friendships, the wider school environment is also important. School ethos has been shown to have a profound effect on children's mental health and self-esteem. Many children do not feel safe at school, and anxiety is an important inhibitor of learning. School-based bullying can cause immense difficulties for children and young people, and its prevalence varies widely between different countries and indeed different schools. School ethos, often measured in terms of engagement and participation, predicts the prevalence of substance misuse in different schools with higher levels in schools with a poor school ethos.

A caring environment and zero tolerance of emotional or physical bullying is important, but the impact of school ethos extends beyond this: for example, the extent to which children are treated with respect at school is important for the development of autonomy. Pupil Councils and pupil representatives on school committees are a potential manifestation of such respect, but can also be 'window dressing'. It is the quality of interactions between staff and pupils that really counts. One key factor in determining school ethos is the emotional and social wellbeing of staff, and current school health promotion programmes (e.g. the national Healthy Schools Scheme and SEAL – see below) include improving staff mental health as an important goal. When things go right with teacher-pupil relationships, schools are able to transcend some of the problems experienced by children from dysfunctional families, but to be able to be helpful with difficult children requires teachers to have robust mental wellbeing.

School mental health programmes

The potential for schools to support children's socio-emotional development and prevent mental health problems has become more widely recognized over the last decade, and a number of evidence-based programmes have been developed in this area. These range from 'emotional literacy' education in classroom settings and anxiety management programmes (sometimes incorporating cognitive behavioural approaches, mindfulness, yoga, and qi gong (a mindful movement originating in China and now popular over much of the Western world)) to whole school approaches to bullying.

The most comprehensive programmes are implemented over the course of several years, involving parents and the local community, and offering parenting support as well as approaches to improving children's mental health. In the UK, the National Institute for Health and Clinical Excellence has now endorsed some such programmes, and the Department for Children, Schools and Families has created the SEAL – the Social and Emotional Learning programmes. These are now being implemented in all primary and secondary schools in the UK. Youth mentoring schemes are also increasingly popular, and have been particularly useful for high risk behaviour in those excluded from school or involved in criminal activities.

Physical environment

The physical environment has important effects on child health. Whilst exposures differ in the developed and developing world, with children in the latter usually being considerably worse off those in the former, the same aspects matter. Aspects which have been shown to influence health include the built environment, exposure to pollutants, and climate change.

Urban (built) environments

Most children now live in cities, but urban environments have not been designed with children's wellbeing in mind. 'Playing out' – spontaneous unregulated play – was a feature of mid-childhood in previous eras and is important for social and cognitive development. Access to green spaces and the natural world are now very limited in cities, and increases in the volume and speed of traffic has rendered most streets unsafe for play. The social environment also plays its part and on many estates children are afraid to walk the streets alone because of the threat of violence. Noise pollution is another constant detrimental feature of many urban children's lives. Children in the developed world are provided with regulated play environments but access to these may be limited to families who can afford to pay. Household congestion and lack of access to private spaces is another limiter on children's personal development. Children are also indirectly affected through the impact of the built environment on their parents' mental wellbeing. Similar factors – neighbour noise, feeling over crowded, lack of access to green spaces and community facilities, and feeling unsafe to go out have been shown to constrain adult mental health. All these factors are exacerbated by poor environments and mitigated by wealth.

Pollution and exposure to chemicals

There has been an enormous increase in the number and type of chemicals to which children are exposed in the last 50 years: it is estimated that 15,000 new synthetic chemicals have been developed during this period. Children are more vulnerable to environmental contaminants. This is because of greater and longer exposure, and the existence of 'windows of susceptibility' during which their neurological, immunological, and endocrine systems are particularly sensitive. Children's exposure to environmental hazards varies across social strata, often due to the overlapping factors of poverty, poor housing conditions, restricted access to education, polluted environment, and lack of information. In 1992, the United Nations Conference on Environment and Development gave prominence to the protection of children from the effects of a deteriorating environment with the development of Agenda 21.

Biological factors, age specific susceptibility, economic, social and psychosocial factors, and vulnerability to global environmental changes all contribute to the impact of environmental exposures on children.

Because cell growth is particularly rapid in the embryo, toxins can have a profound effect in utero. For example, lead or mercury exposure during pregnancy can seriously affect the developing brain.

Adults and children have very different capacities for detoxification and excretion of chemicals. Children are often more heavily exposed, per unit of body weight, to chemicals or radiation. They have a longer 'time at risk' for diseases with a long latency period, for example benzine-induced leukaemia and sunlight-induced skin cancer. Many chemicals cannot be broken down in the body because humans lack the appropriate metabolic pathways. Some substances accumulate and can be passed on to the next generation – for example, dioxins and polychlorinated biphenyls (PCBs). Table 3.7 below shows the effects various exposures may have at different times in a child's life.

Natural environment

There is no longer any doubt that the climate is changing dramatically and that this is caused primarily by the effect of the rise in human induced CO_2; the result of the over-use of fossil fuels. *The Lancet* in 2009 described climate change as the 'biggest global health

Table 3.7 Susceptibility to chemical exposures at different ages

Period	Exposures	Effects
Preconception	Stored maternal PCBs are released in pregnancy	IQ
	Father cigarette smoke	Cancer in offspring
	Occupational exposure to toxins	Increased risk of spontaneous abortion stillbirths and congenital malformations
Embryonic/foetal	Alcohol	Foetal alcohol syndrome
	Tobacco smoke	Llow birthweight
Neonatal	Phthalates (PVC) in bottles and pacifiers	Male reproductive tract cancer
First three years	Lead Inhaled pollutants Toxin ingesting Pesticide vapours	IQ Asthma Allergy
	Tobacco smoke	Glue ear, Sudden infant death syndrome
School-age	Poor air quality Allergens	Asthma
	Toxic arts and craft materials Noise, traffic	Allergies Mental health Injury
Adolescent	Endocrine disruptors Recreational drugs Alcohol substance abuse	Premature puberty Mental health

Source: Data from *Children's health and environment: A review of evidence*, A joint report from the European Environment Agency and the WHO Regional Office for Europe, 2002.

threat of the 21st century', and pointed out that change will have its 'greatest impact on those who are already the poorest in the world; it will deepen inequities and the effects of global warming will shape the future of health among all peoples' (Fig. 3.14).

And yet there is still a lack of urgency in public health circles in tackling this threat, both at a personal level and though advocacy to government.

The likely effects of climate change on child health, as outlined in the Lancet/UCL Commission are listed below:

- Changing patters of disease and mortality e.g. vector borne disease
- Direct effects of heat
- Food insecurity
- Water shortage
- Shelter and human settlements
- Migration

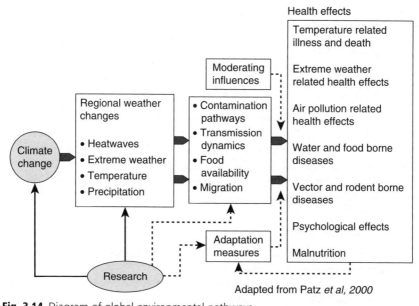

Adapted from Patz *et al, 2000*

Fig. 3.14 Diagram of global environmental pathways.
Source: Adapted from Patz, J. A. et al., 2000. The potential health impacts of climate variability and change for the United States: Executive summary of the report of the health sector of the US National Assessment, *Environmental Health Perspectives*, Vol 108, pp. 367–76, with permission.

Changes in weather patterns due to global climate change can alter local concentrations of air pollutants, particularly ozone. High ozone concentrations can lead to irritable airways, lung inflammation, and other respiratory symptoms, and ozone depletion will increase the risk of skin cancer.

Flooding is another result of climate change, often killing people directly and increasing the risk of waterborne diseases such as cholera. These often affect children disproportionately. Desertification (the degradation of land in arid and dry sub-humid areas) leads to crop failure, which in turn causes famine, hunger, and malnutrition.

Measures to reduce mankind's overuse of fossil fuels and enable humans to reach an ecological balance with our planet and its resources are well known. These are within our grasp but will require a moderation of the lavish lifestyle exhibited by those living in the minority affluent countries, particularly the US and Europe, and a personal commitment to a reduction in carbon footprint by each individual. Time will tell whether health professionals are part of the problem of resource over-use, or part of the solution of moving to a low carbon world.

Policies to protect children from environmental exposures

It is often difficult to know whether a chemical or other environmental insult is going to be harmful to a child. Since 1992 (Rio Declaration on Environment and

Development, as principal 15) there has been an increase in the use of the 'precautionary principle':

> in order to protect the environment, the precautionary approach shall be widely applied by states according to their capabilities. Where there are threats of serious or irreversible damage, lack of full scientific certainty shall not be used as a reason for postponing cost-effective measures to prevent environmental degradation.

This encourages authorities to consider further protective measures even in the face of scientific uncertainty. Many health protection policies aim to reduce exposure of children: for example the regulation and control of landfill sites, environmental tobacco, road traffic control, air quality, building and play materials, pesticide use in foods, injury prevention through environmental alteration, and the provision of information to parents, teachers and children.

Environmental justice

There is increasing evidence that the most disadvantaged groups in society often suffer the worst environmental conditions.

There are over 650 polluting factories in the United Kingdom in areas with average household income of less than £15,000, and only five in postcode areas where average household income is £30,000 or more. The burden of traffic pollution also falls primarily on the social disadvantaged, who may not own cars themselves.

The home environment is another source of inequality. Forty per cent of all fatal accidents happen in the home, and housing in disadvantaged areas is more likely to be unsafe in one or more ways for children.

At an international level, industrialized nations impose disproportionate environmental burdens on the poorest countries, as well as on future generations. Environmental justice has been defined by the US environmental protection agency as 'the fair treatment and meaningful involvement of all people, regardless of race, ethnicity, income, national origin, or educational level, with respect to the development, implementation and enforcement of environmental laws and regulations and policies'.

Children and young people themselves are becoming increasingly aware of the effect that the environment has on their planet and their own health. Child public health professionals need to continue to act as advocates for those living in the poorest circumstances, and to support initiatives that help to address reduction in harmful environmental exposures.

Education

In the developed world, health and longevity are related to educational achievement, and children who drop out of school for any reason tend to fare poorly. Educational opportunities are closely related to socio-economic circumstances, with the better state schools often situated in more well to do areas, and children from the wealthiest backgrounds sent to private schools. Schools with high levels of educational achievement and low drop out rates have not only good academic teaching but a caring school ethos and high student participation and engagement rates. Schools ethos also predicts levels of substance misuse by pupils. So schools which implement policies to improve school ethos also improve academic outcomes and children's mental health and health-related lifestyles.

There is increasing evidence that the quality of pre-school educational provision is improved considerably by having a graduate workforce. Children in these settings are more likely to be emotionally and socially competent, have greater language skills, and to be considered to be ready for school by the appropriate age.

In the developing world, the influence of education is even starker because it is not universally available. Here it is a vital determinant of health. As well as the direct benefits of education (for example, in terms of future earning power), primary education, especially for women, leads to lower infant mortality rates and longer life expectancy. As little as one or two years of schooling for girls can significantly reduce child mortality when these girls reach child-bearing age: a 10% increase in female literacy reduces child mortality by 10% (whereas increases in male literacy have little impact). Yet worldwide, 125 million children are not attending school, two thirds of them girls; half of Africa's children either do not enter primary school or drop out before finishing. Universal primary education is one of the UN's eight anti-poverty goals, and the cost of achieving it is $7–8 billion a year—the equivalent of four days of military spending around the world.

Socio–economic environment

Poverty is perhaps the most important determinant of health worldwide, and the main reason for the differences in health which occur within as well as between countries. Children are more affected by socio-economic circumstances than any other age group in society. There is a strong school of thought that, in the affluent industrialized world where famine and drought are now more or less unheard of, it is *relative* rather than *absolute* poverty which is critical: specifically, the degree of inequality in society. Others believe absolute poverty matters more. The distinction is important because the effects of absolute poverty can be mitigated or abolished by increasing the income and resources available to the very poor. The effects of relative poverty, however, cannot be solved without redistributing income—reducing the income of the rich at the same time as increasing the income of the poor.

Those contributing to the child public health literature in European Union (EU) countries usually base their research on relative measures of poverty. The most common of these assesses the proportion of households with incomes less than 50% of the national average. Chapter 5 discusses different methods of measuring poverty and income inequality in more detail, including comparative and subjective measures.

Poverty in the UK

Using the EU definition of children at risk of poverty (based on a household income threshold of 60% of the national median), the UK does not compare well with other industrialized countries with regard to the extent of child poverty: the level of inequality between rich and poor in this country has been rising steadily for the last 20 years. Figure 3.15 below shows the percentage of children living in poor households (based on the EU definition), showing huge variation between European countries and between regions of England. London, for example, has more than double the child poverty rate of the South East, and only five countries have a worse national rate than the UK.

There are three main reasons for the increase in child poverty in the UK in recent years:

1 Unemployment: over 2 million children in Britain live in households where no adults are in paid work

2 An increase in the number of lone-parent families

3 Changes in the tax and benefits system. Townsend (in *Inequalities in health*: Gordon, D. et al.) identifies as particularly significant the abolition of the link between social security benefits and earnings, the restraints on the value of Child Benefit, the abolition of lone-parent allowances and of the earnings-related addition to Incapacity Benefit, and the substitution of means-tested benefits for universal social insurance and non-contributory benefits for certain groups.

The impact of poverty on child health

The profound effects of socio-economic circumstances on children's health are eloquently demonstrated by the social class differences in childhood mortality illustrated in Fig. 3.16 below. Although the impact on mortality is most marked in the poorest groups, there is a clear trend across all social groups, suggesting that both absolute and relative poverty are important. If absolute poverty were the only problem, we would expect to see increased mortality only in the poorest groups, whereas the trend across all social classes suggests an effect of relative poverty.

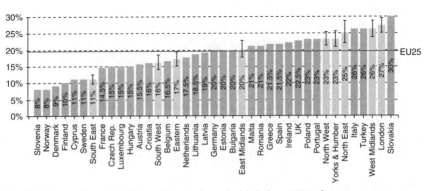

Fig. 3.15 Percentage of children living in households below 60% of contemporary national median income by European nation and English region 2003/04. Source: APHO report 2007.

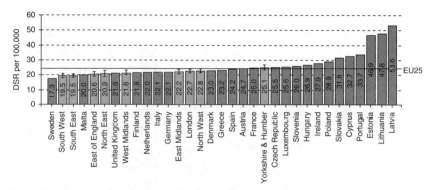

Fig. 3.16 All causes directly standardised mortality rate by European nation/English region 2001–03 (ages 1–19 years).
Source: Reproduced from Indications of Public Health in the English Regions 5: Child Health, Association of Public Health Observatories, 2006, with permission.

Social class differentials in mortality rates are most marked for child pedestrian accidents and deaths from fires, but there is no main cause of death for which children in lower social classes have a lower mortality rate than children in higher classes. Figure 3.17 below shows how the incidence of fractures varies according to deprivation levels (and gender, with boys having a higher risk in all social strata). Social disadvantage effects are also evident in the differential rates of congenital malformations, dental caries, and chronic illness (Fig. 3.18).

Poverty, income inequality, and variations in health

The Black Report, published in 1980, was important in bringing the issue of social inequalities in health back onto the public health agenda (see Chapter 4 for discussion about poverty and health in earlier times). This report, which covered inequalities from cradle to grave, discussed four of the explanations for variations in health across social classes which had been put forward:

1 an artefact of the measurement process

2 natural selection (lower social classes are inevitably made up of weaker people who cannot improve their circumstances)

3 structural problems (poverty and social deprivation affect health adversely)

4 cultural/behavioural (poorer people harm themselves by the excessive consumption of harmful commodities).

The authors presented data that enabled them to discount the first explanation. The second argument, remarkable as it may seem to readers in the twenty-first century, used to inform public health policy in the past (see Chapter 4) but is no longer accepted as a valid argument. The fourth explanation was the one favoured by the Conservative government of the day, but several careful studies have since concluded that differences in health-related lifestyles are insufficient to account for social inequalities in health. Such differences are also now recognized to be heavily influenced by structural factors, since individuals' socio-economic circumstances have a profound effect on

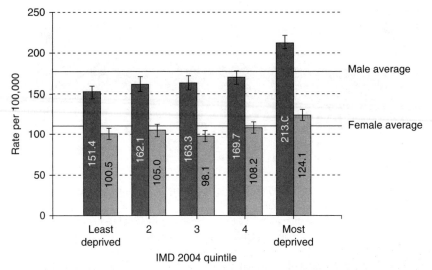

Fig. 3.17 Directly standardised hospital admission rate for long bone fracture by sex (Male is darker grey, female light grey) and deprivation quintile* 2003/04 (0–14 years). Source: Reproduced from Indications of Public Health in the English Regions 5: Child Health, Association of Public Health Observatories, 2006, with permission.

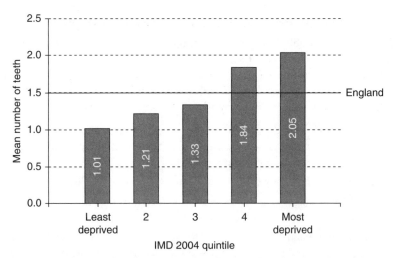

Fig. 3.18 Mean number of decayed, missing or filled teeth in five-year-old children by deprivation quintile 2003/04.
Source: Reproduced from Indications of Public Health in the English Regions 5: Child Health, Association of Public Health Observatories, 2006, with permission.

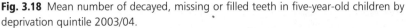

the choices open to them. The authors of the Black Report concluded that the wider issues of class differentials and their impact on living circumstances (structural issues) were the fundamental cause. They did not explicitly touch on the debate about the relative importance of absolute and relative poverty.

The arguments in favour of the importance of relative poverty are well described by Wilkinson. He discusses three interpretations for data showing that countries with wider income disparities have poorer health:

1 the individual income interpretation

2 the neo-material interpretation

3 the psychosocial environment interpretation.

The first suggests that the association between income inequality and health at population level merely reflects the aggregated association at individual level – an argument compatible with the absolute poverty approach. Several studies have, however, shown that national patterns of income distribution have health effects which remain after adjustment for individual income levels within the country, so although individual income is important, something else must explain the observed relationships between income inequality and health.

The neo-material interpretation (favoured by the Black Report) states that health problems among those with low incomes are simply due to lack of provision—of education, health services, transportation, food, housing, and so on. This interpretation is also compatible with an absolute poverty explanation, and remedies for it do not need to involve income redistribution. Improving access to high-quality services and housing should have a beneficial effect.

The psychosocial environment interpretation provides a possible explanation for the mechanisms underlying the impact of relative poverty. It proposes that psychosocial factors are vital in mediating the effect of income inequalities. Those at the lower end of the social scale feel marginalized and excluded, self-esteem suffers, and feelings of powerlessness (both real and imagined) impede lifestyle and environmental change. The distress induced by powerlessness and poor self-esteem may lead to poorer health via a variety of physiological mechanisms, which are currently being explored through research in psychoneuroimmunology. These might include hypertension, lowered immune response, and abnormal clotting mechanisms. If this explanation were the most important, remedies which mitigate the effects of poverty by, for example, providing better education or health services for the poor, would not solve the problem on their own. Redistributive policies which reduce the gap in wealth between rich and poor would be essential. Measures to improve social cohesion might also be helpful, since social cohesion at community level could be expected to mitigate some of these psychosocial effects (see discussion of social capital in Chapter 5).

The priorities for public health action to address the impact of income inequality clearly depend on which of these interpretations is favoured. It is likely that all three contribute, but the exact balance is unclear. Broad based action is indicated, focusing on obtaining a more equitable distribution of public and private resources, improving social cohesion, and improving service provision, and structural barriers to health.

How does poverty affect children's health in practice?

It follows from the arguments above that several mechanisms are likely to be involved in mediating the influence of socio-economic circumstances on children's health, not all of them directly related to lack of money. They include:

the direct effects of low income e.g. insufficient or inappropriate food, lack of heating, and damp housing

the environmental effects of living in a poor neighbourhood e.g. lack of safe play areas and leisure facilities, poor schools, exposure to pollutants and contaminants

the psychosocial effects of poverty e.g. low self-esteem, powerlessness, parental stress precipitating family conflict and domestic violence, parental drug and alcohol abuse, inadequate supervision, parental depression, crime, violence, and lack of social capital in communities (see Chapter 5).

Table 3.8 below illustrates some of these mechanisms and is followed by some practical examples.

Poverty and child health: some examples

Accidents

Accidents to children in the home are strongly influenced by the environment, which is in its turn affected by poverty. Falls and burns are more likely to occur in houses not designed with safety in mind and in the absence of safety equipment such as smoke detectors, stairgates, fireguards, and cooker guards. Safety equipment is expensive and not always easy to obtain, and low-income families are more likely to live in houses that are unsafe, overcrowded, and have old electrical equipment. Motor vehicle accidents are more likely if children have to play in the street. Children may be less well supervised in lone-parent families or where parents both work or have health problems of their own, and older siblings may have to look after younger ones at an earlier age

Table 3.8 Effects of poverty on children's health

Factor	Effect on health
Insufficient or inappropriate food	Undernutrition, malnutrition, obesity
Damp and cold housing	Respiratory infections
Small, overcrowded housing	Increased infection risk
Lack of play space in garden or locally	Increased accident risk (especially road traffic accidents)
Low self-esteem and powerlessness	Difficulty making supportive relationships and lifestyle changes
Parental stress and conflict	Behaviour problems; increased risk of child abuse
Lack of stimulation and play	Poor educational achievement
Lack of supervision	Increased accident risk; behaviour problems
Lack of social capital; crime; violence	Anxiety; bullying; drug abuse; parental illness

than is appropriate. Environmental modification and better provision for children's play is essential if accidental injuries are to be reduced in low-income areas.

Teenage pregnancy

The strong links between teenage pregnancy and low income, as well as other indicators of deprivation, were recognized in the allocation of governmental responsibility for teenage pregnancy in the UK to the government's Social Exclusion Unit. Girls under 16 from deprived areas were shown in a Scottish study to be three times more likely to become pregnant than those from privileged areas, but less likely to have the pregnancy terminated. Overall, rates of teenage pregnancy are up to ten times higher in social class V than social class I. Teenage mothers are six times more likely to have no qualifications than the general population; 'Looked After' children (children in public care) are at greater risk of becoming teenage parents; and one in three male young offenders are fathers. This illustrates the tendency of factors associated with deprivation and poor health to 'cluster'—and since teenage pregnancy itself is a cause of poorer health in both the teenage mother and her baby, it perpetuates inequalities through generations. Possible explanations for the high rate of pregnancy among poorer and deprived teenagers include educational failure and lack of career opportunities, low self-esteem, and the perceived opportunities for independent living resulting from motherhood.

Poverty in the majority world

Poverty is the greatest problem facing children who live in developing countries. The box below illustrates the extent of global poverty, which is severe and worsening, although some countries are succeeding in mitigating its effects. The extent of change is shown by the fact that two centuries ago, income per head in Britain, the world's richest country at that time, was three times higher than that of Africa, then the planet's poorest region. Today, the world's richest country, Switzerland, enjoys per capita income nearly 80 times higher than the world's poorest region, south Asia.

An American having the average income of the bottom US decile is better-off than 2/3 of world population.

(Milanovic 2002, p.50)

The top 10 percent of the US population has an aggregate income equal to the income of the poorest 43 percent of people in the world, or differently put, total income of the richest 25 million Americans is equal to total income of almost 2 billion people.

(Milanovic 2002)

As of May 2005, the three richest people in the world have assets that exceed the combined gross domestic product of the 47 countries with the least GDP (calculation based on data from list of countries by GDP (PPP) and list of billionaires)
http://en.wikipedia.org/wiki/International_inequality
According to UNICEF, 25,000 children die each day due to poverty.
More than 80% of the world's population lives in countries where income differentials are widening.

At least 80% of humanity lives on less than $10 a day.

For the 1.9 billion children from the developing world, there are:

- ◆ 640 million without adequate shelter (1 in 3)

- ◆ 400 million with no access to safe water (1 in 5)

- ◆ 270 million with no access to health services (1 in 7)

http://www.globalissues.org/article/26/poverty-facts-and-stats#src2

As in developed countries, poverty affects health through a wide variety of mechanisms and diseases, although its effects are more stark in countries where absolute poverty is severe.

Lack of access to the basic necessities of life increases susceptibility to ill health (e.g. via malnutrition) and exposure to disease (e.g. via contaminated water supplies), and reduces the capacity to respond to it (including ability to access health care).

In some ways it is better to be poor in a country with a subsistence economy where the majority live in the same situation, than in a country where the majority are well off. However, there are now increasing inequalities within developing countries as well as between rich and poor countries—a relatively new socioeconomic feature which has significantly worsened the situation for the poor. Some of the factors behind this are shown in the box below.

Factors increasing inequalities within developing countries

- ◆ Home government policies such as rapid industrialization, military spending, corruption

- ◆ Urbanization, which increases poverty by moving families from subsistence to cash economy and increases environmental degradation

- ◆ Government debt and structural adjustment policies imposed by the World Bank, reducing the extent of public services and sometimes introducing user charges for health services, which affect the poor more than the rich

- ◆ Marketing of unhealthy products such as infant formula milk by multinational corporations, which the poor cannot afford but feel they need to purchase

- ◆ Rapid population growth and demographic entrapment (when a community's requirements exceed the capacity of the land to support them, as well as exceeding the capacity to migrate to other regions and their economic capacity to buy food and other essentials)

Reference: Carnall, D. (1999)

Poor families, and especially mothers and children, have suffered most in the transition from a labour intensive, agricultural economy to a capital intensive, urban economy.

Education and health services have not kept up with population growth, and infrastructure development has been inadequate to provide for basic needs. Consequently, health has suffered.

Debt

Debts incurred by many developing countries (particularly in Africa) following the boom in oil prices in the 1970s led to a situation where many countries were paying more in interest charges to the developed world than they received in aid and revenue. The World Bank and International Monetary Fund will provide loans but their condition is a structural adjustment policy (see box below) which requires the country to cut back on public spending on health and education, with severely adverse effects on the poor. Attempts are now being made to alleviate the global debt situation, but many very poor countries still face pressure to limit public spending.

World debt and structural adjustment

- In 1970, the world's poorest countries (roughly 60 countries classified as low-income by the World Bank), owed $25 billion in debt.
- By 2002, this was $523 billion
- For Africa, in 1970, it was just under $11 billion
- By 2002, the debt owed by Africa had increased to over half the world total: $295 billion
- Debts owed to the multilateral institutions such as the IMF and World Bank is currently around $153 billion
- For the poorest countries debts to multilateral institutions is around $70 billion.
- $550 billion has been paid in both principal and interest over the last three decades, on $540bn of loans, and yet there is still a $523 billion dollar debt burden.
- The IMF and World Bank provide financial assistance to countries seeking it, but apply a neoliberal economic ideology or agenda as a precondition to receiving the money. For example:
- They prescribe cutbacks, 'liberalization' of the economy and resource extraction/export-oriented open markets as part of their structural adjustment.
- The role of the state is minimized.
- Privatization is encouraged as well as reduced protection of domestic industries.
- Other adjustment policies also include currency devaluation, increased interest rates,'flexibility' of the labour market, and the elimination of subsidies such as food subsidies.
- To be attractive to foreign investors various regulations and standards are reduced or removed.

http://www.globalissues.org/issue/28/third-world-debt-undermines-development

War and conflict

In recent years wars have occurred in most regions of the world—the majority in developing countries, although recently parts of Europe (especially the former Soviet Union and former Yugoslavia) have been substantially affected. War affects children as victims, direct and indirect, and as combatants (child soldiers). Its impact is frequently devastating, and prevention of conflict must rank as a top priority for action to protect children.

In war, children die, are severely disabled, and suffer grave mental health effects as a result of the loss of parents and relatives. Human rights abuses are common, and children may witness (or experience) rape, torture, and murder. Family and community networks are disrupted, and the social and political infrastructure often breaks down, leading to the loss of even basic health care and other services. Any services which remain may be severely overstretched dealing with war casualties, so that preventive services such as immunization are interrupted. Children may be left homeless, orphaned, and having to take care of younger siblings, and the perils may continue beyond the end of the conflict if landmines remain in the area. The box below summarizes recent data on the effects of war on children.

Effects of war and conflict on children worldwide

- Worldwide spending on weapons has risen by 45% between 1999 and 2009 (see Table 3.9)

- In 2009 $1.46 trillion was spent on weapons worldwide

- The UK's spending in Afghanistan and Iraq is projected to be £12bn

- Up to 2 million children were killed in war during the 1990s

- Over 6 million children were permanently disabled or seriously injured

- 1 million children were orphaned

- 20 million children were displaced

- At any given time, more than 300,000 children are being used in hostilities as soldiers

Machel Report update 2000
http://www.un.org/children/conflict/english/machel-reports.html
Useful websites: Medact.org; IPPNW.org; www.icbl.org; www.mag.org.uk

---

Migration and refugees

A further consequence of war and conflict, and also of economic pressure, is migration. The vast majority of those fleeing their homeland seek refuge in neighbouring countries as poor as their own, which can have a serious impact on already overstretched economies and services. In industrialized countries, which (contrary to the prevalent publicity) receive a small proportion of all refugees and asylum seekers, these individuals are often seen as scroungers, labelled as 'bogus' asylum seekers, and are

Table 3.9 Top ten military spenders in 2008 in $bn per year

US	607
China	84.9
France	65.7
UK	65.3
Russia	58.6
Germany	46.8
Japan	46.3
Italy	40.6
Saudi Arabia	38.2
India	30

Source: Adapted from Stockholm International Peace Research Institute (SIPRI), *SIPRI Yearbook 2009: Armaments, Disarmament and International Security* (Oxford University Press: Oxford, 2009), p. 182, with permission from SIPRI

subject to racism and harassment and sometimes, to oppressive government policies. Barriers to entry for asylum seekers are increasing across western Europe, and there is a real risk that the protection and rights offered by the UN Convention on Refugees will be compromised in some countries. Some of the factors affecting the health of refugees and asylum seekers are shown in the box below:

Factors affecting the health of refugees and asylum seekers

- ◆ Previous life experiences e.g. war, torture, bereavement, perilous flight
- ◆ Loss of family networks and community
- ◆ Effects of disrupted health care in home country (e.g. lack of immunizations)
- ◆ For some, increased risk of infectious diseases (including TB and HIV)
- ◆ Impact of poverty and social exclusion in host country
- ◆ Impact of racism and discrimination in host country
- ◆ Effect of being part of ethnic minority in host country
- ◆ Poor access to health care services in host country due to lack of understanding of needs, availability, and entitlements (among staff as well as users), and to language and cultural barriers

The combined health impact of these factors is considerable. Support from health and other services is essential for this vulnerable group in the population. In the UK, asylum seekers and refugees are entitled to receive NHS services in the same way as other residents, and local commissioners have a responsibility to ensure that they have equitable access to appropriate services, including the provision of interpreters, information about NHS services (which may differ substantially from those in their country of origin), and special services (where necessary to cater for particular needs such as mental health problems). Training for health care staff is also essential, and published resources are available to support this.

Children, especially unaccompanied children, are a particularly vulnerable subgroup with high rates of mental health problems as a result of their experiences. The UK has until recently excluded asylum-seeking children from its ratification of the UN Convention on the Rights of the Child, compromising their rights compared to indigenous children. Although they are offered some protection by the Children Act and other legislation, this ceases when they reach eighteen, so their ability to build a new life in this country may be undermined.

Culture and attitudes

It is often said that the UK is not a child-centred society. The examples cited usually relate to negative public attitudes to children and parents, and to negative coverage of children in the media (e.g. the focus on child crime and truancy). Familiar anecdotal evidence includes the lack of welcome given to children in restaurants and other public places compared to other European countries, negative images of teenagers in the press, disapproval of and lack of facilities for breast-feeding in public places, and the low importance and priority UK society accords to parenting (for full-time mothers, but especially full-time fathers).

Perhaps more important is the presence or absence of legislation to protect children and promote their wellbeing. Table 3.10 below gives examples of positive and negative aspects of legislation and planning in the UK.

While we are doing well in some areas, we have some way to go to match our Scandinavian neighbours in recognizing and valuing the contribution of children to our society. A marker of a society's attitude to children's rights is its attitude to child labour.

Child labour

Worldwide, about 250 million children are engaged in work, often over long hours and in hazardous circumstances. Their health suffers from this both directly and indirectly: via loss of schooling, inappropriate physical stresses, inadequate nutrition, and the physical and psychological effects of 'lost childhood' (taking on excessive responsibilities and forgoing opportunities for play and exercise). Many labouring children are employed by corporations based in rich countries, which have a responsibility to curtail the practice and help to develop educational alternatives. It is important to understand that a poor family's income may depend on the working child, so banning work without introducing economic alternatives will be opposed by local people. Solutions should be comprehensive and should entail the elimination of hazardous child labour and the provision of free education, together with wider legal protection for children.

Child prostitution is a particularly damaging practice which is being increasingly recognized in many parts of the world. It has serious adverse effects on both mental and

Table 3.10 Are children protected and supported by government in the UK?

Yes	No
Child labour laws	Physical punishment still legal
Compulsory education	Lack of universally available child care
Child protection legislation	Limited maternity leave
Children Act (England)	Very limited paternity leave
Child Benefit and Sure Start	Legislation against anti-social behaviour stigmatises rather than supporting families
Universal health visitor service	Few facilities for adolescents in NHS
UK has ratified UN Convention on Children's Rights and appointed Children's Rights Commissioners in the devolved countries	No consultation with children on policy matters (but government is committed to improving this)
Minister for Children and the Family (since 2003)	Children in detention are still subject to physical restraint
Increased provision of preschool education	Asylum seeking children face discrimination and services may be withheld
Increased provision of services to support parenting	

physical health, and on life opportunities. The risk of HIV and other sexually transmitted diseases, and also of teenage pregnancy, are particular hazards for child sex workers.

Children's rights

Children's rights are persistently abused in many countries of the world. Even in the UK, a relatively wealthy country, it has proved difficult to implement the UN Convention on the Rights of the Child. The relationship between human rights and health is very close—health workers need to understand and make use of the legal protection provided by the UN Convention (See p.44).

In western cultures, a significant limiter on children's rights is work as unpaid carers. Many children care for disabled or incapacitated parents or siblings, especially in families where parents abuse alcohol and drugs, suffer a mental illness or physical disability. These children's education and development is compromised by the time they spend caring and the need to grow up at too early and age.

Intolerance and stigma

Social exclusion is a feature of all westernized countries and profoundly affects children's health. Social exclusion refers to the handicap imposed on an individual or group as a result of their position in society: it may result from poverty, behaviour, mental health problems, race or religion, gender, or sexual orientation. Several groups of children may suffer from the negative effects of intolerance and stigma. These include the poor, those from minority ethnic groups, asylum seekers, travellers, disabled children, and 'Looked-After' children.

Disability

Although there have been improvements in recent years, there is still discrimination against people with a disability, and access is a vital part of this. How easy is it for a child in a wheelchair to get around the school, to take a bus or train, or to go shopping in town?

The inclusion of children with disabilities in mainstream schools is potentially beneficial both for them and for the wider school population, leading to greater integration, and better understanding and social acceptance of disability. However, there is also the potential for failing to meet such children's educational and social needs: if there is insufficient support in the school, then bullying and isolation are common. This is particularly so for children with learning difficulties, when there are no outward signs to explain why the child is struggling or needs extra help.

Ethnicity and culture

Life is difficult for many ethnic minority children in the UK. Migration around and outside Europe has resulted in a greatly increased mix of ethnic groups especially in large urban areas. In 2006, ethnic minority children (Fig. 3.19) accounted for 10% of the child population in Great Britain (cf. 9% in 1992).

The problems these children face include a higher prevalence of poverty (often exacerbated by poverty in the home country as well as discrimination in the UK that reduces job prospects), racist attitudes, and bullying at school (especially for those for whom English is a second language). In some cases there are difficulties of acculturation

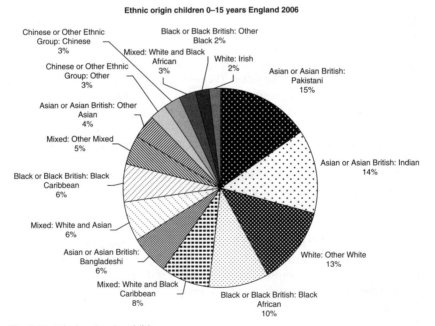

Fig. 3.19 Ethnic minority children.
Source: Data from Office for National Statistics.

(for example, cultural differences in expectation compared to the UK norm, especially for girls in Muslim families, and a lack of continuity in contact with services among traveller families). These collectively confer both physical and mental health risks.

Media

The influence of television is pervasive and often negative. Children are less often allowed to play outside as a result of parental anxiety, and because of the popularity of television as a source of entertainment (as well as a resident 'babysitter' for busy parents), many spend increasing hours in front of a screen either watching television or videos, on the internet, or playing interactive games. In the USA, 9–10 year-old children watch about 15.5 hours of television and 5 hours of videos every week, and play 3 hours of video games. This carries direct health costs as well as opportunity costs. The direct costs come from exposure to the marketing of unhealthy food and drink, to the influence of violence, sexual permissiveness, and alcohol abuse, and to a predominance of male gender values. The opportunity costs are a reduction in physical activity, an increase in obesity, less interactive family life, and less conversation. The latter is especially adverse in young children during the period of language acquisition (Table 3.11).

A new pervasive but subtle influence on children's health has been the rise of reality TV shows. Some have recently filmed babies left in the care of unrelated teenagers for days at a time and children as young as eight years placed in houses together in groups to see how they got on. These shows, created in the name of entertainment, can be frankly abusive to the children involved and raise particular issues about whose responsibility it is to safeguard the 'actors'. Their influence on child health extends much more widely, the programmes apparently endorsing the belief that it is acceptable for babies to be left in the care of unrelated teenagers for long periods or for young children to be left unsupervised. At the same time a spate of programmes on parenting and on child development are spreading healthier messages about parenting and its influence on children for good and ill.

Claims have been made for the educational value of television watching, but they depend on the involvement of active learning, which is rare: television watching is essentially a passive activity. If parents discuss programmes with children after watching together, the benefit is said to be increased, but the extent to which this happens is

Table 3.11 Television: good or bad for children?

Beneficial effects of TV	Adverse effects of TV
Reduced stress on parents	Delays language development
Potential educational benefit	Modelling of violence
Shared family activity	Advertising of junk food + eating it
	Increased levels of obesity
	Reduced activity levels
	Reduced family interaction
	Modelling of sexual activity and alcohol

not known. With increasing awareness, broadcasters are producing more educational materials on child specific channels without advertising content. There are good opportunities for child public health professionals to influence some of the content and shape some universal health promoting messages (see Chapter 7: Social Marketing).

Recent research has shown that reducing the amount of time that primary school children spend watching television and playing video games can make them less aggressive towards their peers, making this an important area for parent and professional education. Reducing television watching has also been shown to contribute to weight loss in overweight children. However, since television is now an integral part of society any public health approach to protect children must be tempered with realism and recognize the importance of market forces. Possible means of controlling the adverse effects of TV on children are shown in the box.

Television: how to curtail its adverse influence on children

+ Public education (e.g. American Academy of Pediatrics 'Media Matters' Campaign, see www.aap.org)
+ School education on media literacy
+ Paediatrician education (as above, not yet evaluated)
+ TV 'limiter' (allows parents to control internet use)
+ State control of media violence
+ Legislation to curb advertising of junk foods to children
+ Complaints to OFCOM (Office for Communications) or equivalent media watchdogs, directly to the channel chief executives, or to Children's Commissioners have succeeded in getting some programmes banned.

Globalization

This term has been coined to describe the universalization of trade, culture, and communication that has developed across the globe in recent years. It has its origins in the worldwide market in commodities, led by multinational corporations, and the explosion of international communication as a result of the spread of TV and the development of the internet. The key elements of globalization, and the impact some aspects of globalization have on children, are illustrated in the Tables 3.12 and 3.13 below.

Key elements of globalization

+ The growth of transnational corporations such as Nike, Nestle, and Esso, many of which are larger in terms of economic productivity than some single countries, and have huge marketing budgets.

Table 3.12 Multinational corporations: good or bad for children?

Beneficial effects	Adverse effects
Reduction in price of consumer goods in industrialized countries	Child labour and poor employment practices
	Marketing of unhealthy products
Wide availability and choice of quality products	Unethical marketing (e.g. infant formula milk)
	Lack of regulation by legislation
	Pressure to buy (fashion)
	Environmental degradation and over-use of scarce resources

- ◆ The domination of the media and communications industry by a few companies such as CNN and News International. This has led to the international dissemination of media icons such as sports and music celebrities and an emphasis on a mainly Western lifestyle in images presented across the world, and increased awareness of their own poverty and disadvantage among those in developing countries.

- ◆ The internet, which has revolutionized communication and access to information.

- ◆ The growth of a global civil society linked by the internet has allowed strong movements to develop, united by a common interest (e.g. the international opposition to the Iraq war, and the campaign to mitigate climate change).

- ◆ It will be a challenge for civil society to develop ways of controlling multinational corporations and ensuring that children are protected from the adverse effects of the internet, in particular pornography and other sexual imagery. Internet safety schemes have begun to address the issue of limiting exposure of children to potentially harmful web content. See http://www.virtualglobaltaskforce.com/

Clustering of problems

This section has reviewed a range of key factors which impact on children's health. Although each exerts independent effects, it is also the case that many of the factors which adversely affect children's health tend to cluster. Thus children with one problem, for example family breakdown, are often at greater risk of experiencing others, for example poverty, and individual adverse factors may potentiate the effects of others. This phenomenon has been called 'social patterning'. We have seen how adverse social circumstances collectively contribute to a higher risk of teenage pregnancy, which in

Table 3.13 The internet: good or bad for children?

Beneficial effects	Adverse effects
Education	As TV
Encourages self-learning	Easy access to pornography
Promotes international networking	Inappropriate cultural images

itself has a negative impact on health for both mother and child, and how children from ethnic minority groups often suffer the effects of poverty as well as intolerance and bullying, while struggling with a new language and culture and difficulties in accessing health and other services. They may also be at greater risk of certain congenital conditions, and possibly of infectious diseases such as HIV and TB which may be prevalent in their country of origin. Similarly, vulnerable children looked after by the local authority are at greater risk of teenage pregnancy, tend to have lower educational achievement, and have often experienced abusive or neglectful family relationships.

Clearly this tendency for clustering of problems compounds the impact on children's health and wellbeing and exaggerates the health inequalities which result. It is important for child public health practitioners to address individual determinants of health, but they also need to be aware of this tendency for adverse factors to cluster and interact, complicating the picture and requiring a more sophisticated approach to tackling child public health problems.

Table 3.14 summarizes the variety of factors impacting on children's health at different ages.

Health and social care services

The perceived importance of health service provision as a determinant of health has waxed and waned. For a period after the foundation of the NHS, it was seen as the single most important influence on the health of the population, and it certainly played a greater part in the second half of the twentieth century than in the first (see Fig. 3.20 below). More recently, growing awareness of the role of social and

Table 3.14 Environmental influences on children

Age	Environmental influences	Outcome
Infant	Parenting sensitivity and attunement to infant needs, nutrition, breast-feeding, housing	Emotional and social development, development of motor skills, speech and language, infections, physical growth, healthy teeth
Preschool child	Parenting style, television exposure, marketing of unhealthy foods, safety of play area, learning environment	Behaviour problems, mental health, language development, accidental injury, cognitive skills, growth, anaemia, abuse, peer group relationships, readiness for school
School-age child	School ethos, parenting style, road safety awareness, television, marketing, sports facilities	Violence, bullying, academic progression, accidental injury, citizenship, physical fitness, depression, behaviour problems, relationship problems
Adolescent	Advertising and media, parental relationships, school ethos, sports facilities, parenting style	Tobacco and substance abuse, relationship problems, sexually transmitted disease, pregnancy, violence, delinquency, criminality

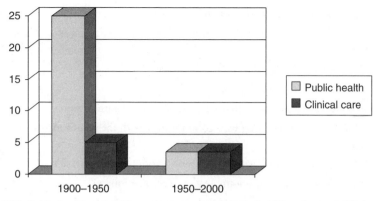

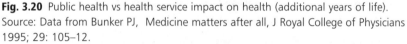

Fig. 3.20 Public health vs health service impact on health (additional years of life). Source: Data from Bunker PJ, Medicine matters after all, J Royal College of Physicians 1995; 29: 105–12.

environmental determinants of health has led to a swing in the opposite direction, with health services seen by many as a minor player in public health terms.

Clearly the truth lies somewhere between these two extremes. It is now well recognized that health services cannot solve the health problems of the population on their own, and that in some areas social and environmental action are of prime importance. Nonetheless, health services do have a vital role to play in maintaining and improving the public's—and not least children's—health. Inequalities in health are exacerbated by inequalities in access to health care, through an unfair geographical distribution of services (the so-called 'inverse care law') and barriers to access such as lack of interpreters or public transport, or limited clinic times.

It is important to be sure that health services—both locally and nationally—promote rather than hinder equity, and that they are effective in meeting the needs of the population. Public health techniques such as health needs assessment and evaluation of services, and the rise in evidence-based medicine, can help to ensure that the country gets best value from the NHS, and that it contributes positively to promoting health and reducing health inequalities.

Recent developments in the NHS point the service in this direction. Historically in the UK there has been an excellent primary care service for children. This is through the provision of health visitors with the potential for home visiting for the preschool child and school health services for the school child, with links to the GP and primary care team to facilitate interdisciplinary working. However, longstanding divisions between the management of preventive and curative services have meant that there is a lack of integration and often inadequate staffing in community child health (as well as limited evidence of effectiveness of some services).

The current trend is to integrate care between various sectors and to ensure that social and health care are commissioned together. Rhetoric does not always match reality in this field, however, and the role of health professionals as advocates to ensure that services meet the needs of children is vitally important.

Current trends in NHS services for children include:

+ 'Joined up thinking' in central government, crossing ministerial and departmental boundaries
+ Greater focus on community and ambulatory care
+ Primary care led commissioning
+ Joint commissioning of children's services with local authorities
+ Local interventions working with communities, with the aim of increasing social capital
+ Emphasis on team work, with no assumption of medical leadership
+ Development of nurse autonomy (e.g. nurse practitioners)
+ Greater partnership with parents and consumer participation in planning
+ More consultation with children and young people
+ Increasing concerns re input of private sector in the delivery of services
+ Excessive emphasis on centrally driven targets

An area of expanding interest in child health services is the role played by complementary and alternative medicine. Increasing numbers of children are now taken to homeopaths, herbalists and nutritionists, particularly for health problems relating to allergies. Many are also taking nutritional supplements which are widely available over the counter. Children from minority ethnic cultures are particularly likely to be using such medicine. The evidence base for such interventions is incomplete and much of what there is suggests lack of efficacy. Parents, however, are voting with their feet and in order to care for children well, health professionals in the Western world need to develop a greater and more sympathetic understanding of these approaches to care.

Problems in health care in developing countries

There are substantial problems with the financing and provision of health care in developing countries. As in the industrialized world, the cost of drugs and hospital care is ever-increasing, while the budgets for health services remain static or shrink. All countries face a conflict over the priorities for health care provision, but this is heightened in low-income countries.

Dilemmas faced by developing countries

+ High cost of drugs and investigations
+ Pressure on doctors to prescribe expensive drugs—drug companies play a role in promoting costly alternatives to simple, cheap drugs and in limiting the availability of low cost generic medicines
+ Pressure from some sections of the population to expand hospital and curative services at the expense of primary and preventive services
+ Pressure from doctors seeking higher salaries

Dilemmas faced by developing countries *(continued)*

- 'Brain drain' of doctors to industrialized countries
- Training of doctors orientates them to curative care rather than to prevention, and to individual consultation rather than teamwork and a population approach
- Relatively low spending on primary care
- Poor management in primary care
- Pressure from the World Bank, IMF, and World Trade Organisation to introduce user charges in health facilities
- Loss of emphasis on primary health care with the introduction of Millennium Development Goals and emphasis by WHO and UNICEF on 'vertical' (top down) services such as immunization, rather than locally delivered 'horizontal' services (see *Lancet* Sept 2008)

As a result of pressure from government officials, doctors, and the general public, a high proportion of health budgets go into the secondary and tertiary sector to the detriment of primary health care, although it is through the latter that the main health benefits for the poor will accrue. This can lead to a situation where basic health care for the majority of the population is poor, but 'high tech' hospitals in the large cities can provide expensive state of the art treatment for a small minority of wealthy citizens. These tensions are present in all countries but are more urgent in poor countries where the health problems are so much more serious. A good example of the ways in which primary care service organizations can impact on health outcomes is in the delivery of vaccinations and the utilization of 'low tech' oral rehydration for diarrhoeal diseases.

Immunization

Table 3.15 below illustrates immunization uptake and the financing of vaccine by governments in different regions of the world (the countries with less support are highlighted). There is not a clear relationship between the two, suggesting that issues other than finance also need to be considered. These include supply and administration, including the disrupting effect of war; insufficiently trained primary care staff; and poor cold chain supply (the essential process by which vaccine is kept sufficiently cold to prevent deterioration between manufacture and delivery to patients). One potential problem is that immunization delivery is often organized centrally and may not be well integrated with primary care systems.

There are also difficult issues to confront in terms of weighing up the benefits and disadvantages of certain interventions. For example, the use of rotavirus vaccine has not been pursued in the US because it carries a risk of complications (intestinal intussusception) which might outweigh the benefits in that country. But in developing countries, where the morbidity and mortality associated with rotaviral gastroenteritis in children are so much greater, the potential health benefits of the vaccine may

Table 3.15 Immunisation coverage and vaccine supply

	% of routine EPI vaccines financed by government	Immunization 2006								% newborns protected against tetanus[λ]
	2006	1-year-old children immunized against								
		TB	DPT		Polio	Measles	HepB	Hib		
	total	corresponding vaccines								
		BCG	DPT1[β]	DPT3[β]	polio3	measles	HepB3	Hib3		
Sub-Saharan Africa	49	82	83	72	74	72	48	24		77
Eastern and Southern Africa	43	85	86	78	77	76	58	36		81
West and Central Africa	55	79	81	67	70	68	38	13		72
Middle East and North Africa	88	92	95	91	91	89	88	24		81
South Asia	91	82	82	63	66	65	25	–		84
East Asia and Pacific	–	91	92	89	89	89	86	2		–
Latin America and Caribbean	96	96	96	92	92	93	89	90		84
CEE/CIS	–	95	96	95	95	97	92	3		–
Industrialized countries[§]	–	–	98	96	94	93	64	82		–
Developing countries[§]	78	86	88	78	79	78	59	17		80
Least developed countries[§]	33	85	87	77	77	74	50	17		82
World	78	87	89	79	80	80	60	22		80

Source: UNICEF Report 2008.

substantially exceed the risk of side-effects. However, there are concerns about the ethics and stigma of promoting interventions and drugs rejected by rich countries in poorer ones.

Pharmaceutical supplies

Pharmaceutical supplies are a major difficulty for developing countries. Much less research is undertaken on the development of new drugs for high prevalence diseases in poor countries than on drugs to alleviate disorders which are common in developed countries. Only 16 out of 1393 new medicines brought to market between 1975 and 1999 were for tropical diseases and TB; it was 13 times more likely that a new drug would be for cancer or a central nervous system disorder than for one of the diseases taking such a toll in poor countries.

Drug supplies may be too expensive for developing countries without their own pharmaceutical industries. The major drug companies resist the use of cheaper generic drugs, which has been a major issue in relation to treatment for HIV and AIDS. There is also a tendency for doctors to prescribe new expensive drugs rather than older cheaper ones, perhaps as a result of the marketing inducements used by pharmaceutical companies. WHO has developed an essential drug list: these drugs should be used in preference to newer and more expensive alternatives. Many countries are introducing legislation to ensure that doctors do not take bribes from pharmaceutical companies to prescribe their products, but these customs are hard to eradicate and there is a great need for self-regulation by the profession itself.

Conclusion

In this chapter we have used the Mandala framework of health determinants to describe the many interweaving factors which influence child health. It forms the basis on which further research to elucidate mechanisms of causation can be formulated, as well as a rational structure on which to base child public health policy and influence both upstream and downstream interventions, as we shall demonstrate in the final chapter of this book.

Further reading

Health promotion in schools

Adi, Y., Killoran, A., Janmohamed, K., and Stewart-Brown, S. (2007) Systematic review of interventions to promote mental wellbeing in children in primary education. A report to National Institute of Health and Clinical Excellence http://www.nice.org.uk/guidance/index.jsp?action=download&o=43911

Living Well in Schools. (2009) Mindfulness-based approached to education health and wellbeing. Breath works, Manchester http://www.doxtop.com/browse/69162f1e/living-well-in-schools.aspx

Stewart-Brown, S.L. (2006) What is the evidence on school health promotion in improving health or preventing disease and, specifically what is the effectiveness of the health promoting schools approach. Copenhagen, WHO Regional Office for Europe's Health Evidence Network (HEN) http://www.euro.who.int/document/e88185.pdf accessed March 2006

Parenting as a determinant

Barlow, J., Coren, E.S., and Stewart-Brown, S. (2004) Parent-training programmes for improving maternal psychosocial health. *Cochrane Database of Systematic Reviews* 2002 (4).

Baumrind, D. (1978) Parental disciplinary patterns and social competence in children. *Youth and Society*, **9**: 239–75.

Conger, R.D., Conger, K., Elder, G., Lorenz, F., Simmons, R., and Whitbeck, L.A. (1992) Family process model of economic hardship and adjustment of early adolescent boys. *Child Development*, **63**: 526–41.

Dawe, S., Harnett, P.H., Rendalls, V., and Staiger, P. (2003) Improving family functioning and child outcomes in methadone maintained families: the parents under pressure programmes. *Drug and Alcohol Review*, **22**: 299–307.

Gerhardt, S. (2004) *Why Love Matters: How affection shapes a baby's brain* Brunner- Routledge, New York.

Ghate, D. and Hazel, N. Parenting in Poor Environments Stress Support and Coping Policy Research Bureau. Jessica Kinglsey: London and Philadelphia.

Lundahl, B., Risser, H., and Lovejoy, M. (2006b). A meta-analysis of parent training: Moderators and follow-up effects. *Clinical Psychology Review*, **26**: 251–262. http://www.pfsc.uq.edu.au/publications/evidence_base.html and http://incredibleyears.com/libray/show_all.asp

MacLeod, J. and Nelson, G. (2000) Programs for the promotion of family wellness and the prevention of child maltreatment: a meta-analytic review. *Child Abuse and Neglect;* **24**: 1127–49.

Madge, N., and Willmott, N. (2007) *Children's Views and Experiences of Parenting.* Joseph Rowntree Foundation and National Children's Bureau. www.jrf.org.uk/bookshop/

Nowak, C. and Heinrichs, N. (2008). A comprehensive meta-analysis of triple positive parenting program using hierarchical linear modeling: effectiveness and moderating variables. *Clinical Child and Family Psychology Review*, **11**(3): 114–144.

Parenting Interventions (for further reading on infant mental health interventions see chapter 8 scenario B).

Patterson, G.R., DeBaryshe, B., and Ramsey, E. (1989) A developmental perspective on antisocial behaviour. *American Journal of Psychology*, **44**: 329–35.

Ramchandani, P. and Stein, A. (2003) The impact of parental psychiatric disorder on children. *British Medical Journal*, **327**: 242–3.

Repetti, R.L., Taylor, S.E., and Seeman, T.E. (2002) Risky families: Family social environments and the mental and physical health of offspring. *Psychological Bulletin*, **128**(2): 330–366.

Shonkoff, J.P.E. and Phillips, D.A.E. (2000) *From neurons to neighbourhoods: The science of early childhood development.* Washington DC, USA: National Academy Press.

Sroufe, L.A. (1996) *Emotional development: The organization of emotional life in the early years.* New York, USA: Cambridge University Press.

Sroufe, E., Egeland, E., and Carlson, E.A. (1999) One social world: intergrated development of parent child and peer relationships. In: WA Collins BL, editor. *Relationships as developmental contexts Minnesota Symposium on Child Psychology.* London: Lawrence Erlbaum Association.

Stewart-Brown, S. (2008) Improving parenting the why and the how. *Archives of Disease in Childhood;* **93**: 102–04.

Waylen, A., Stewart-Brown, S. (2009 in press). Factors influencing parenting in early childhood: a prospective longitudinal study focusing on change. *Child Care Health and Development.*

Werner, E.E. (1993) Risk, resilience and recovery: perspectives from the Kauai longitudinal study. *Development and Psychopathology*, 5: 503–15.

Epigenetics

Caspi, A., McClay, J., Moffitt, T.E., et al. (2002) Role of genotype in the cycle of violence in maltreated children. *Science*; 297(5582): 851–854.

Caspi, A., Sugden, K., Moffitt, T.E., et al. (2003) Influence of Life Stress on Depression: Moderation by a Polymorphism in the 5-HTT Gene. *Science*; 301(5631): 386–389. DOI: 10.1126/science.1083968

McGowan, P.O., Sasaki, A., D'Alessio, A.C., et al. (2009) Epigenetic regulation of the glucocorticoid receptor in human brain associates with childhood abuse. *Nature Neuroscience*; 12(3): 342–348.

O'Connor, T.G., Deater-Deckard, K., Fulker, D., Rutter, M., and Plomin, R. (1998) Genotype-environment correlations in late childhood and early adolescence: antisocial behavioral problems and coercive parenting. *Developmental psychology*; 34(5): 970–81.

Pembrey, M.E., Bygren, L.O., Kaati, G., et al. (2006) Sex-specific, male-line transgenerational responses in humans. *European Journal of Human Genetics*; 14: 159–166.

Spector, T.D. (2003) *Genes unzipped.* Robson Books, London.

Urban environment

Schrader-MacMillan, A., and Barlow, J. (2008) *Promoting the mental health of children through urban renewal: a review of the evidence Institute of Health Sciences Research.* Warwick Medical School.

Day care

Belsky, J. (2006) Early child care and early child development: major findings of the NICHD study of early child care. *European Journal of Developmental Psychology*, 3: 95–110.

Dettling, A., Parker, S., Lane, S. et al. (2000) Quality of care and temperament determine changes in cortisol levels over the day for young children in child care. *Psycohneuroimmunology*, 25: 819–36.

Violence

Pinheiro, P.S. (2006) *World report on violence against children* UN Publishing Services, Geneva.

Obesity

Clark, H.R., Godyer, E., Bissell, P., Blank, L., and Peters, J. (2007) How do parents' feeding behaviours influence childhood obesity. Implications for childhood obesity policy. *Journal of Public Health*; 29: 132–14.

Ericsson, M., Nordgvist, T., and Rasmussen, F. (2008) Associations between parents' and 12-year-old children's sport and vigorous activity: the role of self-esteem and athletic competence. *Journal of Physical Activity and Health*; 5(3): 359–73.

Inequalities

Palmer, G. (2009) *The politics of breast-feeding.* Pinter and Martin, London.

Wilkinson, R. (2005) *The impact of inequality: how to make sick societies healthier.* The New Press, New York.

Wilkinson, R. and Pickett, K.E. (2009) *The spirit level: why more equal societies almost always do better*. Allen Lane, London.

Poverty

Acheson, D. (1998) *Independent Enquiry into Inequalities in Health*. HMSO, London.

Marmot, M. (2008) *Closing the Gap in a Generation: Health Equity Through Action on the Social Determinants of Health*. WHO, Geneva. http://www.who.int/social_determinants/thecommission/finalreport/en/index.html

Spencer, N. (2002) *Poverty and Child Health*, 2nd Edition. Radcliffe Press, Oxford.

Spencer, N. (2008) *Health Consequences of Poverty for Children*. End Child Poverty Coalition, London (www.endchildpoverty.org.uk).

Whitehead, M., Townsend, P., Davidson, N., and Davidsen, N.(1992) *Inequalities in Health: The Black Report and the Health Divide*. Penguin Books, London.

Culture and attitudes

Lorenc, A., Ilan-Clarke, Y., Robinson, N., and Blair, M. (2009) How patients choose to use CAM: A systematic review of theoretical models. *BMC Complementary and Alternative Medicine*; **9** (9) doi:10.1186/1472-6882-9-9

Robinson, N., Blair, M., Lorenc, A., Gully, N., Fox, P., and Mitchell, K. (2008) Complementary medicine use in multi-ethnic paediatric outpatients. *Complementary Therapies in Clinical Practice*; **14**: 17–24.

The People's Health Movement (2008) *Global Health Watch 2: An Alternative World Health Report*. Zed Books, London. http://www.ghwatch.org/ghw2/ghw2pdf/ghw2.pdf

Climate

Costello, A., Abbas, M., Allen, A., Ball, S. et al. (2009) Managing the health effects of climate change. *The Lancet*; **373**: 1693–1733.

UNICEF (2008) Climate change and children: a Human Security Challenge. Unicef, Innocenti Research Centre, Florence.

Advocacy

Aynsley-Green, A., Barker, M. Burr, S., et al. (2000) Who is speaking for children and adolescents and for their health at the policy level? *BMJ*; **321**: 229–232.

Inter-Governmental Panel on Climate Change. Issues authoritative reports on the current status of global warming. www.ipcc.ch/

Milanovic, B. (2002) True world income distribution, 1988 and 1993: first calculation based on household surveys alone. *The Economic Journal*; **112**(476): 51.

Chapter 4

Child public health—lessons from the past

History is important because it can provide explanations for current affairs and also lessons in how things can change. Child health clearly has changed dramatically for the better over the last few centuries, but those who would like to see further improvements can learn a lot from what has gone before. An awareness of previous mistakes can prevent the same mistakes being made again.

The history of child public health is both the history of children's health and the history of society's response to the health problems and diseases of children. As the health of children is an important indicator of the health of society, the history of child public health is closely related to the history of public health in general. Although some childhood diseases and health problems are caused by specific agents (bacteria, pollutants, or genes), child health is also determined by social and environmental conditions. An historical account of child public health therefore needs to address changes in social policy and in the social and physical environment, as well as trends in disease incidence and prevalence. In this chapter, we have primarily focused on an historical context for the country we are most familiar with, namely the UK, without intending to diminish historical perspectives in other nations.

Public health initiatives are easier to implement when philanthropic social attitudes prevail. Many of the public health improvements of previous centuries have been underpinned by changing attitudes towards the health and welfare of vulnerable members of society—the poor, the sick, and children. These have driven legislative regulation of child labour and supported the development of public services such as universal education and child health services. These philanthropic attitudes have also had an impact on children's health by influencing the care babies and children receive from their parents at home. There have been substantial changes over the last two centuries in parenting practices, and in what is regarded as a desirable home environment for children.

Public health reforms may also be driven by self interest and by the interests of the state. Many of the improvements to housing and sanitation in poor areas of cities were introduced, at least in part, to protect the rich from infectious disease. The development of school health services following the Boer War was driven, to some extent, by the need for fit young men to serve in the armed forces to protect the interests of the British Empire. Similar issues arise today in discussions about the purpose of education – is it for the benefit of society, producing adults with skills appropriate for the workforce, or is it for the benefit of the individual, aiming to develop the skills and talents that enhance their lives? These two forces—self interest and philanthropy—while very different philosophically, have frequently acted synergistically to bring about change.

Early times: history relates affairs of state, not so much affairs of the home

The historian tracing the history of child health, and the ways in which societies have tried to improve it, needs to access sources pertaining to childhood. These are scarce. The affairs of the home, where women and children have tended to spend their days, have been regarded as of lesser importance than the affairs of state, and few written records have been preserved. Victorian archivists appear to have selectively destroyed much that was recorded in women's letters or accounts. Historians who have tackled the task of understanding family life in the distant past have therefore worked with snippets of information in records often written for other purposes. Gleaning, collating, and interpreting such information is an arduous task.

Some of the texts which are available paint a pretty dismal picture of childhood in the Western World from the late Middle Ages to the beginning of the eighteenth century. The research of one historian (DeMause 1974 *History of childhood*) documents infanticide, abandonment, neglect, the rigors of swaddling, purposeful starving, beatings, and solitary confinement. He suggests that:

> 'the history of childhood is a nightmare from which we have only recently begun to awake. The further back in history one goes, the lower the level of child care, and the more likely children are to be killed, abandoned, beaten, terrorized, and sexually abused'.

Lawrence Stone (1977 *Family, sex and marriage 1600–1800*), also documents widespread uncaring attitudes towards babies and children, painting pictures of abuse and neglect that include swaddled babies hung up on pegs out of the way of adults. The evidence these historians present makes it clear that the lives of many medieval children were very hard. What we cannot be so sure of is the proportion of children affected. Indeed, later historians (e.g. Pollock 1983 *Forgotten Children*; Hanawalt 1993 *Growing up in Medieval London*) have challenged the views presented above, producing evidence that most children were wanted, that their parents cared about their welfare, and that adults knew that children should and would play.

Today in the UK, we continue to witness the reporting of horrific cases of child abuse and it is estimated that one child still dies each week at the hands of its parents. The difference is that these occurrences are now rare and widely condemned by the rest of society. If, as seems likely, they were quite common and accepted as normal in earlier times, concern for children's health and welfare in social policy and legislation might have seemed quite out of place at that time.

The eighteenth century: the emergence of more humanitarian attitudes

In contrast to material about child care in the home, historians have a wealth of material to work with in the area of social policy. They have been able to demonstrate

Table 4.1 Milestones in child public health 1700–1800

Date	Event
1722	Guy's Hospital admits children to women's ward
1739	Foundling Hospital in London founded by Thomas Coram (Fig. 4.1)
1769	Dispensary for Sick Children of the Poor opened in Red Lion Square, London
1784	A treatise on the diseases of children by M. Underwood, published by the Royal College of Surgeons in Ireland, laid the foundations of paediatrics
1788	1788 Regulation of Chimney Sweepers and their Apprentices Act required apprentices to be at least eight years old; the Act was not well enforced

the emergence of more humanitarian attitudes from the eighteenth century onwards, increasing in prominence and breadth up to the present. These changing attitudes were manifested in legislation regulating child labour and in the establishment of hospitals and health services for poor women and children. At the same time attitudes to vulnerable adults were also softening, resulting in the abolition of slavery and in the extension of the franchise. These developments have been attributed to the endeavours of individual social reformers, such as Thomas Coram and William Wilberforce, but they could not have been achieved without the active interest and backing of a broad section of society. They illustrate the very long timescales between cause and effect in child public health. Although the slave trade was abolished from most of the British Empire in 1833, the legacy of this trade can still be seen in the health and wellbeing of many black children living in the US today.

In the eighteenth century

In the eighteenth century, most children still lived in the country.
Welfare reforms regulating child labour and the establishment of hospitals and health services improved the lot of some children in cities.

The nineteenth century: a time of ups and downs for child health

Philanthropic attitudes were by no means the only driving force in social change, and some policy changes during this era were antithetical to child health. For example, the first half of the nineteenth century saw standards of living rise very greatly in the wealthy sectors of the population. At the same time, the policy of enclosure of the land had made rural existence precarious for the farm servant, and the agricultural slump following the Napoleonic Wars turned many into paupers. During this period of great need, the 1834 Poor Law aimed to withdraw the 'outdoor relief' which had supported poor families during periods of unemployment, and substituted the draconian provision of the workhouse. In practice this law was not fully implemented and outdoor relief continued for some time.

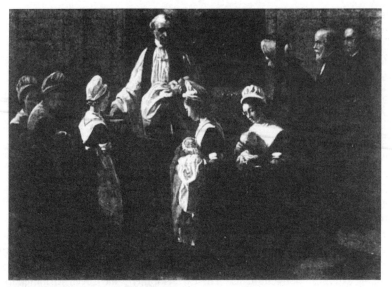

Fig. 4.1 Children in the Foundling Hospital.

Urbanization

Although cities were unpleasant places to live during the nineteenth century, they provided a greater chance of a livelihood than the countryside. As a result, large numbers of people moved to the cities. In 1800, 20% of the population lived in towns and cities; by 1921 this figure had risen to 80%. Rising city populations meant problems with the distribution of food and, in the early nineteenth century, prices were such that the staple diet amongst the poor was bread and tea. A survey in 1841 suggested that only the best paid workers earned enough to achieve an adequate nutritional intake. Both women and children had to work to eat, but the lion's share of the inadequate household food supply went to the men.

In the middle of the nineteenth century, however, the situation changed for the better. The advent of the railways improved supplies to the cities, bringing in cheap fish and coal, and the Corn Laws were repealed, bringing down the price of bread. It has been argued (see Clayton and Rowbotham) that during this period, the nutritional content of the diet of the urban working classes (three quarters of the population) was good, arguably better than the diet we enjoy today. Vegetables, fish and sea food were cheap; watercress was a key and highly nutritious staple; meat was consumed in moderation. Many families grew root vegetables in urban allotments and kept chickens in their back yards, giving them a supply of fresh eggs. These researchers have argued that the remarkably high levels of physical activity sustained by working men and women depended on good nutrition, which was also evident in the relative longevity of those who survived childhood and in the conditions of recruits to the armed forces at that time.

From 1877 onwards food costs fell by as much as 30% due to cheap imports of cereals and meat, but this apparently beneficial change was accompanied by the appearance of processed food and cheap sugar which seems to have had a disastrous effect on population health. The extent of adulteration of foodstuffs during this era is debated, but it certainly occurred. The effect of changing nutrition was most clearly seen in recruits to the armed forces. In 1901 the forces had to lower the minimum height for recruits from 5'4", where it had remained since 1800, to 5'0". Two years later, the poor condition of recruits to the Boer War set off a series of initiatives designed to improve child health (see p. 113). Later in the twentieth century, the second world war also had an effect on the population's diet. Although food scarcity and rationing were a cause of anxiety to mothers in the UK, they paradoxically improved family nutrition. These population level changes suggest solutions to the current nutritional crisis of the developed world, where cheapness and an abundance of processed, sugary food have contributed to the epidemic of obesity. They also suggest, however, that change may require unpopular measures, which may be hard for politicians to make.

Whilst diets fluctuated, the environment in which children lived remained pretty unpleasant. Social reformers and public health doctors like Edwin Chadwick, William Duncan, and William Farr undertook surveys, established hospitals, wrote reports on the conditions of the poor, and voiced their concerns in public. They argued the need for reforms on the basis of enlightened self-interest as well as on the basis of philanthropy. Pointing out that cholera and typhoid from contaminated water supplies were no respecters of social class, they pushed through reforms at national and local level, improving the housing and sanitary conditions of the poor. Social reformers also developed the utilitarian arguments that starving workers were less productive than those who were well fed. From time to time they were able to achieve a sufficient vote in parliament or in the local authorities to achieve the investment or legislation required to improve the lot of children and their families (see Table 4.2).

The 1848 Public Health Act enabled local towns and districts to set up health boards with their own Medical Officers of Health. These new public health doctors supervised the sanitary inspectors whose job it was to notify and prevent infectious diseases and to ensure adequate water supplies. They were well placed to gather and present statistics about epidemics of disease and advance arguments for spending on the infrastructure of the towns and cities. Rural authorities were, however, very reluctant to make such

Table 4.2 Milestones in child public health 1800–1900

Date	Event	Effect
1802	Health and Morals of Apprentices Act	Restricted children's working hours to 12 hours in the daytime, with a requirement for elementary education
1819	Cotton Mills and Factories Act	Prohibited children under nine from working in cotton mills
1831	Local Boards of Health started to be established in the face of cholera epidemics	Boards had responsibility to appoint and oversee district inspectors, to report on sanitary conditions of the poor, and to endeavour to remedy defects

(continued)

Table 4.2 (continued) Milestones in child public health 1800–1900

Date	Event	Effect
1831 & 1833	Mills and Factory Acts	Introduced compulsory holidays and required two hours a day elementary education for younger children
1833	First children's ward opened in a Hospital (Guy's, London)	
1842	Edwin Chadwick reported on the poor state of sanitation in the country and contrasted life expectancy in different social classes	Report led to the establishment of the Royal Commission for Inquiry into the State of Towns and Populous Cities
1847	First Medical Officer of Health Appointed in Liverpool (William Duncan)	
1848	Public Health Act	Created Central Board of Health and required permanent local Boards of Health to be set up outside London
1852	Royal Hospital for Sick Children, Great Ormond Street, founded	
1858	Mines and Collieries Act	Prohibited employment underground of children under 10
1862	Manchester and Salford Ladies Health Society appointed the first health visitors	These visitors 'being women of working class to visit the poor and teach them the rules of health and child care'.
1867	Vaccination Act (later rescinded)	Made vaccination with cow pox compulsory for all infants
1870	Education Act	Attempted to provide elementary education for all children; many local school boards did not use their powers to compel children to attend
1872	Infant Life Protection Act	Required all those who took in two or more children for reward to be registered
1874	Births and Deaths Registration Act	Introduced a penalty for failure to notify and required medical certificate of cause of death
1875	Public Health Act	Consolidated and amended previous Acts; empowered local authorities to provide hospitals and medicines and medical assistance to the poor
1876	Elementary Education Act	Placed a duty on parents to ensure that their children received elementary education
1899	First Infant Welfare Centre opened in St Helen's, Liverpool	
1900	First free milk supplied to nursing mothers	

appointments, knowing that they were likely to result in increased expenditure on sanitation and isolation hospitals. It was not until 1910 that the Town and Housing Act made Medical Officer of Health appointments compulsory. It was recognized that the new public health doctors were likely to make themselves unpopular with the wealthy burghers who dominated the committees of the county councils, and their appointments were protected by a measure of independence. They could not be dismissed from their posts by a decision of the local authority alone. In theory, therefore, they were free to speak out about health and social problems, making the case for reform. While many did do so and, in this way, contributed to important improvements in the living conditions of the poor, many others kowtowed to prevalent 'victim blaming' attitudes which were used to justify lack of investment in health infrastructure.

The history of child public health has thus been dictated by ebbs and flows. Against a backdrop of gradual progress, there have been many setbacks. Powerful advocates have needed to gather data, establish alliances, and make the case for reform. They have often been opposed by those who saw no need to change the status quo and might bear the brunt of the financial consequences of reform.

Changes in child care practices among the wealthy

Such records as do exist suggest that life for many children in the nineteenth century was a definite improvement on life in the eighteenth. The practice of swaddling (which renders babies passive, quiet, and easy to care for at the cost of their physical development) had been largely abandoned during the eighteenth century. The practice, amongst the wealthy, of putting children out to wet nurses had begun to disappear when Georgiana, Duchess of Devonshire, an influential trend-setter of her time, elected in 1783 to breast-feed her own daughter.

Although boarding schools developed and flourished in this era, the younger children of the rich were often cared for in their own homes by mothers or servants. They seem to have been beaten and whipped less frequently, but it was still common during the nineteenth century for small children to be punished with food restriction or to be shut in dark closets for long periods.

Child care amongst the poor

The life of most children in the labouring classes continued to be grim. Mothers needed to work up to and straight after childbirth to bring in sufficient income, but the industrial revolution had separated the world of work from the world of the home, so children were often abandoned to the care of someone else from a very young age. Maternal mortality was high, so many children were brought up in motherless households. Babies were frequently fed gin and narcotics to allay their fretfulness for want of food. Many children thus grew up supervised by children little older than themselves in a hazardous environment, fed, in some eras, on inadequate quantities of bread and tea, and, in many families, subjected to frequent physical abuse. Survival was often rewarded with a move into the relentless, monotonous, and dangerous world of factory work at the age of six or seven. During the nineteenth century, a series of Factory Acts set out to limit the age at which children could be employed and to improve the conditions for child workers.

The 1870 Education Act, and several subsequent Acts, attempted to establish universal elementary education. It was some time before these Acts took full effect.

The writings of Charles Dickens in the 1830s and 1840s have provided an enduring image of life in boarding schools during that period (Fig. 4.2).

In the nineteenth century

- ◆ The populations of cities grew dramatically and conditions deteriorated.
- ◆ Sanitation was poor, food availability, price and quality variable and child labour the norm.
- ◆ The practice among the rich of putting babies out to wet nurses disappeared, but children were still sent away to boarding school at young ages.
- ◆ A series of cholera outbreaks led to a number of sanitary reforms and the gradual establishment of effective sanitation and public health services.
- ◆ A series of Education Acts aimed to establish universal elementary education and Factory Acts restricted the employment of children, but neither took effect for some time.
- ◆ Childhood mortality rates started to fall in the latter half of the century.

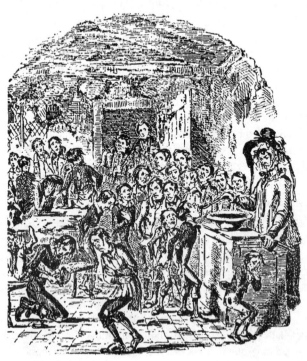

Fig. 4.2 Cartoon of Dotheboys Hall.
Source: Reproduced from Charles Dickens, The life and adventures of Nicholas Nickleby (1987). Oxford University Press, Oxford, with permission.

The twentieth century: interest in child public health waxes and wanes

Although the medical profession played a role in advocating and enabling change, the improvements in child public health that occurred in the eighteenth and nineteenth centuries were achieved almost entirely through changes to the social and environmental conditions in which children lived. During the twentieth century, particularly the latter half, public health was also informed by advances in understanding of the causes of disease and the development of medical practice. Indeed, public health practice became increasingly dominated by the provision of medical services and by attempts to prevent or treat specific diseases and conditions.

The emergence of epidemiology

By the beginning of the twentieth century, routine monitoring of death rates in different age groups and from different causes was practicable, and the discipline of epidemiology developed. It was possible to demonstrate quantitative improvements in public health by charting reductions in mortality rates. Fig. 4.3 shows the mortality rates amongst males in three age groups – under 1 year of age, 1–4 years of age, and 5–14 years (rates in girls are very similar). The data are presented as a logarithmic plot which allows changes in the very different rates in the three groups to be compared on the same graph. The graph shows rates to be falling amongst older children from 1850 onwards and those in 1–4 year olds from 1870. Infant death rates however remained high, only beginning to fall in 1905.

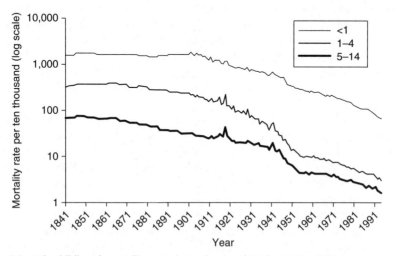

Fig. 4.3 Male childhood mortality rates in England and Wales 1841–1991.
Source: Drawn from data provided by Dr John Charlton, Office for National Statistics, London.

Services to reduce infant mortality

Infant mortality rates, apparently resistant to the social and environmental improvements which had reduced mortality rates in older children, were a cause of concern. Public health interest therefore focused on reducing the common causes of infant deaths as recorded on death certificates – infection, poor nutrition, and 'overlaying'.

Charitable societies were the first to develop services to support mothers, paying for midwives, health visitors, and infant welfare centres. Charitable provision continued to be an important source of health care for the poor throughout the first half of the twentieth century. Several Medical Officers of Health and many of those involved in the local charitable societies proposed that the social and physical environment— inadequate nutrition, sickness, overwork, insanitary housing, and overcrowding— were to blame for high infant mortality rates. They made the case for the provision of monetary benefits to mothers, and provided them with free milk and meals in infant welfare centres. Some local authorities also started to develop preventive services, appointing community health doctors and midwives. There was, however, a widespread reluctance to accept that poverty was the key problem, with much discussion in the policy literature about the 'ignorance and fecklessness of mothers'. In the main therefore, public health policy and local authority provision continued to concentrate on services to 'educate' mothers.

From 1905 onwards, infant mortality rates started to fall. Whether this change can be attributed entirely to the new child public health services is doubtful, but the public health doctors of the day were quick to claim that this was the case. Maternal mortality rates, however, continued to give cause for concern. These concerns led to the passing of the Maternity and Child Welfare Act (1918) which required local authorities to appoint a committee 'to be concerned with the health of expectant and nursing mothers and of children under 5 years', and encouraged the development of infant welfare clinics and health visiting. For mothers this Act was a mixed blessing. The availability of health care free of the stigma of the Poor Law, the provision of milk and food to mothers, and the setting up of child health surveillance programmes are likely to have made a valuable contribution to mothers' and children's health. However, in order to avail themselves of these services many mothers would have had to run the gauntlet of patronizing advice, and disapproval of a lifestyle over which they had little control.

Some of the advice which was provided to mothers by health professionals during the early part of the twentieth century went beyond that designed to improve nutrition and reduce infection. In 1921, the Society for the Health of Women and Children published the child care manual of the paediatrician Truby King. This advised mothers: 'In the interests of their babies' health and welfare, to feed them by the clock, to ensure that their bowels moved every morning, to avoid fond and foolish overindulgence and spoiling' (said to be more damaging than intentional cruelty or callous neglect), and to note that 'obedience in infancy is the foundation for all later powers of self control'. This advice, as can be seen in Chapter 5, had a pervasive and detrimental effect on the nurture of babies in the UK and on their mental and physical health in later life.

School health services

The Boer War (1899–1902) played an interesting part in the development of twentieth-century child health services. The low level of fitness amongst recruits to the armed forces in this war so alarmed the establishment that an Interdepartmental Committee on Physical Deterioration was established to investigate the health of school children. The committee heard evidence from teachers, school inspectors, and local public health doctors, which suggested that a high proportion of children were undernourished and suffering from recurrent illness, to the extent that they could not benefit from education. There was increasing concern about the health of the urban poor and discussion about whether this was improving or declining.

> The low level of fitness of recruits to the armed forces in the Boer War led to a health survey of school children which showed a high proportion of children to be undernourished and suffering from recurrent illness.

The report of this committee in 1904 made recommendations on a wide spectrum of health matters, many of which were incorporated into health and education legislation in 1907 and 1918. Recommendations included the establishment of the school health service, appointment of health visitors and full-time medical officers in every local authority, periodic medical examination of all school children, health education classes in schools, and the provision of school meals.

The 1907 Act made no provision for children found during inspections to be in need of treatment, and few families had the money to pay for this. Lucky children lived in cities where charitable hospitals or dispensaries made some provision for the treatment of children, either through subscriptions schemes or private donations, but rural children fared less well. The 1918 Education Act enabled, but did not require, local authorities to offer free treatment for 'defects' found. Local authorities varied in the alacrity with which they availed themselves of this opportunity to spend local taxes. The provision of free school meals, which legislation also permitted but did not require, was similarly patchy. Thus, while the legislation which enabled the development of the school health service marks an important milestone in the history of child public health, it did not necessarily improve the lot of children throughout the country. Indeed, for many it meant little more than the requirement to submit to somewhat unpleasant medical inspections and enforced delousing.

School medical inspections did, however, make a contribution to epidemiology, providing the first statistics on the level of disease in living populations, and many believed that they made an important contribution to child health. By the time of the Second World war, some Directors of Public Health were claiming that

the child of 1938–9 was bigger, more resistant to disease, better nourished, cleaner and in every way fitter to bear the strain of wartime than his predecessor in 1914 and much of the credit for this can be unhesitatingly given to the school health service.

Dr J. Alison Glover in Chadwick lecture, May 1942

Others, however, noted that all was not yet quite perfect.

> The evacuation of our cities and the findings of our Medical Recruitment Boards have laid
> bare such a mass of preventable disability that we are ashamed.
>
> Ministry of Health Hospital Survey, The Hospital Services of Berkshire,
> Buckinghamshire, Oxfordshire HMSO 1954

The years of the Second World War, with the introduction of rationing and high rates of employment, were widely regarded as good for children's physical health. Growth rates continued to rise and dental health showed a marked improvement. Children's emotional health, which must have suffered greatly as a result of absence of fathers, bereavement, evacuation, and bombing, does not appear to have attracted interest at the time.

In the first half of the twentieth century

- ◆ Public health interest focused on infant and maternal mortality rates and led to the setting up of maternal and infant welfare services by charitable organizations and city public health departments.

- ◆ Although many believed that the poor health of mothers and infants was attributable to poverty, officials often blamed the fecklessness and ignorance of mothers.

- ◆ Recruitment for the Boer War led to recognition of the high levels of disability and disease among children.

- ◆ The school meals and school health services were established, and regular statistics on levels of disease were generated by medical inspections.

Declining interest in child public health

Around the beginning of the twentieth century, public health policy was informed by the belief that health in childhood plays an important part in determining health in adulthood. This belief led public health officials to anticipate a drop in adult mortality rates commensurate with the improvement in childhood mortality rates (Fig. 4.3) that had occurred at the end of the nineteenth century. Figure 4.4 contrasts the continuing decline in mortality rates in 1–4 and 5–14 year olds from 1870 to 1950 with the relatively constant mortality rate in the same generations as adults. It shows that people who were born at the end of the nineteenth century experienced lower childhood mortality rates than those born earlier, but that adult mortality rates in the same generation (age 55–64 years) did not show a decline to the extent which was expected in the period 1925–1975. Death rates in this age group only began to decline from 1970 onwards.

Longitudinal observations like these on mortality rates across generations seem to have alarmed public health officials of the time and led to speculation about the cause. The theories of eugenicists such as Karl Pearson, who believed that the public health reforms were leading to the survival of 'degenerate and enfeebled stock', seemed to some to offer an attractive explanation of the unexpected trends. Statistics showing an increase in deaths due to cancer and heart disease fuelled the belief that these new

Table 4.3 Milestones in child public health 1900–50

Date	Event	Effect
1904	Report of the Interdepartmental Committee on Physical Deterioration	Recommended a wide range of public health measures which were gradually implemented over the next 50 years, including: establishment of the school health service, appointment of full-time medical officers of health and health visitors in every local authority, medical inspections and health education classes in schools, provision of free school meals, registration of stillbirths
1907	Education Act	Local authorities given duty to inspect and attend to the health of children at elementary schools
1908	Children Act	Gave powers for the removal of children from undesirable situations and placing children in care
1915	Compulsory birth notification by midwives to medical officers of health introduced	
1918	Maternal and Child Welfare Act	Required local authorities to appoint committees to be concerned with maternity and child welfare, and suggested full-time health visitors, free hospital care for complicated pregnancies, and maternal and child welfare clinics up to five years
1918	Education Act	Raised school leaving age to 14 years (not implemented immediately) and abolished elementary school fees
1927	Tetanus toxoid and BCG vaccine first introduced	
1928	British Paediatric Association founded	
1929	Abolition of the Poor Law and conversion of workhouses into hospitals	
1944	Education Act	Secondary education to be provided free for all children (1947 Act—up to 15 years; 1973 Act—up to 16 years); free milk, subsidized meals, and free medical and dental inspection; special education for handicapped children
1947	National Health Service Act	
1948	Universal Family Allowance introduced	Beginning of welfare state

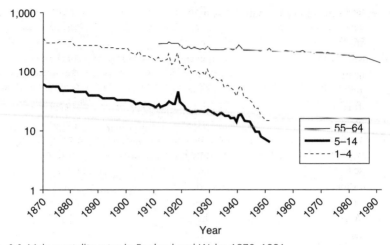

Fig. 4.4 Male mortality rates in England and Wales 1870–1991.
Source: Drawn from data provided by Dr John Charlton, Office for National Statistics, London.

epidemics were indeed caused by survival of 'degenerate stock', as a result of the new public health services for mothers and children.

The impact and aftermath of the First World War and the depression of the 1930s are likely to have contributed to the static adult mortality rates in that era, but do not seem to have been considered a sufficient cause. Instead, the juxtaposition of these relatively static adult mortality rates in a generation for whom childhood mortality rates suggested greatly improved childhood health, together with apparent epidemics of heart disease and cancer, seem to have led public health officials to discard theories relating adult health to child health, and to focus on contemporary causes of disease in adulthood. The epidemic of heart disease appeared at the time to be more of a problem in those from the upper social classes than the lower social classes, diverting attention away from the social environment as a cause.

The middle of the twentieth century therefore saw a shift in focus of public health research and policy away from concerns with child health, the assumption being made that any gains to public health which could be achieved through improving child health had already been achieved. Demonstration of the critical role that smoking played in the development of lung cancer and subsequently heart disease must have fuelled the belief that adult lifestyle was the field in which solutions to contemporary public health problems were to be found.

As a result, child public health more or less disappeared from the research agenda of those practicing in the new medical specialty of public health. Policy developments in public health concentrated on encouraging adults to adopt healthy lifestyles and, subsequently, on the early identification and treatment of disease through screening. The policy developments with an impact on child public health which did occur during this period, for example in child protection, were largely driven from outside public health. Child public health became the concern of community child health doctors and health visitors.

With the 1974 local government and NHS reorganization, community child health services were transferred to the NHS, and with NHS reorganizations in 1990 and 1997, from health authorities to general practice. The 1974 reorganization saw the abolition of the post of Medical Officer of Health and the separation of medical public health from community child health services. Although for a decade expertise in child public health continued to be provided by consultants in public health at area health authority level, further NHS reforms and developments in the medical specialty of public health have resulted in less and less expertise in child public health amongst doctors trained in public health. This situation is now gradually changing for the better.

The low professional status of community child health doctors and the poor academic base for the specialty meant that they had little influence on policy development. Although there were attempts to restate the importance of community child health services—for example, the Court Report in 1974—they had only a limited impact at the time. A delayed effect was the establishment of the medical specialty of community paediatrics, the appointment of consultant community paediatricians, and the establishment of university departments of community child health. These changes are now having a gradual impact on the status of community child health services and on research and development in child public health.

Vaccination and immunization

Although the latter half of the twentieth century was an inactive period in terms of child health policy, child health itself witnessed great advances as a result of the introduction of new vaccinations and immunizations. Childhood vaccination has a long history, but most important developments took place in the twentieth century (Fig. 4.5). The first Vaccination Act of 1867, which was never fully implemented and was later withdrawn, made vaccination of children against smallpox compulsory. The interwar period witnessed the development and introduction of vaccines against the toxins produced by diphtheria and tetanus and against tuberculosis. In the 1950s, vaccines were developed against polio and pertussis and introduced nationwide. BCG vaccination was offered to all school leavers. Measles vaccination was introduced in 1968, rubella vaccination of schoolgirls in 1970, and the combined measles, mumps, rubella vaccine to one-year-olds in1988. The last decade of the twentieth and first decade of the twenty-first centuries have witnessed the introduction of three further vaccines, one against Haemophilus influenza, one against meningitis C and one against the human papilloma virus; the latter to protect teenage girls against cervical cancer in later life. BCG vaccination of school leavers has now been discontinued in most parts of the UK as the risk of contracting TB is now lower than the risks from the vaccine. A programme of immunization of high risk neonates is provided in its place, protecting children in high risk families from contracting TB in childhood.

Together these vaccines have played a part in the dramatic reduction in health problems attributable to infectious diseases in childhood, but they have also brought some problems in their wake. As vaccines take effect, the circulation of wild viruses in the population declines, so children who were not vaccinated or who were inadequately vaccinated (amounting to 10–20% of the population) grow into adulthood without

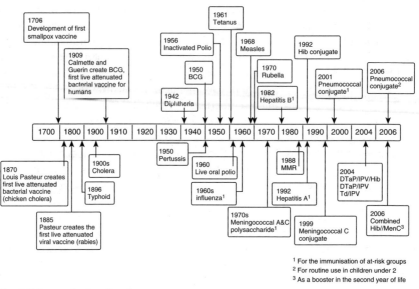

Fig. 4.5 Immunization timeline.
Source: Reproduced from http://www.immunisation.nhs.uk/Library/Research/Historical_vaccine_developments, with permission.

developing immunity. As result, epidemics of childhood infectious diseases now occur in adults, particularly the student population, with greater risk to health from, for example, mumps orchitis. Vaccines have also come in for very bad press from time to time. The original injected Salk killed-virus polio vaccine inadvertently caused disease and disability. This led to a switch to a more effective oral vaccine (Sabin, introduced in 1963), in which the virulent portion is inactivated (attenuated). More recently, there have been spurious claims that vaccines cause disease: for example, whooping cough vaccine and brain damage, and more recently MMR vaccine and autism (Fig. 4.6). Despite scientific evidence of the falseness of such claims, they made significant numbers of educated parents sceptical about the benefit-to-risk ratio of certain vaccines, and lowered the take up of MMR to the extent that outbreaks of measles became very likely. This scepticism challenges paediatricians and child public health professionals to communicate the messages of science much more effectively and sensitively.

The effect of these 'scares' on vaccination rates can be marked, and it can take some years for adequate protective levels in the community to be restored.

Screening programmes

Another key development in twentieth century child health has been the introduction of screening programmes. Childhood screening programmes evolved from the routine medical inspections required for all school children by the 1918 Education Act. The inspection of pre-school children in child health clinics, with the aim of identifying

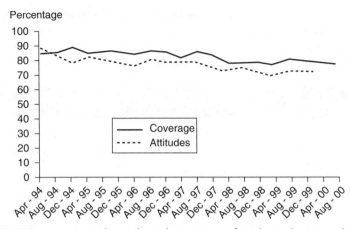

Fig. 4.6 MMR coverage at 16 months and percentage of mothers who report that MMR vaccine is safe or contains only a slight risk.
Source: Adapted from Ramsay ME, Yarwood J, Lewis D, Campbell H, White JM. Parental confidence in measles, mumps and rubella vaccine: evidence from vaccine coverage and attitudinal surveys. Br J Gen Pract 2002; 52(484): 912–6.

those likely to need special education, followed. These programmes were not screening programmes in the precise current sense, but they did identify children with health needs that were not being met, and led to treatment for some problems. It was not, however, until the establishment of the NHS and the medical specialties of paediatrics, ear, nose, and throat surgery, and ophthalmology that these childhood screening programmes really took off. By the 1980s a very large number of children were being referred for treatment of minor childhood illnesses and developmental abnormalities (e.g. glue ear, tonsillitis, and amblyopia).

In the late 1980s, paediatricians and public health specialists working in community child health started to examine the benefits of such programmes and suggested that some were resulting in overtreatment. (See Chapter 5 for information on the evaluation of screening programmes.) Some of the programmes offered to parents and children in the 1980s raised parental concerns about problems which were likely to resolve spontaneously and for which no useful intervention could be offered. A series of reports—the Hall Reports—identified the components of such programmes that were beneficial, and recommended the discontinuation of those which were not. A national standard programme of child health surveillance and monitoring was recommended and endorsed by the new National Screening Committee. The current National Healthy Child Programme (2008) is an umbrella programme which includes health promotion, screening, surveillance, and immunization for all pre-school and school-aged children.

Many of the current screening tests, such as physical examination for developmental hip (acetabular) dysplasia or congenital heart disease, vision, and developmental screening, remain under scrutiny. The imprecision of screening tests, bringing with it problems associated with false positive and false negative results, and uncertainty about the extent of benefit from treatment, mean that it is difficult to demonstrate that overall these programmes do more good than harm. Other programmes—antenatal screening for spina bifida and Down's syndrome, neonatal screening for phenylketonuria and neonatal hearing screening—have had an important impact on the incidence of disability attributable to these health problems.

In the second half of the twentieth century

- ◆ There was a general lack of interest in child public health.
- ◆ Hospital and health services for children continued to be developed but public health services concentrated on adults.
- ◆ There were important developments in immunization.

The development of hospital paediatric services

Until the twentieth century, sick people who could afford it were looked after in their homes. Lying-in hospitals (maternity), hospitals for the mentally ill, for foundlings, and for people who were dying had been built in the eighteenth century on charitable donations, but provision was patchy and these hospitals were dangerous places. Until Semmelweiss and Nightingale identified measures to control the spread of infection in the mid-nineteenth century, mortality was very high. In the second half of the nineteenth century, concerns about the spread of infectious diseases led to the establishment by local authorities of municipal hospitals, separate from workhouses, and by 1911 there were over a thousand of these hospitals. Children suffering from diphtheria and other infectious diseases would be sent to such hospitals, where they existed. In areas where they did not exist, the diagnosis of a case of diphtheria would usually herald the closure of the local school and the suspension of education until the epidemic had passed.

In 1921, the newly established Ministry of Health recommended that hospitals should be overseen by a Hospital's Commission and should receive a block grant from Parliament in addition to their charitable funding. This was the beginning of a national hospital service and heralded the rapid development of effective medical care. With the abolition of the Poor Law in 1929, large numbers of workhouses were turned into hospitals and hospital stock increased. The establishment of the NHS in 1947 accelerated the process (Table 4.4).

Although the Royal College of Surgeons in Ireland had published *A treatise on the diseases of children* in 1784, laying the foundation for the establishment of the speciality of paediatrics, the training of paediatric doctors and nurses did not begin until 1931 in Edinburgh—somewhat later than in other European countries. Special medical services for children began to be developed widely from 1945 onwards. Antibiotics were introduced in 1936, and surgery and anaesthetics gradually became safer.

By the 1960s, surgery on children was commonplace, and a high proportion were hospitalized for tonsillectomy and adenoidectomy. As obstetric care became safer and more sophisticated, more and more babies were born in hospital. Paediatricians began

Table 4.4 Milestones in child public health 1950–2008

Date	Event	Effect
1957	Universal immunization with Salk polio vaccine recommended	
1966	Measles vaccine became available	
1970	Rubella immunization available	
1971	Faculty of Community Medicine established (became Faculty of Public Health Medicine in 1989 and Faculty of Public Health in 2003)	
1974	Local government and NHS reorganization	Local authority child health services to be provided by the NHS; NHS organized into regional, area and district authorities; post of Medical Officer of Health abolished; community physician posts introduced into NHS
1976	Court Report, 'Fit for the Future' published	Appointment of consultant community paediatricians, integration of child health services and development of child disability teams
1980	Abolition of area health authorities	
1983	Griffiths Report on the NHS	Recommends general management at every level of the NHS and major cost improvement programmes and commercial orientation introduced
1988	Measles, mumps, rubella vaccine introduced	
1989	Children Act	Provided a radical reform of the law on children; abolished concepts of custody and access; brought in notions of parental responsibility and rights of children to be heard
1990	NHS Act	Established the purchaser-provided split in which health authorities purchased health care from hospital trusts; enabled general practice fundholding
1997	The New NHS—Modern and Dependable	Enables the development of primary care trusts and the abolition of health authorities
1998	Establishment of the Royal College of Paediatrics and Child Health	
1999	Vaccination against Meningococcus C introduced	

(continued)

Table 4.4 (continued) Milestones in child public health 1950–2008

Date	Event	Effect
2001	Vaccination against Pneumococcus introduced	
2003	Every Child Matters	A blueprint to improve children's life chances with five key areas of activity: be healthy, staying safe, enjoying and achieving, making a positive contribution and economic wellbeing
2004	Children Act	The formation of Childrens Trusts to formalize cooperation between health, education and social care to cooperate to improve childrens lives
2004	Sure Start Childrens Centres	Over 2500 centres developed in socially disadvantaged communities to provide child care, parental support and integrated child services
2008	Human Papilloma Virus vaccination introduced	For prevention of later cervical cancer
2008	National Healthy Child Programme	A programme of screening, surveillance, immunisation and health promotion for all children

to research the newborn and develop ways of supporting babies born preterm. Successful treatments for childhood cancer were identified.

These advances made an important contribution to children's health, but as with so many important advances in health care, the story is not one of unmitigated success. In the middle of the century, children who were sick with rheumatic fever, TB, renal disease, or Perthes' disease were hospitalized for very long periods of time in strictly regimented wards with very little visiting from their parents, leaving, for many, long-lasting emotional scars. Children with mental and physical disabilities were incarcerated in hospitals where they lived under very cramped conditions, with no privacy, and no access to the outdoors. More and more severely preterm babies survived, but many had disabilities. In the 1950s, paediatricians started to recommend, on what turned out to be a spurious basis, that all babies should be nursed prone, causing, as can be seen in Fig. 4.7, a 20-year epidemic of Sudden Infant Death Syndrome.

Some of these problems have now been rectified—the time children spend in hospital and away from their families is kept to a minimum; children with disabilities are cared for in their own homes or in the homes of foster parents, with support from the government; and public education campaigns have ensured that few babies are now nursed prone.

Changes in child care in the twentieth century

Lack of interest in children's health amongst policy makers was accompanied by remarkable changes in child care in the home during the late twentieth century. The practices recommended by Truby King and adopted by many parents have now been largely discontinued, fuelled in part by the research of the paediatricians, John Bowlby and Donald Winnicott, and also by the books of Benjamin Spock and,

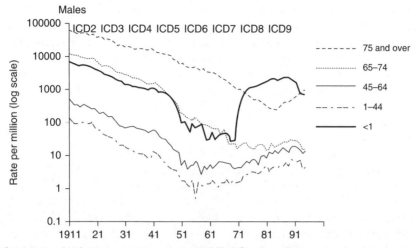

Fig. 4.7 Deaths due to symptoms, signs, and ill-defined conditions. Cot death is the commonest cause of this group of deaths in infancy.
Source: Reproduced from Charlton, J. and Murphy, M. The Health of Adult Britain in 1841–1994. Stationery Office, London, 1997, with permission.

subsequently, by those of Penelope Leach. A much more nurturing attitude now prevails in most families, but accompanying this change, discipline and boundary-setting have become lax in some families, creating problems of a different sort. The majority of parents also take very seriously their role in stimulating children's cognitive, social, and physical development and devote time and energy to this. At the same time, dramatic increases in the number of married women in paid employment has meant that babies and children now spend much of their early life outside the home in nurseries and pre-school educational facilities.

Parents have also had an effect on children's social and educational environment in other ways. Collectively in the 1960s and 70s, through charitable organizations such as the Pre-school Playgroups Association, parents developed a network of inexpensive pre-school playgroups which by the late 1980s was supporting the social and educational development of 80% of the country's children. More recently in a similar social movement, parents started to disseminate to other parents the implications of research on the impact of common parenting practices on children's mental and social health. Through parenting education and support, parents are helped to learn new ways of responding to children's distress and difficult behaviour, and abandoning unhelpful practices such as physical punishment (see Chapter 3). There are now free nursery school places for all four-year olds and many three-year olds, and provision of support for parenting is a major plank of the government's child policy (see below and Scenario B, Chapter 8).

The rediscovery of child public health

Although the lack of interest in child public health at academic and policy level during the last half of the twentieth century has had a detrimental effect on research and development, a small number of multidisciplinary academic groups continued to take an interest in child health and in the impact of early life experiences on adult health. The setting up of cohort studies such as the 1000 families study in Newcastle-upon-Tyne in 1947 and the National Birth Cohort Studies in 1946, 1958, 1970, and 2001 are witness to lasting interest in child health. These studies have continued to point to the social and environmental causes of illness and disease in childhood and to provide evidence on the influence of child health on health in adulthood. As a result there is now a large body of literature attesting to the importance of child health and pointing to approaches to improvement.

At the same time, public health research on the impact of lifestyle on health has failed to explain the pervasive influence of social inequalities on the most common health problems of adulthood—heart disease and cancer. As can be seen in Chapter 6, the child health literature appears to hold many of the answers, and public health interest in child health is now being rekindled. This, together with the election of a government which espoused somewhat more egalitarian social attitudes than those of governments at the end of the twentieth century, brought about a resurgence of interest both in social inequalities and in child public health.

Some of the child health problems of today are similar to those of the past—for example, the general susceptibility to ill health attributable to living in poverty and to inadequate or inappropriate nutrition—but, as Chapters 1 and 3 make clear, many are different. The key problems are now mental health, delinquency and violence, obesity, substance misuse, injuries, asthma, and lack of exercise. Child health is also threatened by the pervasive influence of television, advertising, and marketing, the influence of globalization, and the threat of environmental deterioration. These are important for public health in general, but are especially important for children because of their increased susceptibility and their future expectations of life.

Later in the twentieth century

- Public health officials focused more on preventing the new epidemics of cancer and heart disease in adults.

- Public health interest in child health declined and child health services were transferred to the NHS

- Attempts to restate the importance of community child health services, such as the Court Report in 1976, had a limited impact.

- Vaccination and immunization services developed and had a dramatic effect on childhood infectious disease rates.

- Pre-school child health surveillance services were developed and hospital services for children flourished. These services contributed significantly to child health, but created some unforeseen problems.

- Interest in child public health and addressing social inequalities have recently been rekindled.

Changes in society's view of the importance of childhood

Accompanying the rekindling of public health interest in children has been the development of more egalitarian social policy towards very young children. Research on the family origins of adult social problems, particularly violence, crime, antisocial behaviour, and mental health problems more generally (see chapters 3 and 6), and on the pervasive influence of poverty on child development, has persuaded policy makers to invest in the pre-school period. In the US, the Head Start initiative introduced high quality day care and family support for 0–4's in deprived areas. The UK developed multidisciplinary pre-school services in a major nationwide initiative called Sure Start. These services were available only in selected deprived areas, but the concept is now being rolled out across the UK and by 2012 every family with a 0–3 year old will have access to a Children's Centre which will provide family services, including support for the development of parenting, child care and health, social and educational services. Local authorities in the UK are now required to appoint Parenting Commissioners whose job it is to develop parenting services in the locality, and there have been several high-profile government initiatives to support the development of parenting services to families with school age children. These changes augur well for the future of child health.

The last two decades have also witnessed the emergence of social scientists' interest in childhood. Prior to that time, studies of childhood were rare. Social scientists who wrote about children adopted the traditional view of childhood as a time when families shaped children to fit in with the society into which they were born, a view which was compatible with the prevailing 'behaviourist model' of child psychological development. More recently social scientists have begun to emphasize the role that children themselves play in their families and in their own development. This concept is linked with the increasing understanding that children are rights-holders and should not just be the subject of protection by society, but also have a significant role in participation in decision-making and in discussions on service provision (see pp 43–44). Studies have illuminated the importance of peer culture in learning about sharing, gaining control, communicating, making sense of the world, developing identity, and gaining autonomy.

They have also fuelled interest in the need for policy makers to listen to children. An important step forward in the lives of children has been the appointment of Children's Commissioners in the now devolved countries of the UK, independent advocates whose role is to speak on behalf of children, and to uphold the provisions of the UN Convention on the Rights of the Child. Finding ways of listening to children and young people and working with them has been an important part of the work of many Commissioners Offices. These initiatives have strengthened interest not only in the early years, but also in the development of appropriate high quality adolescent services, including transition-to-adulthood services for those with disability and chronic longstanding illnesses.

Reflections from the past and lessons for child public health practice today

Approaches to the practice of child public health have also changed. It is now rarely important for those practising public health to know a great deal about drains. On the other hand, the ability to make use of information technology is a key skill. Many of the approaches pertinent in the past remain, however, and are still important today. One of these is the need to accept long timescales. Although there have been dramatic improvements in child public health over the last few centuries, the process has not been one of consistent improvement, but rather of ebbs and flows. There will have been times when it seemed as though things were getting worse. The recommendations of the Report of the Committee on Physical Deterioration took almost 50 years to be implemented. In the end, however, persistence has paid off.

Leadership and advocacy is still very important in bringing about change. However, the influential leaders of the past could not have achieved what they did without widespread support. Developing alliances between different professional groups and with charitable organizations, and gaining the support of the public, is still necessary for success in the long term.

Information is a vital adjunct to advocacy and can influence public attitudes. The gathering and presentation of epidemiological data has played an important part in bringing about child health reforms. But the gathering of quantitative data is not enough to improve health. These data can identify the problems but not necessarily the solutions, and solutions developed in the absence of insight from those with the problem can go disastrously wrong. In order to avoid some of the mistakes made around the turn of the last century, the development of solutions to child public health problems needs to involve parents and children; data need to be gathered by qualitative as well as quantitative methods. It is also important for those practising child public health to bear in mind the possibility that well-intentioned interventions could do more harm than good, and to continually review what they are providing and why.

Child health remains critically dependent on parents and what they are able to provide for their children. Very major changes in the way parents care for children have taken place over the last three centuries and these have played a very important part in improvements in child health. Health professionals have clearly demonstrated that they can have an influence over the way babies are cared for, but some of their interventions have been unhelpful. Enabling parents to support their children's health and development is an important but not an easy task, and it needs to be undertaken in partnership with parents. In Chapter 8 we explore some of the ways in which this can be achieved using lessons from the past together with current insights into the origins of child health and wellbeing.

Key messages from the past for practice today

- The prevention of infection and maintenance of food hygiene and purity remain important
- Leadership and advocacy is still important
- Patience and long timescales are essential
- Epidemiological information is vital and influential
- Child health remains critically dependent on parents, and supporting parents remains a key task for those concerned with child public health

Further reading

Bowlby, J. (1953) *Childcare and the growth of love*. Penguin Books Limited, Harmonsworth, Middlesex.

Charlton, J. and Murphy, M. (1997) *The health of adult Britain 1841–1994*. Volume 1. Office of National Statistics. The Stationery Office, London.

Clayton, P. and Rowbotham, J. An unsuitable and degraded diet? Parts 1–3 *Journal of the Royal Society of Medicine;* **101**: 282–289,350–357,454–462.

Cosler, R. (1992) *In the name of the child: Health and welfare 1880–1940*. Routledge, London.

Cosaro, W.A. (2005) *The Sociology of Childhood*. Pine Forge Press (an imprint of Sage Publications), London.

Court, S.D.M. (1976) *Fit for the future: the Committee on Child Health Services Court Report*. (Chairman S.D.M. Court) HMSO, London.

Field, K. (2001) *'Children of the nation?' A study of the health and well-being of Oxfordshire children 1891–1939*. DPhil Thesis, University of Oxford.

Hardyment, C. (1995) *Perfect Parents – Baby care post and present*. Oxford University Press, Oxford.

Harris, B. (1995) *The health of the school child: a history of the school medical service in England and Wales*. Open University Press, Buckingham.

King, T.T. (1821) *Feeding and care of baby*. Macmillan, London.

Kuh, D. and Davey Smith, G. (1997) The life course approach: an historical perspective with particular reference to coronary heart disease. In *A life course approach to chronic disease epidemiology* (eds. Kuh, D. and Ben–Schlomo, Y.). Oxford University Press, Oxford.

Leach, P. (1978) *Babyhood. Infant development from birth to two years*. Knopf, New York.

Lewis, J. (1980) *The politics of motherhood. Child and maternal welfare in England 1900–1939*. Croom Helm, London.

Manning, A. and Ball, M. (2008) *Improving services for young children. From Sure Start to Children's Centres*. Sage Publications, London.

Payne, L. (2009) Twenty years on: the implementation of the UN Convention of the Rights of the Child in the UK. *Children and Society;* **23**: 149–155.

Pugh, G. (2007) *London's Forgotten Children: Thomas Coram and the Foundling Hospital*. Tempus Publishing Ltd, Stroud, UK.

Spock, B.M. (1955) *Baby and child care*. Bodley Head, London.

Warren, M.D. (2000) *A chronology of state medicine. Public health, welfare and related services in Britain, 1066–1999*. Faculty of Public Health Medicine, London.

Winnicott, D.Y. (1965) *The family and individual development*. Tavistock Publications, London.

Winnicott, D.Y. (1965) *The maturational processes and the facilitating environment. Studies in the theory of emotional development*. Hogarth Press; Institute of Psycho-Analysis, London.

Winnicott, D.Y. (1975) *Through paediatrics to psychoanalysis*. Hogarth Press; Institute of Psycho-Analysis, London.

See www.dh.gov.uk for details of Legislation and Policy.

Chapter 5

Key concepts and definitions

In this chapter, we present a number of concepts from the fields of public health and child health which we have personally found useful in our exploration of child public health.

It is by no means an exhaustive survey; and some concepts will be more familiar than others, depending on the reader's own knowledge and background. In many cases there are whole textbooks covering a particular subject, and signposts to relevant reading are provided.

The chapter is divided into four broad themes:

a) **epidemiological concepts**

b) **concepts related to health improvement**

c) **concepts relating to disease prevention and**

d) **concepts relating to the practice of public health and health promotion.**

Epidemiological concepts

Epidemiology is the study of disease in populations. Epidemiologists measure the frequency with which disease occurs in populations and population subgroups, and trends in disease prevalence over time. Our ability to intervene and to effect changes in the health of a population relies on an understanding of the factors associated with disease, and those factors that are involved in triggering or protecting against ill health. Causality and risk are key concepts here, and they are worth exploring in some detail.

Causality

Causality can be defined as 'the operation or relation of cause and effect'. The idea of a single agent causing a single disease has been prevalent in medical thinking since the development of the 'germ theory' of disease in the nineteenth century, but it turns out that there is rarely a single cause–effect relationship in triggering disease. Why is it, for example, that one child in a nursery appears to catch every infection he or she encounters, while others escape many of them, despite having the same exposure to infectious agents?

Rothman defines a cause of a specific disease event as

an antecedent event, condition, or characteristic that was necessary for the occurrence of the disease at the moment that it occurred.

Recognizing the interaction of several different factors, he uses the term 'sufficient cause' to describe a complete causal mechanism, or a set of minimal conditions and events, that are necessary in order to produce disease.

> There is rarely a single cause–effect relationship in triggering disease; usually several factors are involved. It is easier to demonstrate *association* with a disease then causality.

It is often easier, however, to show which factors are *associated* with a disease or illness than to say which *cause* it. Bradford Hill proposed a set of criteria which can help us to distinguish the two, and to determine whether the relationship between exposure to a particular factor and developing a particular disease is causal or coincidental. These criteria are set out in Table 5.1.

These have been reviewed recently by Howick et al. and usefully simplified into Direct (experiment, strength, and temporality), Mechanistic (biological gradient, plausibility) and Parallel (coherence, consistency, and analogy) types of evidence.

One key point is that it is not always necessary to understand the *mechanisms* involved in a causal relationship in order to be sure it exists and to act on it. Famous examples of important public health interventions in which the mechanism behind a causal association was (or is) incompletely understood include the removal of the handle from the Broad Street pump to halt the spread of cholera in Victorian London, the recommendation to stop smoking in order to reduce the risk of lung cancer, and the 'Back to Sleep' campaign in the prevention of sudden infant death syndrome. These examples arguably illustrate separate phases of our understanding of causality and its link with preventive action, which Susser has described as different 'eras' in the evolution of epidemiology. We are now entering the era of eco-epidemiology which takes advantage of combining emerging biomedical technologies (genetic, imaging, etc.) and information technology (see Table 5.2).

It is worth noting that causality can be considered both in epidemiological and in socio-anthropological terms. The epidemiological approach consists of the scientific study of patterns of disease and of cause and effect, as outlined above, whereas the socio-anthropological perspective reflects the beliefs and understanding of parents and children about the causes of disease and ill health. An extension of the eco-epidemiological methodology involves including the privileged epistemological perspective of community members in the definition of variables, the design of measurements and interventions, the data collection, and the analysis. This aims to ensure that research design reflects the way people in the study population experience life. The child public health professional and researcher alike will find a rich source of emerging data with respect to service redesign based on these interrelated perspectives.

> Causality can be considered both in epidemiological and in socio-anthropological terms the latter reflecting the beliefs and understanding of parents and children about the causes of disease and ill health.

Table 5.1 Bradford Hill criteria for causation

Criteria	Comments
Strength—the ratio of incidence to exposure, or the relative risk (see below) (e.g. passive smoking and childhood asthma)	The stronger the association is, the less likely it is to be due to some other coincidental factor (a 'confounder')
Consistency—the repeated observation of an association in different populations (e.g. vitamin D deficiency and rickets)	This again makes it unlikely that the association is due to another factor, which might well vary between different populations
Specificity—a particular cause leads to the same particular event in all cases (e.g. congenital limb malformations seen in babies exposed to thalidomide in *utero*)	This criterion has been criticized on the grounds that single exposures may lead to many effects (e.g. smoking leads to a myriad of diseases as well as being a 'cause' of lung cancer)
Temporality—the cause precedes the effect (e.g. an inflamed arm following immunization)	Logically, effect must follow cause
Biological gradient—a dose-response relationship, where higher levels of exposure lead to greater risk or more serious disease (e.g. lower iron intake leads to more severe anaemia)	There are two criticisms of this criterion: (a) some relationships are *threshold* effects as opposed to gradients (e.g. the association of diethylstilboestrol in pregnancy and vaginal cancer in the offspring) (b) A confounding factor may also have a dose–response relationship: e.g. the non-causal association between birth order and risk of Down's syndrome, which is really due to maternal age
Coherence—the proposed cause–effect relationship does not conflict with what is already known of the natural history and biology of the disease	This is a similar concept to plausibility. The presence of conflicting information may be useful in refuting a hypothetical causal link, but this information may itself be mistaken or misinterpreted, so care is needed here
Experimental evidence—evidence from laboratory experiments on animals or intervention studies in humans shows that removing the exposure reduces the incidence of the disease	This is a *test* of causality as opposed to a criterion for establishing it, and in many instances evidence of this kind is unavailable
Analogy—a similar causal relationship is already well-established (e.g. smoking is known to cause lung cancer, which strengthens the case for a causal association with other kinds of cancer)	As for plausibility, the absence of analogies may only reflect a lack of imagination or experience, not the falsity of the hypothesis
Plausibility—the existence of a biological explanation for the association (e.g. effects on specific organs at cellular level or on cell division)	This depends on possible mechanisms having been identified and tested, which is not always the case even for relationships which do turn out to be causal—but it is still a useful criterion

Source: Data adapted from the Oxford textbook of Public Health Third Edition (1997); 15:626–7.

Table 5.2 Different eras in the evolution of epidemiology

Era	Paradigm	Analytic approach	Preventive approach
Sanitary statistics (first half of 19th century)	Miasma: poisoning by foul emanations from soil, air, and water	Demonstrate clustering of morbidity and mortality	Introduce drainage, sewage, sanitation
Infectious disease (late 19th century through first half of 20th century)	Germ theory: single agents relate one to one to specific diseases	Laboratory isolation and culture from disease sites, experimental transmission and reproduction of lesions	Interrupt transmission (vaccines, isolation of the affected through quarantine and fever hospitals and ultimately antibiotics)
Chronic diseases epidemiology (latter half of the 20th century)	Black box: exposure related to outcome, without necessity for intervening factors or pathogenesis	Risk ratio of exposure to outcome at individual level in populations	Control risk factor by modifying lifestyle (diet, exercise, etc.), agent (guns, food, etc.), or environment (pollution, passive smoking, etc.)
Eco-epidemiology (emerging)	Chinese boxes: relations within and between localized structures organized in a hierarchy of levels	Analysis of determinants and outcomes at different levels of organization: within and across contexts (using new information systems) and in depth (using biomedical techniques)	Apply both information and biomedical technology to find leverage at efficacious levels from contextual to new molecular

Source: Reproduced from Susser, M. and Susser, E. Choosing a future for epidemiology: II. From black box to chinese boxes and eco-epidemiology. *American Journal of Public Health Medicine*; 1996; 86:5, 674–7, with permission from the American Public Health Association.

Risk

Risk can be defined as 'a chance or possibility of danger, loss, injury, or other adverse consequences'. In health terms, a risk factor is one which exposes an individual or population to the chance or possibility of disease or ill health. Risk factors may be factors in the environment, or chemical, psychological, physiological, or genetic elements which predispose an individual to the development of a disease.

The nature, measurement, and communication of risk is a complex area in public health. Exposure to a risk factor does not necessarily lead to the development of the disease it 'causes', nor can we usually explain why some exposed people develop the disease and others do not, because we do not usually know precisely which factors are involved and how these different factors interact. For the unlucky toddler already described, who catches every infection 'going round' the nursery, there must be other factors apart from exposure to viruses which increase his or her risk of succumbing to infection. Although we are uncertain exactly what these factors are, they might include his or her home environment, the adequacy of nursery staff handwashing, emotional stress, whether the parents smoke, sleep patterns, exercise, environmental temperature and humidity, and nutritional factors.

> Risk factors predispose individuals to disease, but do not necessarily lead to the development of the disease. Often the best we can do is to work out the average risk for a group of people with the same level of exposure to a particular factor.

What we can do, however, is to work out the average risk posed to people exposed to a certain hazard or agent by looking at the incidence of disease in all those exposed and comparing it with the incidence in those not exposed (see further discussion of statistical descriptors below). For hazards which are not 'all or nothing' (e.g. factors such as poor nutrition or lack of exercise, rather than exposure to the rubella virus), a graded approach may be used, categorizing people according to their level of exposure and the level of risk this carries. Risks assessed in this way can be described as 'indicators' in predicting ill health among certain groups.

In essence, therefore, this approach involves assigning the same average risk to every member of a particular group or population. It has important shortcomings, one of which is the so-called 'ecological fallacy', which applies to any situation where people are considered in groups and conclusions are drawn about the group as a whole without examining the individuals. The argument goes that the features of the individuals who are affected by the condition in question may differ from those of others in the group. The group's 'defining characteristic' (the reason we have grouped them together—e.g. the risk factor we are looking at) may not after all be the key causal factor.

For example, suppose there is a high incidence of congenital abnormalities in babies born in a town near a chemical plant where many of the local population are employed. Comparing the incidence of abnormalities in this town with those in other local towns, and relating them to the proportion of parents employed in the chemical factory, a local investigator concludes that there is good evidence to suggest that the chemical factory is the cause of the abnormalities, and the population of factory workers is identified as at increased risk of having babies with congenital abnormalities. However, when the actual cases are examined, it turns out that very few of their parents work at the factory, and a totally different explanation presents itself—perhaps they are members of the same extended family and share a genetic mutation. In this example, it would be relatively simple to study the individuals concerned and expose the ecological fallacy, but where larger populations or more common conditions are involved—or where the 'risk' is harder to define individually or consists not of black and white but shades of grey—then it can be much harder to detect the flaw in the supposed cause–effect relationship.

The explosion of genetic phenotyping may allow us to assign more precise risk estimates to individuals, as some of the 'hidden' factors involved in mediating cause and effect relationships may turn out to be genetic and measurable. For now, however, group effects are often the best we can do, and much of the science of epidemiology relies upon them. They have been good enough to determine much of what we know about the determinants of public health today.

Statistical descriptors of risk

Various different terms and concepts can be useful in describing and quantifying risk.

Absolute risk: This is the incidence of a condition in a certain population. It is usually expressed as a decimal or a percentage, e.g. 2% or 0.02. The absolute risk of a condition may vary between different populations, e.g. those living in different countries or areas, or those who are or are not exposed to a risk factor.

Relative risk: This is the ratio of the incidence of a condition in an exposed population to its incidence in an unexposed population. The 'strength' of association described in Table 5.1 above is greater when this figure is higher. For example, if 20% of children whose diets contain less than the recommended daily allowance of vitamin A develop nightblindness, compared to 0.1% of children consuming the recommended amount, then the relative risk associated with inadequate intake would be 20 ÷ 0.1, or 200. Because it is a ratio, relative risk does not have units.

Another name for relative risk is the **risk ratio**. The **odds ratio** and **rate ratio** are similar concepts, measured in slightly different ways, which can be used as an approximation of the relative risk. Risk, odds, and rate use the same *numerator* (the number of new cases seen in a population in a given time), but different *denominators*. For risk, the denominator is the size of the population (e.g., the number of disease-free people at the start of a cohort study). For odds, it is the number of people who do NOT become cases within the given time. For rate, it is the total person time at risk (i.e. the number of disease-free people multiplied by the time period).

It is often important to know both the absolute and the relative risk in order to make a meaningful assessment of risk. For example, suppose the relative risk for those exposed to a particular hazard was 20. If the absolute risk in the general (unexposed) population was 2%, this would give the exposed group a 40% (20×2) chance of developing the disease or condition. If, however, the absolute risk in the unexposed population was 0.002%, or 2 per hundred thousand, then the exposed group's chance of developing the disease would only be 0.04%, or 40 per hundred thousand—a much less worrying statistic.

Attributable risk: This is the amount of risk in an exposed population which can be attributed to their exposure to the risk factor concerned. For example, suppose the risk of Brown's disease in a population of children exposed to a certain environmental agent is 20%, and the risk in the unexposed population is 2%. We can say that of the 20 cases per hundred children seen in the exposed population, 2 would be expected anyway because of the background risk in the general population, and an additional 18 occur as a result of being exposed. The attributable risk is therefore 18%. It can be calculated as the risk in the exposed group (R_e) minus the risk in the unexposed group (R_o): here, $20\% - 2\% = 18\%$.

Sometimes attributable risk is expressed as a proportion of the overall risk in the exposed population—in this example, $18 \div 20 = 0.9$, or 90%. This is called the attributable risk percentage or *aetiologic fraction*—the proportion of the exposed population's risk which is due to their exposure. It can be calculated as $(R_e - R_o) \div R_e$.

As the baseline incidence of a condition in the general (unexposed) population goes up, the aetiologic fraction goes down, because a higher proportion of cases in the exposed population are attributable to their background risk rather than to exposure to the risk factor. In the example above, if the risk of Brown's disease in the unexposed population was 12% and the risk in the population exposed to the hazard was 30%, the attributable risk would still be 18% but the aetiologic fraction would be $18 \div 30 = 0.6$, or 60%.

Population attributable risk: This is the amount of risk in the total population that is attributable to the exposure. It reflects the attributable risk in the exposed population and the proportion of the total population who are exposed. Using the Brown's disease example again, let us suppose that 10% of the population are exposed to the environmental risk factor. Using the initial figures of 2% risk in the unexposed population and 20% risk in the exposed population, we can examine the overall incidence of Brown's disease in a hypothetical representative sample of, say, 1000 people. Of these, 900 will be unexposed, and 2% of 900 = 18 of them will develop the disease. The remaining 100 will be exposed, and 20% of 100 = 20 of them will develop the disease. The total across the population is therefore 18 + 20 = 38 cases in 1000 people (or 3.8%), of which we know 18 are due to exposure to the risk factor (the attributable risk calculated above). The *population* attributable risk is therefore 18 cases per 1000 people, or 1.8%.

Again, rather than working out from first principles each time, there are mathematical formulae for calculating the population attributable risk. It can be calculated *either* as the risk in the population as a whole (R_t) minus the risk in the unexposed population (R_0) *or* as the attributable risk multiplied by the proportion of the population exposed. Here, the first calculation would give us 3.8%–2% = 1.8%, and the second method would give us 18% × 0.1 (which is also 1.8%).

Number needed to harm: This is a related concept. It is the number of people who would need to be exposed to a risk factor in order for one additional person to be harmed or to develop the condition concerned. In the example above, we know that exposing 100 people to the risk factor results in 18 additional cases of Brown's disease. The number of people who would need to be exposed to result in one additional case is therefore $100 \div 18 = 5.5$. This is the number needed to harm.

Perception of risk

The public at large may not always perceive risk in the same way as professionals. Hazards over which people have no control (such as landfill sites or nuclear installations) may be perceived as more threatening, as may new or unfamiliar threats (such as Bovine Spongiform Encephalitis). Although far more children are killed by a parent or carer than by a stranger—and very many more by cars than by any human being—the publicity and distress which follows a child murder by an unknown assailant reflects and feeds intense public fear of such events.

Children's perceptions of risk may be influenced by the views of their parents, teachers, or others, but may also differ significantly from them. Risks which children can visualize (again, the dangerous stranger) are often more worrying, and they tend to perceive living things (e.g. people or dogs) as more threatening than inanimate objects such as cars. However, unseen dangers ('germs', poisons, or aliens under the bed) can also capture the imagination and be perceived as a serious risk. Children may also connect events to generate their own causal theories in a way adults may not expect: 'grandpa died in hospital, so if I have to go there I'll die too'.

Communicating risk

As well as measuring and evaluating risk using the methods described above, public health practitioners also have an important role in communicating risk to the population and helping them to understand and to respond to it—for example, by changing their behaviour (e.g. altering their babies' sleeping position to reduce the risk of SIDS) or by lobbying for action by others (e.g. adding fluoride to drinking water to reduce the incidence of dental caries in local children). To do this effectively they need to be aware of public perceptions as well as measurable levels of risk.

> Public health practitioners have an important role in communicating risk to the public and helping them to understand and to respond to it.

Risk communication can be defined as the open two-way exchange of information and opinion about risk, leading to a better understanding and better decisions being made. This definition acknowledges the two-way nature of the process as opposed to the unidirectional doctor to patient route. As noted above, the context of risk is important: risks may be voluntary or imposed; they may be familiar or unknown (which may affect the degree of dread); and they may be concentrated or dispersed over time. An example which neonatal intensive care specialists and parents regularly face is how best to weigh up the intensity of resuscitative and maintenance measures for an extremely premature infant and the risks of later serious handicap. This dilemma is extended to the population level when rationing decisions have to be made about health care services.

One of the most common dilemmas facing GPs is communicating the risks of a certain intervention – for example, the benefits of antibiotics for acute otitis media in children – against possible harm or no effect. The use of diagrams can be very helpful in communicating such ideas (see Fig. 5.1).

Some evidence-based approaches in communicating risk

- ◆ Avoid using areas or volumes to depict quantities.
- ◆ Absolute risks (with appropriate scales) should be given greater prominence than relative risks – in both information for patients and journals for professionals.
- ◆ Comparison with everyday tasks is valuable, such as where the risk can be compared with other well-known risks (car accident).
- ◆ The influence of 'framing' of risk should be countered by using dual representations (loss and gain, mortality and survival).

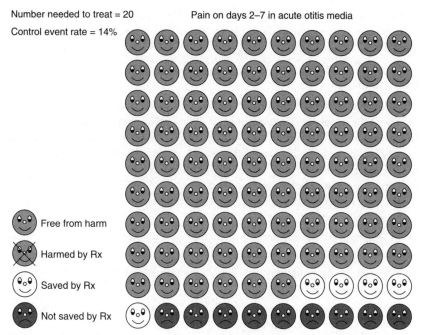

Fig. 5.1 Portrayal of risks and benefits of treatment with antibiotics for otitis media designed with Rx, a program that calculates numbers needed to treat from the pooled results of a meta-analysis and produces a graphical display of the result.
Source: Reproduced from Edwards, A., Elwyn, G., and Mulley, A. *BMJ* (2002) 324: 827–30 with permission from BMJ Publishing Group Ltd.

General susceptibility

One of the problems with the application of the risk model is that, because it has been developed with disease prevention in mind, risks are determined with respect to individual diseases. So for example, we can describe the level of risk of lung cancer for people who smoke compared to those who do not. We can even describe different levels of risk of lung cancer for different numbers of cigarettes smoked per day. However, smoking is a risk factor not just for lung cancer, but also for a host of other diseases, including other cancers, heart disease, and even osteoporosis. Smoking therefore creates susceptibility to a wide range of diseases – and can be said to create general susceptibility to ill health.

In the field of international child health, we have seen that malnutrition is associated with a huge range of diseases. The idea that a single agent or factor can cause many health problems, like the idea that most diseases have a range of different causes, runs counter to the belief that there is a single cause for a single disease.

Some risk factors – such as smoking or malnutrition – do not just predispose to one disease but create general susceptibility to a range of conditions.

It is clear from the discussion above that certain groups or populations of individuals may be at different risk of disease from others. This is explored further in the next section.

Populations

The science of epidemiology is based on the study of populations. Knowledge about the size of the populations is essential in providing *denominators* with which to calculate rates or risks of certain conditions (see above). We can find out from the cancer registry how many cases there are of childhood leukaemia in a local population, but in order to compare this incidence with that in other areas, we need to know the size of the population in which the cases occurred.

There are many types of population to which children belong, and which might be useful as denominators. Examples include:

◆ *geographical* or spatially defined populations – a borough or locality, or a health visitor's 'patch'

◆ *administrative* populations – such as a GP caseload, a school, or a primary care organization population

◆ *at risk* populations e.g. those on the child protection register, unimmunized children, or those from traveller families

◆ *target populations* for screening or preventive programmes

Children can also be divided into *age groups* e.g. neonatal, infant, pre-school, school-age, adolescent. These populations are clearly not mutually exclusive.

Populations are used to establish denominators, which are needed to calculate rates or risks of disease. Examples include geographical populations, practitioner caseloads, schools, and age groups.

The focus of a child health professional's interest, or of a specific intervention, might be aimed at several overlapping categories.

Geographical populations

It is possible to relate health data to population data within different geographical areas in order to assess the health of a given small-area population and make comparisons between different areas. This can be done at a number of levels:

Enumerator districts are the areas within which a single census enumerator is responsible for distributing and collecting census forms.

Local authority 'wards' are commonly used: census data can be converted automatically to this unit, which has more meaning for individuals and service planners. Ward data can then be aggregated into larger areas, such as local authority districts – but only where the boundaries of the larger area correspond to those of the wards. This can cause difficulty if, say, a primary care organization's population is required, and its boundaries cut across ward boundaries.

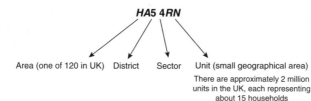

Fig. 5.2 'Anatomy' of a postcode.

Super output areas (SOAs) are more commonly used as their boundaries are less likely to change than wards, each lower level SOA covering between 1000 and 2000 people. They are used extensively with the Index of Multiple Deprivation (IMD) (see below).

Postcodes are increasingly being used as a means of defining and counting populations. Because they represent smaller areas than wards or enumerator districts, they offer greater flexibility in 'reconstituting' larger populations (such as those within PCTs or other primary care organizations). If all the postcodes within a particular population area are known, then the size and composition of that population can be calculated (Fig. 5.2).

Other kinds of population

It is often useful to be able to divide children into different populations or categories in order to analyse the different level of risk experienced by each group. This helps us to understand the role and significance of risk factors in child health, and ultimately to devise interventions designed to promote the health of children. The examples below illustrate this.

Categorization by birth weight

Birth registration is a key source of information about the number of children in an area. It was first established as a statutory duty in the UK in 1874, and parents are still required to register the infant's name and other details within six weeks of delivery. Hospitals also supply data about each birth, which is combined with the registration data by the Office of National Statistics (ONS). One way in which this information is used is to categorize births into different weight bands, which include:

- Low birth weight (LBW) <2500 g
- Very low birth weight (VLBW) <1500 g
- Extremely low birth weight (ELBW) <1000 g

The risk of certain conditions such as cerebral palsy (CP) among babies in different groups can then be compared. The graph (Fig. 5.3) clearly shows the increasing risk of CP with lower birth weight. Using the concepts described above, low birth weight is a risk factor for CP, and the relative risk of CP increases with each decrease in birth weight. These sort of data are invaluable when planning services for high-risk groups of children leaving the neonatal intensive care unit. There have been considerable improvements in survival at the expense of increased rates of disability especially in extremely low birth weight infants. The data are also useful in promoting preventive measures designed to reduce the incidence of low birth weight, such as good antenatal care and maternal nutrition.

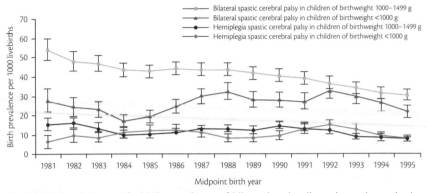

Fig. 5.3 Birthweight-specific birth prevalence of bilateral and unilateral spastic cerebral palsy (3-year moving average) from nine European centres, 1980–96.
Error bars=SE.
Source: *Mary Jane Platt, Christine Cans, Ann Johnson, Geraldine Surman, Monica Topp, Maria Giulia Torrioli, Inge Krageloh-Mann*
Trends in cerebral palsy among infants of very low birthweight (<1500 g) or born prematurely (<32 weeks) in 16 European centres: a database study *Lancet* 2007; 369: 43–50.

Categorization by social class

Since the 1921 Census, the UK has used a system of five (or six) social class categories based on the occupation of the 'head of household'. The rankings were intended to reflect wealth and culture, the latter being equated with a 'combination of knowledge and skill which enables a person to use his purchasing power wisely' (T.H.C. Stevenson, Statistical Superintendent of the General Registrar's Office). For children, social class is obviously ascribed in terms of their parents' (almost always father's) occupation. The categories are illustrated in Table 5.3a.

These categories were initially used to describe the large differences in infant mortality rates between different strata in society. Even today, there are still major differences in mortality, morbidity, and behaviour patterns in both children and parents belonging to different social classes, as we saw in Chapter 3.

Table 5.3a Social class categorization (until 2001)

Social class I	Professionals e.g. doctors and lawyers
Social class II	Intermediate e.g. teachers, nurses, managers
Social class IIIN	Skilled non manual e.g. clerks
Social class IIIM	Skilled manual e.g. coalminers, technicians, ambulance drivers
Social class IV	Partly skilled manual e.g. postmen, bus conductors
Social class V	Unskilled manual e.g. porters, ticket collectors, general labourers

Source: Data from Office for National Statistics.

Table 5.3b National Statistics Socioeconomic classification (NS SEC)

8 classes	5 classes	*3 classes
1. Higher managerial and professional occupations 1.1 Large employers and higher managerial occupations 1.2 Higher professional occupation 2. Lower managerial and professional occupations	1. Managerial and professional occupations	1. Managerial and professional occupations
3. Intermediate occupations	2. Intermediate occupations	2. Intermediate occupations
4. Small employers and own account workers	3. Small employers and own account workers	
5. Lower supervisory and technical occupations	4. Lower supervisory and technical occupations	3. Routine and manual occupations
6. Semi-routine occupations 7. Routine occupations 8. Never worked and long-term unemployed	5. Semi-routine and routine occupations Never worked and long-term unemployed	Never worked and long-term unemployed

* 3-classes names revised 5 October 2001.
Source: Data from Office for National Statistics.

A further example concerns consulting ratios in general practice, which are higher among children living in council housing than those living in owner-occupied housing, for most major causes of consultation. The differences are largest for conditions classed as serious, where consulting ratios among children in council housing are 20% higher than those in owner-occupied housing. Consulting ratios for diseases of the nervous system, however, show a reversed social class trend, with higher consultation rates among higher social classes.

Data on differentials between social classes is crucial in driving the important public health agenda aimed at reducing inequalities in health, and in monitoring the impact of interventions designed to improve the health of the worst off. However, the traditional social class classification system has important disadvantages: it is based on the occupation of the head of household (normally male) – thus children whose parents have never worked do not have a social class, and women whose partners are unemployed or have a job which belongs to a lower category than their own may be inappropriately classified. There may also be wide variations of income within one social class. A new system, the National Statistics Socio-economic Classification, was introduced in the UK in 2001 to replace social class classification, and is designed to overcome some of these problems. The Table 5.3b above shows the three different classifications in the new system, involving 8, 5 and 3 different classes respectively.

Many of the examples we have used in this edition of the book use the older classification as data were more readily available in that format. Further approaches to assessing social inequalities are discussed below.

Categorization by poverty and social deprivation

The importance of poverty as a determinant of health has been well described in chapter 3, but poverty has been defined in different ways and it is important to recognize which is appropriate for which situation.

Townsend defined poverty in this way:

> Individuals, families and groups can be said to be in poverty if they lack the resources to obtain the types of diet, participate in the activities and have the living conditions and amenities which are customary, or at least widely encouraged or approved, in the societies to which they belong.

(Townsend, 1979, p.31)

This is a relative definition which takes into account material deprivation and potential social exclusion. Townsend developed an index of deprivation, which can be calculated for a given geographical area and takes account of measures such as the proportion of the local population who are unemployed, living in overcrowded households, and who own a house and/or car. The Townsend Index was used for many years to examine the relationship between health events such as admission rates to hospital and material deprivation. Brian Jarman, Professor of Primary Care in London, developed a similar scoring system (the Jarman Index) which aimed to explain GP workload variation in relation to social factors. The more recent Index of Multiple Deprivation and its child-specific measure (IDACI) and the Child Wellbeing Index are described below.

The Index of Multiple Deprivation 2007 (IMD 2007) aims to capture the various elements of deprivation and produce a score which can be used to compare areas. It is based on the small area geography known as Lower Super Output Areas (LSOAs). In most cases, these are smaller than electoral wards, thus allowing the identification of small pockets of deprivation. There are 32,482 LSOAs in England. The LSOA ranked 1 by the IMD 2007 is the most deprived and that ranked 32,482 is the least deprived.

The LSOAs are often presented as ranked quintiles (splitting the population into fifths) so that health and other indices can be compared and presented across different levels of social disadvantage.

The IMD 2007 consists of 38 indicators arranged in seven deprivation domains:

Income

– including income support and family credit recipients

Employment

– including those claiming unemployment benefit, incapacity, or disablement allowance

Access

– to a post office, food shop, GP, and primary school

Education

– including qualifications among adults and school attendance / college enrolment among children and young people

Health deprivation and disability

- including mortality ratios for men and women, limiting longstanding illness, and infant mortality

Living environment deprivation

- including indoors (housing in poor condition; lack of central heating) and outdoors (air quality; road traffic accidents involving pedestrians and cyclists)

Crime

- including burglary, theft, criminal damage, and violence

IMD analyses have been applied at Regional Government Office, County Council, and Local District Authority levels in England.

Some examples are shown below.

The map (Fig. 5.4) demonstrates the concentration of high deprivation in the central and eastern parts of London.

Table 5.4 illustrates the numbers and proportions of the local population in each region of England who live in most deprived 20% (quintile) of LSOAs in England.

A measure of deprivation has been specifically constructed for children, the Income Deprivation Affecting Children Index (IDACI), which is defined as the proportion of children 0–15 years living in income-deprived households as a proportion of all children 0–15 years. This index (Figs. 5.5 and 5.6) is useful in highlighting the variation in children's experiences of poverty across the country.

Categorization by income inequality

As we saw in chapter 3, income inequality is arguably a more important determinant of health than absolute income or poverty. The Gini coefficient is the most commonly used measure of income inequality, particularly for comparing inequality in different countries.

The Gini coefficient The Gini coefficient is derived from a Lorenz curve, which is a graph plotting (a) the cumulative income distribution in a particular country, divided into population groups ranked from smallest to largest share of the national income, and (b) a straight diagonal line which represents a hypothetical cumulative distribution where incomes are identical throughout society (see Fig. 5.7). The further the 'actual' curve sags away from the 'hypothetical' straight line, the greater the inequality of income distribution. The Gini coefficient is derived by comparing the area between the two lines with the total area under the straight line, obtaining a value between 0 and 1. The nearer the figure is to one, the more unequal the income distribution within the country.

Key concepts in health improvement

As we shall see later in this chapter, improvements in health can be achieved by preventing and treating disease and by improving the health of the whole population. The latter is, perhaps, less intuitive for those trained in treatment and prevention, partly because it requires an understanding of the concept of positive health or wellbeing, a subject which is not on the curriculum in most medical or nursing schools.

London GOR
Index of Multiple Deprivation 2007

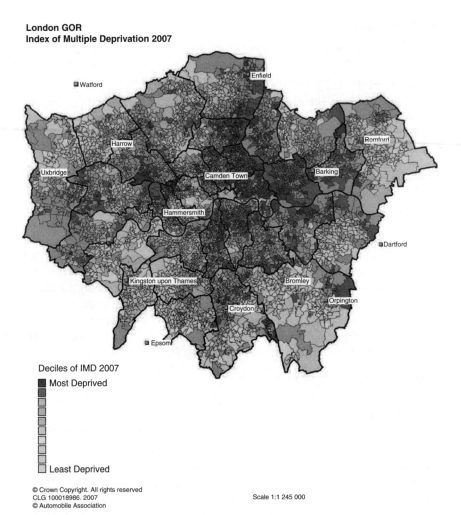

Deciles of IMD 2007

■ Most Deprived

□ Least Deprived

Scale 1:1 245 000

Fig. 5.4 London IMD map.
Source: Reproduced from The English Indices of Deprivation, Department for
Communities and Local Government, March 2008, with permission.

The nature of health and wellbeing has been the subject of much writing and debate
over the millennia, but it did not attract much interest in the twentieth century. Holistic
thinking was much more the norm in earlier times, when the boundaries between
medicine, art, religion, and philosophy were less clear than they are now. Mental,
social, and indeed spiritual health were regarded as integral to physical health, and
disease was often seen as an imbalance between the functioning of the body, mind and
spirit and the physical environment. In Hippocratic times, disease was framed in terms
of the imbalance of the four humours (blood, phlegm, and black and yellow bile). In
China disease was considered to be caused by an imbalance or lack of harmony between
Yin and Yang and between the five elements of earth, fire, water, metal, and wood.

Table 5.4 People living in the most deprived 20% of LSOAs

	Population in most deprived 20% of LSOAs in England (thousands)	Regional Population (thousands)	% of Regional population living in most deprived 20% of LSOAs in England	% of England population living in most deprived 20% of LSOAs in England	Proportion of people living in the most deprived 20% of LSOAs in England, by Region
East Midlands	717	4,322	16.6	1.4	7.2
East of England	345	5,559	6.2	0.7	3.4
London	2,128	7,455	28.5	4.2	21.2
North East	858	2,547	33.7	1.7	8.6
North West	2,170	6,834	31.8	4.3	21.6
South East	485	8,178	5.9	1.0	4.8
South West	468	5,083	9.2	0.9	4.7
West Midlands	1,464	5,347	27.4	2.9	14.6
Yorkshire and The Humber	1,389	5,103	27.2	2.8	13.9
Total	10,023	50,428	–	19.9	100.0

Source: Reproduced from The English Indices of Deprivation, Department for Communities and Local Government, March 2008, with permission.

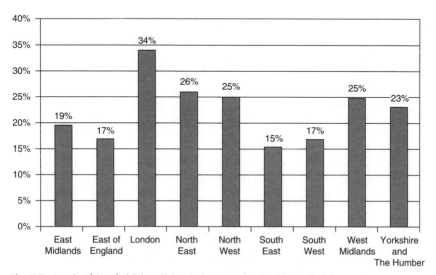

Fig. 5.5 Graph of % of children living in income deprived households.
Source: Reproduced from The English Indices of Deprivation, Department for Communities and Local Government, March 2008, with permission.

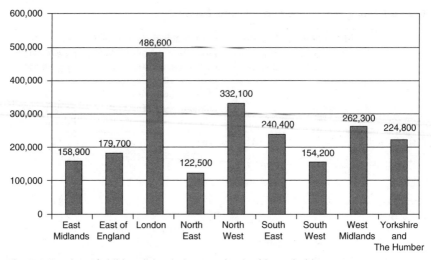

Fig. 5.6 Number of children living in income deprived households.
Source: Reproduced from The English Indices of Deprivation, Department for Communities and Local Government, March 2008, with permission.

Whilst wellbeing is now very much on the public and policy agenda in the UK and Europe, the science of wellbeing is still relatively new. There are very few epidemiological studies of wellbeing and its determinants and even fewer evidence-based interventions to promote wellbeing. As this situation is likely to change in the twenty-first century, we have devoted this section of the chapter to exploring what is known about positive health and wellbeing.

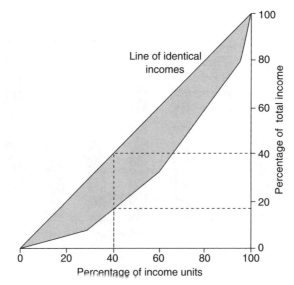

Fig. 5.7 The Lorenz curve.
Source: From Pete Alcock and Jo Campling, Understanding Poverty, published 1993, reproduced with permission of Palgrave Macmillan.

Definitions of health and wellbeing

Health has traditionally been defined by the medical establishment as the lack of disease – the so-called 'deficit model', which dichotomizes health and disease as opposing and mutually exclusive states and fails to acknowledge any positive aspects of health. This definition has not satisfied those interested in promoting optimal health, who have, over the years, given much thought to alternative definitions. Perhaps the earliest attempt, in recent history, was that published by the World Health Organisation in 1948:

> Health is a state of complete physical, mental and social wellbeing and not merely the absence of disease or infirmity.

This definition remains seminal as a statement of 'holism' and is still widely referred to. But it was ahead of its time in many ways, and is still criticized for being over-idealistic and unattainable. Further definitions have been attempted which are more of a half way house.

For example, Lalonde's 'health field' concept, first described in 1974, defines health as a function of individual lifestyle and the environment, influenced by human biology and health-care provision. This model was used implicitly by the UK government in the 1999 White Paper *Saving Lives: Our Healthier Nation* as the basis for action to promote health.

Health has also been defined in functional terms. The Ottawa Charter for Health Promotion in 1986 produced the following definition:

> 'Health is a resource for living, not the object of living. It is a positive concept emphasizing social and personal resources as well as physical capabilities'.

This perspective was also evident in the resolution of the 30th World Health Assembly at Alma Ata in 1977 which declared that:

> The main social target of governments and of the World Health Organisation in the coming decades should be the attainment by all citizens of the world ... of a level of health that will permit them to lead socially and economically productive lives.

In this context, health is considered as a resource for living, which in turn requires certain conditions to ensure its maintenance. These were defined in the Ottawa Charter as:

- Peace
- Shelter
- Education
- Food
- Income
- Stable ecosystem
- Sustainable resources
- Social justice
- Equity

Public perceptions of health and wellbeing

In the UK the 'wellbeing' agenda is being driven partly by the general public. The requirement for public and patients' voices to be represented in policy-making has revealed a demand for the NHS to concern itself with the promotion of wellbeing as well as the treatment and prevention of disease. Most government policy documents now present wellbeing as an NHS goal; few, however, define what is meant by the term.

For an idea of what the public mean by health and wellbeing we need to look to academics and philosophers. In the 1980s the renowned social scientist Mildred Blaxter sought the views of ordinary people in the UK about what health meant to them. Their answers fell into ten main groups, reflecting the different definitions of health discussed above:

1 Don't know or don't think about it – only know what illness is
2 Health as 'not ill' – lack of symptoms; never having to see the doctor
3 Health as the absence of disease or being well despite disease
4 Health as a reserve – recovering quickly or taking risks and not suffering the effects
5 Health as behaviour – the 'healthy life' (no smoking, no drinking, etc.)
6 Health as physical fitness or athletic prowess
7 Health as energy and vitality
8 Health in terms of social relationships – ability to help and support others
9 Health as function – ability to do things
10 Health as psychosocial wellbeing – a holistic view of health as 'a state of mind'

The results of this research reflect the range of views about health still held across society, from absence of illness at one end to wellbeing at the other. It is possible that the proportion of people holding each view has changed over time, and the results of the study might have been different if it had been carried out in different countries or different cultures.

In a book on child public health, it is also important to consider what children think health is. A small study in Oxford in the early twenty-first century found that children defined health and wellbeing in similar ways, but with more of an emphasis on holistic health and wellbeing. The aspects they described included:

- Being myself
- Absence of illness
- Body working well
- Behaviours that promote health (e.g. cleaning teeth, eating well, running)
- Positive feelings
- Absence of negative feelings
- Being normal
- Being involved – having opportunities and experiences
- Achievement

- ◆ Independence and choice
- ◆ A sense of security
- ◆ Good relationships with others (parents, friends, siblings)

In preparing the recent cross-government policy statement Every Child Matters, the government undertook further research with children which endeavoured to identify the outcomes on which children value. Their responses, like those in the Oxford study, indicate a predominantly holistic view of wellbeing. They have been used by the government to developed the five aspects of children's wellbeing now enshrined in much recent UK policy relating to children:

- ◆ Be Healthy
  - physical, mental, and emotional health,
  - healthy lifestyles,
  - sexually healthy,
  - choose not to take illegal drugs
- ◆ Stay safe
  - Safe from maltreatment, neglect, violence, sexual exploitation, accidental injury, death, bullying discrimination, crime, antisocial behaviour.
  - Security
  - Stability
  - Feeling cared for
- ◆ Enjoy and achieve
  - Be ready for school, attend and enjoy school,
  - Achieve educationally, personally and socially
  - Enjoy recreation
- ◆ Make a positive contribution
  - Engage in decision making and support the community and environment
  - Engage in law abiding, positive behaviour
  - Develop positive relationships and choose not to bully and discriminate
  - Develop self confidence and successfully deal with significant life changes and challenges
  - Develop enterprising behaviour
- ◆ Achieve economic wellbeing
  - Engage in further education, employment, or training on leaving school
  - Be ready for employment
  - Live in decent homes in sustainable communities
  - Have access to transport and material goods
  - Live in households free from low income

From: Every Child Matters. London, HM Government 2004. © Crown copyright, with permission.

Thinking about what would make a difference to children's wellbeing, the Children's Commissioner's office carried out a survey of 3000 London children and identified five areas that children perceived as priorities for action to improve health and wellbeing: violence and safe streets, child abuse, drugs, bullying, and racism.

Mental wellbeing

Physical wellbeing is a familiar concept to most of us, even if, as the studies cited above demonstrate, it has been defined in a variety of ways. Mental and social wellbeing are perhaps less familiar. Mental wellbeing has been described by the Mental Health Foundation as positive or good mental health. As the box below makes clear, that encompasses much more than the absence of mental illness:

Good mental health is not just the absence of mental health problems. Individuals with good mental health:

- ◆ Develop emotionally, creatively, intellectually, and spiritually
- ◆ Initiate, develop, and sustain mutually satisfying relationships
- ◆ Face problems, resolve them, and learn from them
- ◆ Are confident and assertive
- ◆ Are aware of others' needs and empathize with them
- ◆ Use and enjoy solitude
- ◆ Play and have fun
- ◆ Laugh both at themselves and at the world

Mental Health Foundation (2002)

Psychologists who have debated the meaning of mental wellbeing describe two distinct components: emotional or subjective wellbeing, and psychological wellbeing. The former equates to 'hedonic' wellbeing as described by Aristotle (concern for one's own happiness and wellbeing as the key drivers) and eudaemonic wellbeing, which he described as leading the good life – one in which concern for others dominated. Psychological wellbeing covers such concepts as confidence, autonomy, purpose in life, personal growth and development, clarity of thinking, creativity, flow, and good relationships with others. The links to social wellbeing are therefore strong. Many now feel that mental wellbeing includes both psychological and emotional wellbeing, noting that both are compromised in mental illness.

In the literature, mental wellbeing in children is often described as emotional and social wellbeing, and the concept of emotional literacy is seen as key. The latter is the capacity to understand one's own and other people's emotions and the influence they have on behaviour, and to use emotional knowledge to support positive relations with others. At the operational level, it has to be acknowledged, emotional and social wellbeing is often considered in much more limited terms, principally as a lack of behaviour problems.

A wide range of studies show that those with a spiritual or religious life have better mental (and indeed physical and social) wellbeing than those without, and the philosophies, approaches and practices of the ancient spiritual traditions, particularly Buddhism, are increasingly informing the mental wellbeing agenda in the West. However, a significant section of the general public remains sceptical of spirituality, pointing to the myriad of problems that religions have caused – and still are causing – across the globe. This is an active area of debate, and things are likely to change over the next decade, but spiritual wellbeing is somewhat in the background of the mental wellbeing agenda in the UK at present.

Social wellbeing

Social wellbeing is dependent on the capacity to function as a social being, to form healthy supportive relationships, and to participate positively in community affairs. It is also determined in part by the norms of behaviour in particular societies or communities.

Social wellbeing has been envisaged in several different ways. One approach focuses on social networks, and regards the existence of positive social networks to support the individual, and the ability of the individual to contribute positively to those networks, as the key attributes. Both the giving and receiving seem to be important. John Helliwell has analysed several global surveys and found that the *general* level of group membership (e.g. the number of people belonging to social clubs, churches, and religious institutions) in a community can contribute to individuals' wellbeing, even if they do not participate themselves. Conversely, when individuals participate in groups they benefit the community's wellbeing as well as their own wellbeing. Whilst Helliwell's research did not yield significant findings in every survey, overall he found that community-level social wellbeing (i.e. effects that remain after individual-level effects have been accounted for) were always either positive or neutral. In contrast, results from the same studies relating to income showed that what Helliwell calls the 'externalities of material advantage' (the effect of increasing my income on your wellbeing) were always negative.

Social capital

Another approach to defining social wellbeing involves the related concept of social capital. The term has its origins in economics and the concept of financial capital – the accrual of money which can be used to make more money. This concept appealed to social scientists as a way to describe attributes of communities where there is co-operation for mutual benefit, trust in civic institutions, and participation in community affairs. It has been found that people living in such communities experience a number of benefits, including improved health (as measured by life expectancy and rates of heart disease and cancer). Most of the studies relating social capital to health have been carried out in adults, not children. Social capital may therefore be more important for parents than for their children.

> Social capital has become an important concept in public health. It describes attributes of communities where there is co-operation for mutual benefit, trust in civic institutions, and participation in community affairs. Social capital can have a positive impact on health—although it is not clear how this happens.

Social cohesion and connectedness are terms which have been included in definitions of social capital. They describe the invisible glue which binds communities of people together, gives them a shared sense of identity, and enables them to work together for the benefit of the whole community. They are generated by social network interaction and can be characterized by feelings of trust and belonging to the community or society, and of interaction and interrelationship. Social capital thus principally reflects attributes of relationships between community members collectively, and to a lesser extent as individuals. There is good evidence from detailed studies in Chicago that the social or organizational characteristics of neighbourhoods explain variations in crime rates that are not attributable to the aggregated demographic characteristics of the individuals within them. In this case, it is the 'collective efficacy' (the linkage of mutual trust and willingness to intervene for the common good) of the community in not tolerating crime that acts as a form of informal social control.

Communities with low average income are more likely to have low levels of social capital, but these two determinants of health are independent of one another, and it would seem that high social capital may protect members of economically deprived communities from some of the health effects of poverty.

Mechanisms The impact of social wellbeing on health is an example of an epidemiological phenomenon being identified before the mechanisms are clear (see p. 132), and there has been much debate about precisely how it affects health. Mechanisms which have been proposed include promotion of the economy through networking and collaborative ventures (economic capital), and the development of skills and competencies (human capital) in the community or group. Social capital may also represent a resource for further development of the community, in that new networks may be built upon older networks, using social relationships, norms and values, trust and information that have already developed. At the simplest level, however, social capital can be seen as a description of supportive, respectful relationships between community members. Such relationships could have a direct effect on health by enhancing emotional wellbeing and by reducing the stress generated by day-to-day life events. Destructive relationships – those characterized by suspiciousness, exclusion, and fear – could have a direct deleterious effect on health. We have seen in Chapter 3 that there is good evidence that the quality of relationships between parents and their children has a powerful effect on children's health, and like these relationships, social capital appears to offer a measure of protection from the deleterious effects of poverty. Studies of social capital and adult health may therefore be capturing a similar phenomenon amongst adults.

The box shows one tool which has been developed for measuring social capital.

Measuring social capital

The WHO Health Behaviour of School Children survey in 2001/2002 used a social capital 'package' with four components:

1 Social networks and social support
2 Power and control through engagement
3 Local identity
4 Perception of resources

Although most of the social capital literature focuses on adults, there are some studies relating to children. Coleman found that low social cohesion was the strongest predictor for high school students dropping out of school, and Runyan showed that children from low-income areas who scored high on a social capital index performed consistently better on developmental and behavioural testing than their peers. An ecological model proposed by Earls and Carlson ties family relationships and community relationships together, seeing family processes and individual development as embedded in community and other macrosocial structures (Fig. 5.8).

This might be considered a somewhat reductionist model of child wellbeing. It implies that all that society – and families – need to do to promote children's wellbeing is to supervise and control their behaviour, and that self-efficacy is the only aspect of mental health that matters. Earls derived his model from work in violent or disruptive neighbourhoods, but warmth and affection, positive regard, and approval within the family are also important for emotional wellbeing, along with the traditional 'limit setting', supervisory parental role.

> Despite criticisms of the literature on social capital, there is no doubt that it is an important concept for health promotion and may modify the impact of poverty on health.

There has been criticism of the term 'social capital' on the grounds that it has a poor theoretical framework and that it simplifies a range of social phenomena to 'one true

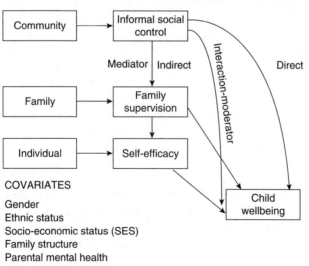

Fig. 5.8 Multilevel analytical model of child wellbeing.
Source: Reproduced from Ravens-Seiberer et al., (2008) Health-related quality of life in children and adolescents in Germany: results of the BELLA study, *Eur Child Adolesc Psychiatry* [Suppl 1], 17: 148–156, with kind permission of Springer Science+Business Media.

measure' which can be substituted for the social understanding required for humane social policy and public health practice. Others have suggested that the concept is just not applicable to children, especially as in some guises social capital emphasizes civic institutions and public affairs, and these are social activities from which children are often excluded.

In spite of these criticisms and a lack of precise understanding of the mechanisms involved, the phenomena described in the social wellbeing literature are undoubtedly of importance to health promotion. In the context of social inequalities, health promotion practitioners need to address the question: is it most effective to foster social capital and social cohesion in disadvantaged communities with poor levels of 'connectedness', or should interventions be aimed at improving income equality? This is an important question for everyone concerned with tackling health inequalities and improving the lot of the worst off in society. Most of those working with disadvantaged communities would consider that both approaches are important – that interventions should be directed both at income improvement and at developing local networks and facilities, trust, and support. The latter approach depends on harnessing the close co-operation and involvement of members of the community, through activities such as community participation or community development.

Measuring wellbeing

For wellbeing to be taken seriously in government policy it is important that it can be measured, but measurement demands a degree of consensus about the concept and is thus a relatively recent endeavour. Early attempts in the health world to measure wellbeing described what they measured as 'quality of life', particularly health-related quality of life. Health-related quality of life instruments have been important in the context of the 'evidence base' for medical interventions, bringing holistic outcomes to studies which had previously focused exclusively on levels of disease. Such measures have been developed both for the general population (generic measures) and for those who are suffering from a particular condition or have undergone some intervention or treatment (disease-specific measures). All measures are necessarily subjective, reflecting the perspective of the individual completing them about their own health. The best known examples of generic measures for adults include the SF-36, which measures eight dimensions of health covering physical and psychosocial health, and the EuroQOL, which reduces health to a single dimension and is therefore important for economic studies.

Psychologists have made a number of attempts to measure wellbeing itself. Measures range from single items capturing 'happiness' or 'satisfaction with life', which are favoured by economists in their studies of the determinants of wellbeing (see Helliwell above), to long inventories capturing specific concepts such as psychological wellbeing and emotional literacy. A recent measure developed for the UK population, the Warwick Edinburgh Mental Wellbeing Scale (WEMWBS) is proving very popular because of its brevity and positive contents. This measure has been adopted by the Scottish government to monitor mental wellbeing at a national level, and is likely to be adopted by other UK countries. It is valid for use in young people age 13 years and over.

Measurement is important because it provides the basis for studies of the determinants of wellbeing. These may turn out to be the inverse of the determinants of mental illness, but may also include other factors. Measurement of wellbeing can also enable studies of the impact of wellbeing on health. Whilst these are few and far between at present, those that exist show, for example, that positive mood is associated in prospective studies with reduced mortality (Chida and Steptoe 2008) and, in cross-sectional studies, with lower levels of salivary cortisol and inflammatory markers (Steptoe et al. 2008).

The New Economics Foundation has argued strongly that wellbeing should be monitored by governments, and that as much attention should be given to wellbeing as to GDP. Their publication 'National Accounts of Wellbeing' shows how wellbeing varies between countries and in different age groups. It shows that wellbeing is less clearly related to income and GDP than are disease measures. The NEF measure of wellbeing covers positive feelings, absence of negative feelings, satisfaction with life, vitality, resilience, self esteem, positive functioning, supportive relationships, and trust and belonging.

A number of child-specific quality of life measures have been developed in recent years, and these are being used to examine the relationship between specific health conditions and children's perceptions of their physical and psychological health. The PEDsQL is perhaps the most widely known. This has a generic module which can be used alone or in combination with a range of disease-specific modules, covering, for example, diabetes and asthma. Children with chronic pain, special educational needs or mental health problems tend to have lower scores on these measures. Kidscreen is a European measure which has been used in large scale surveys in many European countries.

Figure 5.9 below shows scores on yet another measure, the KINDL-R; high scores indicate a higher perceived quality of life. The figure compares the scores of children with and without special needs (CSHCN: Children with Special Health Care Needs), chronic pain, asthma and mental health problems.

Parent report is the only way of measuring wellbeing in from preliterate children, and even amongst older children parent reported responses are common. Parent and child scores often differ, however, and it is now regarded as important that children's views are sought directly when ascertaining the outcome of a specific clinical intervention or service reconfiguration.

Emotional and social wellbeing have traditionally been measured in children with instruments that cover behaviour problems and internalizing disorders. The Strengths and Difficulties Questionnaire (SDQ) is the most recent, and currently the most popular measure. The SDQ can serve as a screening tool for children with mental health problems, and most of the items focus on negative behaviours and attributes, but the measure does include one prosocial scale. The Kidscreen instrument covers a wide range of aspects of mental and social wellbeing. In a study of 8–12 year olds with cerebral palsy, Kidscreen scores showed, reassuringly, that these children's self-reported quality of life was similar to the general population (Fig. 5.10).

UNICEF recently sponsored a project which aimed to measure and compare children's wellbeing in economically advanced nations (Fig. 5.11). The measure used in this study included a subjective rating of wellbeing, but overall it focused on

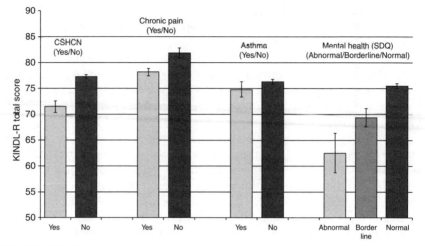

Fig. 5.9 KINDL-R scores.
Source: Ravens-Sieberer et al., (2008). Health-related quality of life in children and adolescents in Germany: results of the BELLA study, Eur Child Adolesc Psychiatry [Suppl 1],17: 148–156, with kind permission of Springer Science and Business Media.

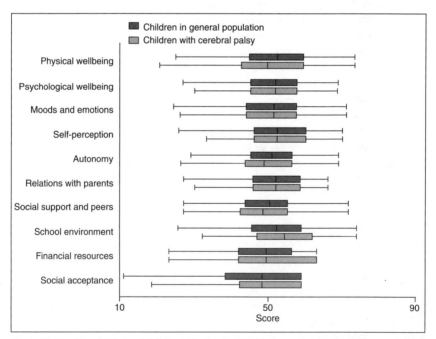

Fig. 5.10 Quality of Life in Children with Cerebral Palsy (measured using Kidscreen). Source: Reprinted from The Lancet, 369, Dickinson et al. Self-reported quality of life of 8–12-year-old children with cerebral palsy: a cross-sectional European study (2007), 2171–78, with permission from Elsevier.

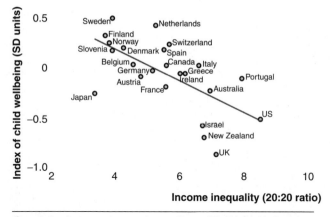

Correlation between income inequality and the Unicef index of child wellbeing in 23 rich countries

Fig. 5.11 Index of child wellbeing in the EU -25.
Source: Reproduced from Pickett, K. & Wilkinson, R. (2007), BMJ 335: 1080–5, with permission from BMJ Publishing Group Ltd.

problems and material and social conditions. It is thus not a true measure of child wellbeing in the sense in which we have used the term here. However, as the study found children in the UK to have the lowest levels of wellbeing amongst all countries studied, it has played a key role in stimulating the child wellbeing agenda in the UK. The components of the UNICEF measure were based on currently available data and included material wellbeing (poverty, unemployment, deprivation); health and safety (infant mortality, immunization levels, injury mortality); educational achievement (reading, maths and science at age 15, proportion of 15–19 year-olds not in education, training or employment); relationships (family structure, family relationships, peer relationships); health behaviours (diet, smoking, fighting and bullying); and subjective wellbeing (rating of own health, liking school a lot, life satisfaction).

Although there has been criticism about the use of this data, because different years of data collection compromised direct comparability between countries, there is still a trend that supports the hypothesis that objective and subjective measures of wellbeing are closely related to relative poverty in a society.

Local Authorities in England have recently produced an index of child wellbeing which covers:

Material Wellbeing (receipt of income support and other state benefits)

Health (derived from emergency and outpatient appointments and receipt of disability living allowance)

Education (examination scores, absence rates, and further education enrollment)

Crime (including burglary, violence, and criminal damage)

Housing (overcrowding, sharing, and homelessness)

Environment (see Table 5.5)

Children In Need

Table 5.5 Detail of environment domain of the Children's Wellbeing index

The Indicators

Environmental quality
- Air quality: *combined air quality indicator*. Source: Geography Department at Staffordshire University
- The natural environment: *percentage of green space and woodland*
- The number of bird species. Source: European Environment Agency's CORINE Land Cover (CLC) database; British Trust for Ornithology bird breeding atlas
- Road safety: *severity-weighted accidents per 1000 children aged under-16*. Source: Department for Transport.

Environmental access
- Availability of opportunities for sports and leisure: *average number of different types of sports and leisure facility within waking distance for children aged 11 to 16*. Source: Ordnance Survey Points of Interest
- Distance to school: *average road distances to primary and secondary schools for children aged 4 to 10 years and 11 to 16 years*. Source: PLASC (2005) and Edubase (2005).

Source: Reproduced from Local Index of Child Wellbeing Summary Report, Communities and Local Government, 2009, with permission.

This index covers important determinants of children's health and wellbeing not captured in other measures and is a useful indicator for comparing performance at local authority level (see Table 5.6 below), but it does not capture either subjective wellbeing or the social environment. This sort of measure is necessarily based on routinely available data and such data take some time to catch up with changes in thinking.

Wellbeing and health improvement programmes

Health improvement programmes are based on the relatively new concepts and definitions presented in this section. The approaches to health improvement to which they have given rise, such as community development, are described in Chapter 7. Because these concepts are new and because approaches to measurement are still in their infancy, epidemiological studies quantifying their impact are relatively rare. In this respect health improvement contrasts strongly with disease prevention, where epidemiological studies abound and quantification is common.

Table 5.6 Child wellbeing in English cities. Table comparing highest and lowest ranking cities for Children's Wellbeing Index (CWI) in England.

Lowest wellbeing		Highest wellbeing	
354	Manchester	1	Hart
353	Tower Hamlets	2	Ribble Valley
352	Liverpool	3	Mid Sussex
351	Islington	4	East Hertfordshire
350	Hackney	5	Rutland

(continued)

Table 5.6 (continued) Child wellbeing in English cities. Table comparing highest and lowest ranking cities for Child Wellbeing Index (CWI) England.

Lowest wellbeing		Highest wellbeing	
349	Kingston upon Hull, City of	6	Waverley
348	Southwark	7	Wokingham
347	Birmingham	8	South Northamptonshire
346	Nottingham	9	Surrey Heath
345	Middlesbrough	10	Horsharn
344	Lambeth	11	Chiltern
343	Leicester	12	Elmbridge
342	Newcastle upon Tyne	13	Mid Bedfordshire
341	Haringey	14	South Cambridgeshire
340	Sandwell	15	West Oxfordshire
339	Knowsley	16	St Albans
338	Barking and Dagenham	17	Fareham
337	Lewisham	18	Congleton
336	Newham	19	Rushcliffe
335	Bradford	20	Uttlesford

Source: Reproduced from Local Index of Child Wellbeing Summary Report, Communities and Local Government, 2009, with permission.

Concepts of disease prevention

Disease represents a deviation from the 'normal' or healthy state and is a much more familiar concept than wellbeing. Disease can be considered on many different levels: explanations in terms of cellular and organ dysfunction are the most familiar to doctors, but social scientists and anthropologists have shown that disease is also a social and cultural phenomenon which may be defined differently in different societies.

> Disease is a deviation from the 'normal' or healthy state – but it is also a culturally-determined phenomenon.

In Western society, the development of germ theory in the nineteenth century led to the concept of 'a single cause for a single disease', which was reinforced by the subsequent success of immunization in preventing disease. However, as non-infectious diseases increased in significance, it became evident that this model had serious limitations. It has now been largely replaced with a multifactorial model of causation which is relevant even to infectious diseases, since it is now recognized that the host and the environment play a significant part in their causation, as well as the infective agent.

As discussed above, Susser has described the various shifts in epidemiological paradigms over the last 100 years (Fig. 5.12). We are currently in the eco-epidemiological era, where disease causation is considered in terms of multiple levels of influence (like the Mandala approach set out in Chapter 3). In some ways, therefore, understanding of disease and its causes is creeping closer to a holistic model reminiscent of the causes of wellbeing examined in the previous section.

Disease prevention, however, remains concerned primarily with preventing specific diseases. It includes, for example, not only immunization programmes and infection control policies, but also a wide range of other activities, including measures such as risk factor reduction which often have a more general benefit for health. A useful diagram produced by Tannahill describes the close interrelationship between prevention, health education, and health protection, seen in Fig. 5.13 as overlapping circles.

The three approaches are often synergistic, each increasing the effectiveness of the others. For instance, consider the introduction of a programme aimed at reducing injury and death in road accidents through increased use of seat belts – an example of a prevention programme. This could be assisted by passing legislation to make seat belts compulsory (health protection) and by explaining the benefits of seat belt use to the public (health education).

Disease prevention is often described as comprising three levels of activity: primary, secondary, and tertiary prevention.

Primary, secondary, and tertiary prevention

Primary prevention

Primary prevention involves stopping a disease or condition from occurring in the first place. Examples in the field of child health include immunization, fluoridation of water to prevent dental decay, legislation aimed at preventing accidents (health protection), and the 'Back to Sleep' campaign to reduce cot death. Primary prevention measures usually aim to increase resistance to ill health – for example, healthy eating programmes which help prevent obesity and diabetes, or interventions to reduce the uptake of smoking among young people. Primary prevention is often

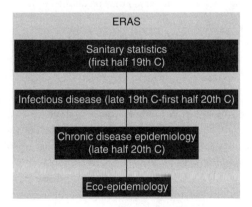

Fig. 5.12 Eras of epidemiology and disease understanding (after Susser).

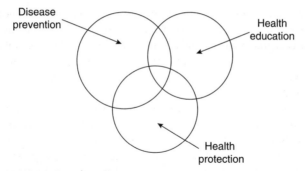

Fig. 5.13 Tannahill overlapping circles.
Source: Adapted from Downie, R.S., Tannahill, C., Tannahill, A. (1996). Health
Promotion: Models and Values. Oxford University Press, Oxford, with permission.

aimed at a whole population, such as a community, school, or general practice caseload. In this way it is similar to the promotion of positive health and wellbeing. The difference lies in the different goals of the two activities, and this difference is important. The success of disease prevention programmes is measured in the extent to which they prevent a specific disease; the success of wellbeing promotion programmes in the extent to which they improve health and wellbeing in a holistic sense.

Secondary prevention

Secondary prevention refers to the early identification of disease or impairment so that it can be reversed, or its effects mitigated, through treatment. Screening programmes are examples of secondary prevention, such as the neonatal blood spot ('Guthrie') test for congenital metabolic disorders. This includes hypothyroidism, the impact of which can be all but eliminated by early intervention. Another example is interventions to prevent the recurrence of events or illnesses, including instituting child protection measures for abused children.

Tertiary prevention

Tertiary prevention involves slowing the progress and managing the consequences of established disease or disability, with the aim of alleviating its impact on the lives of the sufferer and his or her family. Examples include the use of inhalers to reduce the frequency and severity of a child's asthma attacks, supplying a wheelchair to a child with severe cerebral palsy to aid mobility, or teaching an adolescent with spina bifida self-catheterization to enable independent toileting.

Universal and targeted approaches

Whenever interventions are being considered, whether they are preventive or therapeutic, some thought needs to be given to who should receive them. Some interventions, such as healthy eating advice, are appropriate for a whole population; others may apply only to some members – perhaps a particular age group (e.g. the child health immunization programme) or ethnic group (e.g. screening for thalassaemia or sickle cell disease). But we also need to consider the fact that interventions which could benefit everyone in the population to some extent may have greater advantages for some members than others. For example, although increasing levels of exercise would do everyone some good, the health benefits are more marked for those who are sedentary than for those who already exercise regularly. Should we, then, be aiming interventions (and the limited resources available to support them) at those who have the greatest need, or are at greatest risk? In some cases this approach is appropriate, but the argument is not as clear as one might first imagine.

In *The Strategy of Preventive Medicine*, the late Geoffrey Rose argued that the population cannot be neatly divided into the sick and the healthy. For most diseases or health problems there is a continuum of severity rather than an absolute distinction between those with the disease and those without. The 'case definition' of a disease often involves a convenient, conventional, but more or less arbitrary cut off – for example, of body mass index for obesity, blood glucose for diabetes mellitus, or peak flow for asthma. This is even more pertinent when considering those at risk of disease. There is no clear dividing line between individuals 'at risk' and those 'not at risk' (see the detailed discussion of risk earlier in the chapter), even when we know that a particular indicator is an important risk factor. The risk of heart disease or stroke, for example, is not confined to those with the highest blood pressure; instead, there is a continuous distribution of risk throughout the entire population, with higher blood pressure tending to correlate to increasing risk, but some risk attached even to those with average or 'normal' blood pressure. In the maternal and child health setting, the same applies to defining those at risk of Down's syndrome, speech and language delay, emotional and behavioural problems, or child abuse.

> There are good arguments both for universal approaches to health promotion and disease prevention, and approaches which target high risk groups. Much depends on the aim of the programme and the nature of the intervention.

In looking at the total 'burden' of a particular disease or condition within a population, it is important to consider the actual numbers of individuals at each level of risk. As Fig. 5.14 shows, for many risk factors there are usually relatively few individuals at the extreme end of the risk distribution, and increasing numbers as we move down through the spectrum.

What implications does this 'bell curve' distribution have for disease prevention? Crucially, most cases of disease will occur among the many who are not at especially high risk, rather than among the few who are at very high risk. The majority of infants with Down's syndrome, for example, are born to mothers in younger age groups, although we know the individual risk is greater for the older mothers who make up a small proportion of the total pregnant population (Fig. 5.15).

Another example is illustrated in the Figs. 5.16 and 5.17.

The *prevalence* of behaviour problems in 5–15 years-olds in the lowest social groupings is nearly three times that in the highest, but in any representative group of

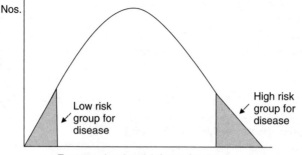

Exposure level to risk factor for disease

Fig. 5.14 Bell curve – low and high risk groups.

children the actual *numbers* affected are low at both extremes of the socioeconomic groups. Interventions targeted at the highest risk group (children of those who never worked or are long term employed) are therefore bound to miss a high proportion of children with problems.

Going back to the question posed earlier about whom interventions should be aimed at, it can be shown that in many situations a greater reduction in morbidity will be achieved by including the whole population, rather than by attempting only to influence those at the upper end of the risk distribution. Examples might include child corporal punishment legislation in Scandinavia, which has substantially reduced exposure to physical violence across the entire child population, or school-based programmes to deliver free fruit to all children and thus increase average consumption of fruit and vegetables in the school-aged population. The impact of this kind of intervention is illustrated in Fig. 5.18. The broken curve shows the new lower distribution of exposure after a population-wide control measure (reducing exposure from level A to B), which succeeds in shifting the entire population risk distribution to the left, thus reducing the prevalence of the disease being targeted. The total population risk (the area under the curve) is clearly much lower as a result – whereas merely eliminating the 'tail' at the top end of the risk distribution would have a much lesser impact.

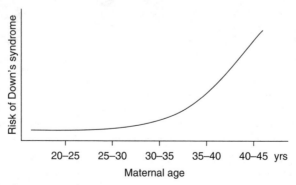

Fig. 5.15 Risk of Down's syndrome.

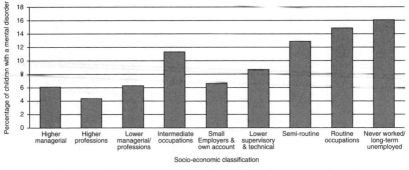

Fig. 5.16 Prevalence with behaviour problems in children (5–15 years) in each socioeconomic classification.
Source: Reproduced from Mental Health of children and Young People in Great Britain 2004, ONS 2005, with permission.

It can be argued, therefore, that targeting interventions at those sections of the population with the highest risk, or the highest prevalence of problems, may not be the best way to reduce the burden of disease or problems in society as a whole. This is known as the **population paradox**. As Rose put it

the visible tip of the iceberg of disease can be neither understood nor properly controlled if it is thought to constitute the entire problem.

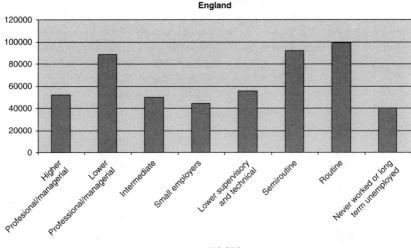

Fig. 5.17 Numbers of children 5–15 years in each socioeconomic group.
Source: Data from 2001 census, www.nomisweb.co.uk, Office for National Statistics (data extracted 17 June 2009).

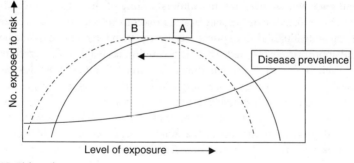

Fig. 5.18 Risk and exposure.

This constitutes a strong argument, then, for universal interventions. The elimination of infectious diseases by the development of herd immunity is one good example of an effective population approach: in this case, immunization of one group of people can protect others who cannot be immunized. Further arguments for the universal approach have been advanced by those interested in mental health promotion, since the mental health of the 'well' has an impact on the prevalence and severity of illness in the 'ill'. Racism, bullying, stigma, domestic violence, and child abuse are all important causes of mental health problems, but they are also indicators of less than optimal mental health among the perpetrators. Thus interventions to improve the mental health of the population as a whole arguably have an important role to play in reducing mental ill health amongst those most susceptible to it.

> Reducing risk across a whole population can have a much greater impact than concentrating on high risk individuals. This is known as the population paradox.

On the other hand, the argument for a targeted strategy, focusing on those at greater risk, is that this approach is more efficient, yielding the most benefit given that resources are limited and may not stretch to cover a whole population. It is also the case that individuals who perceive themselves as being at lower risk are less likely to alter their behaviour and thus their risk profile, so that 'shifting the distribution downwards' may not be an easy outcome to achieve.

The efficiency argument in favour of targeted prevention has had a major impact on health visiting services in the UK, where caseloads are often 'profiled' according to various child and social risk factors, and divided into groups which receive different intensities of intervention according to their perceived level of need or risk. It is important here to point out the distinction between a *universal* and a *uniform* service. It is quite possible to provide universal coverage of a population in a preventive programme but to devote more time and resources to those in greatest need – and this is essentially what health visitors do in prioritizing their time.

It has been argued, moreover, that Rose's approach is not based on adequate scientific evidence. Also, risk can currently only be imprecisely defined according to broad bands or groups. Targeted interventions are clearly more appropriate, the argument goes, but we need a fuller understanding of the actual mechanisms of causation rather than descriptive statistical associations between risk and disease. If we could define individuals' risks of disease accurately, then interventions could he effectively and appropriately targeted. There is no doubt that many of the screening tools currently used for selecting the population to be 'targeted' (for example, assessment of mental health problems using the Edinburgh Postnatal Depression Scale) are imprecise, and may incorrectly classify individuals to receive – or not to receive – services.

There are persuasive arguments, then, in favour of both universal and targeted approaches to prevention. In practice, the choice of approach often reflects political or pragmatic considerations: the main aim of fluoridating water may be to reduce dental decay among disadvantaged children, but the most practical approach must be to treat the water supply for an entire area. Sometimes it is stigmatizing to select some individuals in a group to receive an intervention, and in order to improve uptake among those who most need it, it is better to offer a universal programme – health visiting services, as opposed to, e.g., social services involvement with a family. There is also an increasing recognition that the effectiveness of certain interventions is greatly increased by attempting to alter the behaviour or ethos of an entire group, via a 'settings' approach. This may involve promoting healthy schools, workplaces, even prisons or young offenders' institutes. It reflects the fact that the social environment can be a powerful (positive or negative) influence on health, and that behaviour – especially among children and young people – is strongly influenced by the peer group.

Often, however, a combination of universal and targeted approaches is most appropriate. In seeking to reduce teenage pregnancy, we need to consider services for the whole teenage population (such as effective sex education programmes and easy availability of emergency contraception) and special interventions for those we know are at highest risk (including looked-after children and those from disadvantaged backgrounds).

Finally, it is important to be clear about what a particular disease prevention programme hopes to achieve. One crucial distinction is between two different aims: a general decrease in morbidity across the whole population, or a reduction in health inequalities achieved by improving the health of the worst off and least healthy more than the better off and more healthy. It has become clear that general improvements in health often occur at the expense of widening gaps between the two extremes, and a targeted approach is often promoted as a way of reducing inequalities in health. The UK government has set a target for infant mortality that clearly sets the objective of reducing the difference between 'manual groups and the population as a whole'. Although many of the interventions and services which might contribute to this are universal (such as improvements in antenatal and neonatal care), others are aimed specifically at disadvantaged groups (such as the Family Nurse Partnership programme, see Chapter 8, scenario B). It is important to bear in mind the issues raised in the discussion above when shaping health policy.

Screening

We have defined secondary prevention as the early identification of disease or impairment. There are two approaches to early diagnosis: one depends on prompt attention to the earliest symptoms of disease, the other to detection of latent or early disease in an apparently healthy, asymptomatic individual. The latter requires the administration of a *screening test*, usually as part of an organized screening programme, in order to identify individuals who:

- definitely have the disease or condition in question
- or, more commonly, have a result which indicates that they have a high chance of having the disease or condition

In the latter case, a second *diagnostic test* is required to confirm or refute the possible diagnosis. This might range from a relatively innocuous procedure, such as a more precise audiological test in the case of neonatal hearing screening, to an invasive procedure, such as amniocentesis in the case of Down's syndrome screening.

> Screening tests and programmes aim to reduce risk – and thus prevent ill health – by detecting conditions at an early stage when interventions can be more effective.

In order for screening programmes to be appropriate and effective, certain conditions must be met. Wilson and Jungner first established a set of criteria against which proposed screening programmes could be assessed. A modified version of these is illustrated below, adapted by Hall and Michel specifically for neonatal screening programmes for liver disease and extra-hepatic biliary atresia, but equally applicable to other childhood screening programmes.

1 The condition should be an important public health problem as judged by the potential for heath gain achievable by early diagnosis.
2 There should be an accepted treatment or other beneficial intervention for patients with recognized or occult disease.
3 Facilities for diagnosis and treatment should be available and shown to be working effectively for classic cases of the condition in question.
4 There should be a latent or early symptomatic stage and the extent to which this can be recognized by parents and professionals should be known.
5 There should be a suitable test or examination. It should be simple, valid for the condition in question, reasonably priced, repeatable in different trials or circumstances, sensitive, and specific. The test should also be acceptable to the majority of the population.
6 The natural history of the condition and of conditions that may mimic it should be understood.
7 There should be an agreed definition of what is meant by a case of the target disorder; also an agreement as to (i) which other conditions are likely to be detected by the screening programme, (ii) whether their detection will be an advantage or a disadvantage.
8 Treatment at the early, latent, or presymptomatic phase should favourably influence prognosis, or improve outcome for the family as a whole.
9 The cost of screening should be economically balanced in relation to expenditure on the care and treatment of persons with the disorder and to medical care as a whole.

10 Case finding may need to be a continuous process and not a once and for all project, but there should be explicit justification for repeated screening procedures or stages.

More recently, the UK National Screening Committee has updated Wilson and Jungner's criteria to reflect a range of factors: recognition that screening is not infallible, that it can lead to harm as well as benefit (specifically in terms of its psychological impact, and in some cases the need for risky or invasive diagnostic procedures after a positive screening test), that it must be seen in the context of the entire range of service provision for the disease in question, and must be subject to strict quality controls to ensure it is effective. Their list of criteria is shown below.

UK National screening committee criteria

The condition

- The condition should be an important health problem.
- The epidemiology and natural history of the condition, including development from latent to declared disease, should be adequately understood and there should be a detectable risk factor, disease marker, latent period, or early symptomatic stage.
- All the cost effective primary prevention interventions should have been implemented as far as possible.

The test

- There should be a simple, safe, precise, and validated test.
- The distribution of the test values in the target population should be known and a suitable cut-off level defined.
- The test should be acceptable to the population.
- There should be an agreed policy on the further diagnostic investigation of individuals with a positive test result and on the choices available to those individuals.

The treatment

- There should be an effective treatment or intervention for patients identified through early detection, with evidence of early treatment leading to better outcomes than late treatment.
- There should be agreed evidence-based policies covering which individuals should be offered treatment and the appropriate treatment to be offered.
- Clinical management of the condition and patient outcomes should be optimized by all health care providers prior to participation in a screening programme.

The screening programme

- There should be evidence from high-quality randomized controlled trials that the screening programme is effective in reducing mortality or morbidity.
- There should be evidence that the complete screening programme (test, diagnostic procedures, treatment/intervention) is clinically, socially, and ethically acceptable to health professionals and the public.

- The benefit from the screening programme should outweigh the physical and psychological harm (caused by the test, diagnostic procedures, and treatment).

- The opportunity cost of the screening programme (including testing, diagnosis, and treatment) should be economically balanced in relation to expenditure on medical care as a whole.

- There should be a plan for managing and monitoring the screening programme and an agreed set of quality assurance standards.

- Adequate staffing and facilities for testing, diagnosis, treatment, and programme management should be available prior to the commencement of the screening programme.

- All other options for managing the condition should have been considered (e.g. improving treatment, providing other services).

Screening test properties

The ideal screening test has the ability to detect all those with the condition in question and exclude all those without it. This is rarely the case, and there are therefore almost invariably 'false positives' and 'false negatives' from the initial screening test – both of which have economic, psychological, and social costs attached. False positives (those with a positive screening test who turn out not to have the disease) are usually identified once the second diagnostic test has been applied, but false negatives (those with a negative result on the screening test, but who *do* have the disease) often do not emerge until later, when the disease or condition reaches its overt stage. A useful framework for identifying false positives and negatives is given in the box below:

| | *Disease* | |
Screening test	Present	Absent
Positive	a	b
Negative	c	d

a True Positive; b false positive; c false negative; d true negative

The performance of a screening test depends on the number of false positives and negatives it produces and is usually described in terms of its *sensitivity* and *specificity* – essentially, how good the test is at picking up cases and not picking up non-cases. Sensitivity refers to the proportion of cases of disease which are accurately detected by the test (and is lower if there are many false negatives); specificity refers to the proportion of those without the disease who are accurately detected by the test (and is lower if there are many false positives).

Another way of looking at a screening test's performance is to assess its *positive predictive value* and *negative predictive value* – or how useful a positive or negative test is in predicting the presence or absence of disease. Positive predictive value refers to the proportion of those testing positive who turn out to have the disease (lower if there are many false positives); negative predictive value refers to the proportion of those

Table 5.7 Mathematical definitions of sensitivity, specificity, positive and negative predictive values

Term	Definition	Formula
Sensitivity	The proportion of those with the condition *who test positive*	a/a + c
Specificity	Proportion without condition *who test negative*	d/b + d
Positive predictive value	Proportion with positive test *who have condition*	a/a + b
Negative predictive value	Proportion with negative test *who do not have conditon*	d/c + d

testing negative who turn out not to have the disease (lower if there are many false negatives). These concepts are defined mathematically in Table 5.7 using the letters from the box above.

The performance of a test is influenced not only by its own properties, but also by the prevalence of the condition in a particular population: although sensitivity and specificity depend only on the test, the positive and negative predictive values vary. Suppose the prevalence of Shergar's disease is 1% in a population of 100,000, and the sensitivity and specificity of the screening test designed to detect latent cases are both 90% (quite a reasonable assumption). There will be 1000 true cases, of which the test will detect 900; and there will be 99,000 healthy individuals of whom 9900 will also have positive results. Thus, out of a total of 10,800 positive results, only 900 will turn out to have Shergar's disease. The positive predictive value is therefore 900 ÷ 10,800 (a/a + b), which is 8.3%, and there will be 12 false positives for every true positive. If the prevalence is lower, say 0.1%, the positive predictive value will be 0.89% and there will be 112 false positives picked up for every true positive. In addition, in either case 10% of those with Shergar's disease will be missed by the screening test and falsely reassured, although this will be a larger number when the prevalence is higher. The decision as to whether the cost in economic or social terms is acceptable is an important area for debate with the target population and their families or carers.

> The performance of a screening test is influenced by its sensitivity and specificity, and also by the prevalence of the disease in the population.

It is clear that screening programmes are not infallible, and may on balance do more harm than good if they are not carefully thought through. This is a concept which the general public finds hard to accept, especially when screening programmes are presented as beneficial services and there is a certain amount of pressure to accept testing. The National Screening Committee recognizes that screening programmes must be presented in an appropriate way if they are to be acceptable and comprehensible to the population. It stresses the importance of promoting individual choice about whether or not to undergo screening tests, and redefines screening as a risk reduction programme rather than as a reliable means of early diagnosis.

Table 5.8 Advantage and disadvantages of screening programme

Benefits	Disadvantages
◆ Improved prognosis for some cases detected by screening	◆ Longer morbidity for cases whose prognosis is unaltered
◆ Less radical treatment which cures some early cases	◆ Possible overtreatment of questionable abnormalities
◆ Reassurance for those with true negative test results	◆ False reassurance for those with false negative results
◆ Lower resource costs for early treatment	◆ Anxiety and sometimes morbidity for those with false positive results
◆ May reduce overall incidence and prevalence of disease in population	◆ Hazard of screening test e.g. venepuncture, radiation
	◆ Resource costs: scarce resources diverted to screening programme
	◆ Unnecessary medical intervention for those with false positive results

Advantages and disadvantages of screening programmes

A summary of the benefits and disadvantages of screening programmes is given in Table 5.8.

Systems approaches

There has been a shift in recent years from a focus on the development of individual services and prevention programmes for children to synergy between programmes, or the development of 'systems'. Systems-based approaches look at how all services and organizations in an area can be involved and aligned with the wider determinants of health and disease, based on shared goals, partnership arrangements and strategies. This approach has been well described by Halfon and others in the US as part of the Early Childhood Systems Building tool. It focuses on access to primary care, mental health and social development, parenting education, early child care and education, and family support, and has introduced the concept of the 'medical home' (a US term which refers to the place where a child and family would receive their medical care on a continuing basis in contrast to in emergency departments). The organizations responsible for these different elements of the 'system' work closely together to develop joint goals and strategies for delivery. Fig. 5.19 shows how these components interact.

In the UK, the Every Child Matters programme and the development of Children and Young Persons Strategic Partnership Plans both adopt a systems approach (Title V refers to a US Government maternal and child health block grant).

The approach is best illustrated with an example (Fig. 5.20). In the context of parent support for healthy child development, seven steps are described:

1 **Setting the goal:** parents have access to the knowledge, skill development and resources they need to support their children's healthy development.

2 **Identify the environment for the goal:** for example, a family resource centre (Children's Centre in England). Positive features: one-stop entry point; community

health workers present. Negative features: not available in all communities; fragmented funding system.

3 **Measurable outcomes and data sources:** e.g. availability and use of home visiting
programmes; parent knowledge and parent-child relationship before and after
participation in parenting education programmes; breastfeeding rates.

4 **Generic strategies:** e.g. measurement, communications, organizational capacity-
building and family development.

5 **Key partners:** parents, private providers, community health centres, Children's
Centres, child care centres and preschools, hospital maternity units, large businesses
in the area.

6 **Specific activities:** e.g. media campaign on literacy or parenting, information
packs for parents, and development of locality website.

7 **Plan for monitoring:** this might involve routine data sources or a specific survey
of local households.

Patient pathways

Another framework that is used increasingly when developing services is the concept
of the 'patient pathway'. This describes all the components of service provision for a

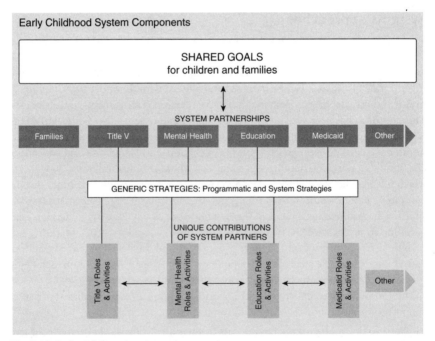

Fig. 5.19 Early childhood system components.
Source: Reproduced from Ruderman, M., Gruson, H. Early Childhood System Building
Tool. Baltimore, MD: Johns Hopkins Bloomberg School of Public Health. Los Angeles, CA:
The National Center for Infant and Early Childhood Health Policy; 2004, with permission.

GOAL	MEASURABLE OUTCOME	GENERIC STRATEGY	PARTNERS	ACTIVITY
Parents have access to the training and resources they need to support their children's healthy development	Number and percentage of parents who report having received information on early literacy and reading to their children	Communications	Large businesses Media organizations Hospitals Health plans Governor's Office	Media campaign on literacy Packets to new parents State website on literacy and reading

Fig. 5.20 System building steps diagram.
Source: Reproduced from Ruderman, M., Grason, H. Early Childhood System Building Tool. Baltimore, MD: Johns Hopkins Bloomberg School of Public Health. Los Angeles, CA: The National Center for Infant and Early Childhood Health Policy; 2004, with permission.

specific health condition (including prevention, early identification, assessment, treatment, and long term support if necessary) by considering the 'journey' of an individual patient through the course of the disease or condition. This is shown schematically in Fig. 5.21 below, within the structure of a pyramid of services.

An example illustrating the different components is given below for meningococcal septicaemia.

Meningococcal septicaemia

Component	Action/output	Measurable indicators
Prevention	Immunization	Population uptake of immunization
Identification	Adolescent awareness	Proportion of 16-year olds receiving health education
Assessment	First contact	% GPs with paediatric training
	Second contact	% emergency department staff with APLS training
Interventions	Antibiotic access	Time between rash recognition and antibiotics
Long-term support	Hearing impairment	% assessed at discharge
	Speech and language therapy	% access within 6 weeks

Concepts and definitions in public health and health promotion practice

There have been many different definitions of public health and health promotion. The most widely accepted definition of public health is now that of Acheson:

> Public health is 'the science and art of promoting health, preventing disease and prolonging life through the organized efforts of society'.

> Acheson (1986)

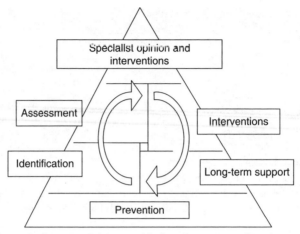

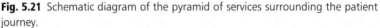

Fig. 5.21 Schematic diagram of the pyramid of services surrounding the patient journey.
Source: Modelling the future, RCPCH 2007 p. 73. © 2007 Royal College of Paediatrics and Child Health.

This definition underpins our definition of child public health, which was presented in the introduction (see p. 2).

Public health typically addresses health at the population level rather than at the individual level and is broadly-based and multidisciplinary in its approach. In the UK, public health practitioners are supported by the Faculty of Public Health, which was until recently a solely medical body. At the beginning of the twenty-first century, the Faculty opened its registration procedures to practitioners from a wide range of other backgrounds, including health promotion. This change is gradually having an influence on the practice of public health, moving from a primarily preventive focus to one in which the promotion of wellbeing plays a greater part.

The UK Faculty has identified nine key areas of practice which demonstrate the scope of the discipline. They are listed in Table 5.9, with examples to illustrate how each area of practice might relate to child health. Further details of many of the activities listed can be found in later chapters.

Public health had its origins in the nineteenth century and is grounded in the recognition that health is affected by environmental and social conditions, with adverse conditions and lifestyles interacting to create susceptibility to disease. As well as protecting individuals from specific disease-causing agents, public health interventions often aim to make general improvements to social and environmental conditions in order to prevent disease. The distinction between public health reforms and more general social reforms is not always clear, as improved health may be one of many social goods which are delivered through social reforms such as laws to limit child labour. See Chapter 4 for a fuller discussion of the history of public health and lessons from the past.

Table 5.9 Nine key areas of public health practice in the UK

Area of practice	Child health examples
Surveillance and assessment of the public's health and wellbeing	Overseeing routine child health surveillance; collecting health data on special groups such as looked-after children or those with disabilities; developing shared databases with other agencies
Assessing the evidence base for health and health care interventions, programmes and services	Undertaking systematic reviews to synthesise the results of trials of treatments or preventive interventions
Policy and strategy development and implementation	Working in local strategic partnerships to examine ways of preventing teenage pregnancy; membership of a Children's Task Force at National level
Strategic leadership and collaborative working for health	Advising commissioners of health care on priorities for development within child health; input to service planning as a member of local Children's Partnership Group; helping service providers make use of pooled budgets to deliver more effective respite care services for families
Health Improvement	Healthy Schools' initiatives; advocating for children's rights; working with other organisations to persuade the government to introduce a ban on smacking
Health Protection	Managing communicable disease outbreaks (e.g. meningococcal disease, Hepatitis A) in schools or colleges; overseeing immunization programmes
Health and social service quality	Effective co-ordination of multi-agency projects, such as developing innovative child and adolescent mental health services in conjunction with local social services
Public health intelligence	Developing a local child health profile/public health report Linking data from local authority on parks, roads and injury data
Academic Public Health	Teaching of epidemiology and public health principles to health care students and practitioners; research on the efficacy of interventions or health services

These competencies show the broad spectrum of public health practice. Public health practitioners are a relatively rare species and the agenda is very large. At present in the UK, a high proportion of the available public health resource is devoted to assessing the effectiveness of health care interventions, commissioning effective and high quality services, and protecting the public from environmental and communicable diseases. In this book we have concentrated on the health improvement, surveillance, strategy, and leadership functions, giving less room to commissioning and health protection, both of which are well covered elsewhere.

Health promotion

The aims of health promotion

Health promotion aims to improve health in the positive, holistic sense enshrined in the WHO definition cited at the beginning of this chapter, and in the discussion of wellbeing on p. 156. Tackling social inequalities in health is another key goal, and this may be oriented more towards disease prevention. These aims are illustrated in the WHO European Region's main areas for action in health promotion: first, to reduce health inequalities between and within countries, and second, to strengthen health as much as to reduce disease. The four principles of 'Health for all in Europe' reflect this agenda:

1 *Ensure equity in health* by reducing the present gap in health status between countries, and between groups within countries.

2 *Add life to years* by ensuring the full development and use of people's integral or residual physical and mental capacity to derive full benefit from and to cope with life in a healthy way.

3 *Add health to life* by reducing disease and disability.

4 *Add years to life* by reducing premature deaths and thereby increasing life expectancy.

Approaches to health promotion

Health promotion aims to work both at the individual and at the community level and there is sometimes a tension between these approaches. Definitions of health promotion have shifted over the years from those that leant more towards the individual to those that leant more towards societal change. Some examples are shown in Table 5.10.

The differences of accentuation implicit in these definitions reflect both different belief systems and also change over time. The individual focus derives from the belief that individuals have control over their health-related behaviour and that societal constraints are less important.

The concept of empowerment is important here. This term was first used by health promotion practitioners who recognized that powerlessness prevented people from acting on health knowledge. Powerlessness can be an individual or a collective phenomenon and has both subjective and objective components. Different individuals in the same situation will differ in the extent to which they are able to change the way they live, but some groups of individuals (an extreme example would be those living in totalitarian societies) have less power than others over their lifestyle. Empowerment describes the process of enabling people to develop a sense of personal power, which is manifested as *agency* (the ability to have an influence on the world), *self-efficacy* (belief in the capacity to exert influence), and personal *autonomy* (the ability to speak and act independently of others). Empowerment has been practised most commonly at community level, for example as a fundamental feature of community development projects. The development of agency, self efficacy and autonomy are also goals of

Table 5.10 Some key definitions of health promotion

Lalonde (1974)
Lalonde, M. A new perspective on the health of Canadians: a working document. Ottawa, Canada Information, 1974.
A **strategy** 'aimed at informing, influencing and assisting both individuals and organisations so that they will accept more responsibility and be more active in matters affecting mental and physical health'

US Department of Health, Education, and Welfare (1979)
Green, L.W. National policy in the promotion of health. *International journey of health education,* **22**: 161–168 (1979).
'A **combination** of health education and related organisational, political and economic programs designed to support changes in behavior and in the environment that will improve health'

Perry and Jessor (1985)
Perry, C.L. & Jessor, R. The concept of health promotion and the prevention of adolescent drug abuse. *Health education quarterly,* **12**(2): 169–184 (1985).
'The implementation of **efforts** to foster improved health and wellbeing in all four domains of health'

WHO (1984, 1986); Epp (1986)
Discussion document on the concept and principles of health promotion. Copenhagen, WHO Regional Office for Europe, 1984 (document).
Ottawa Charter for Health Promotion. *Health promotion,* **1**(4): iii–v (1986).
Epp, J. Achieving health for all: a framework for health promotion. Ottawa, Health and Welfare Canada, 1986.
'The **process** of enabling people to increase control over, and to improve, their health'

Goodstadt *et al.* (1987)
Goodstadt, M.S. et al. Health promotion: a conceptual integration. *American Journal of health promotion,* **1**(3): 58–63 (1987).
'The maintenance and enhancement of existing levels of health through the implementation of **effective programs, services, and policies**'

O'Donnell (1989)
O'Donnell, M.P. Definition of health promotion. Part III. Expanding the definition. *American journal of health promotion,* **3**(3): 5 (1989).
'The **science** and **art** of helping people choose their lifestyles to move toward a state of optimal health'

Labonté and Little (1992)
Labonté, R. and Little, S. *Determinants of health: empowering strategies for nurses.* Vancouver, Registered Nurses Association of British Columbia, 1992.
'Any **activity** or **program** designed to improve social and environmental living conditions such that people's experience of wellbeing is increased'

Source: Adapted From Rootman, I. et al. (ed.) (2001). *Evaluation in health promotion. Principles and perspectives.* WHO Regional Publications, European Series, No. 92, p.10. WHO Office for Europe, Copenhagen, with permission.

many individual psychotherapeutic programmes, because these are key components of mental wellbeing. The 1984 WHO definition (Table 5.10.) encapsulates the idea that individual empowerment is an important 'tool' and is also important in itself for mental and social wellbeing and therefore health, especially when a lack of empowerment means that a person feels powerless to influence the way they live. Labonte's definition, (Table 5.10) on the other hand, recognizes that an individual's capacity to change the way in which he or she lives is constrained by the social and physical fabric of society – they may not merely *feel* powerless, but *be* relatively powerless to effect change.

These different definitions have implications for the way health promotion programmes are conceived and implemented. There are generally thought to be at least three levels at which such programmes may operate:

1 the individual level (e.g. health education and individual empowerment)

2 the social or community level (e.g. social action and community empowerment)

3 the policy level (e.g. lobbying and advocacy directed at healthy public policy)

It is usually more effective to combine action at two or three different levels rather than to focus on one. Each is discussed further in the following sections.

Many health promotion activities and programmes include, or are specifically directed at, children and young people: they may seek to promote health and wellbeing both in the children of the present and for the adults of the future. For example, promoting exercise in young people may both increase their current self-esteem, sporting prowess, and social interactions, and improve their long-term health and life expectancy. A different approach is often needed to ensure that interventions or services are relevant, accessible, and acceptable to the age groups concerned.

The latest international charter for health promotion – the Bangkok Charter (2005) focused almost exclusively on the societal component of health promotion, encouraging those working in all sectors and settings to:

◆ Advocate for health based on human rights and solidarity

◆ Invest in sustainable policies, actions and infrastructure to address the determinants of health

◆ Build capacity for policy development, leadership, health promotion practice, knowledge transfer and research, and health literacy

◆ Regulate and legislate to ensure a high level of protection from harm and enable equal opportunity for health and wellbeing for all people

◆ Partner and build alliances with public, private, non-governmental and international organizations, and civil society to create sustainable actions

Settings are an important concept in health promotion practice. Settings typically include institutions such as schools and workplaces, geographical settings such as communities, and social groups such as the family. The settings approach can be contrasted with the topics approach in which, for example, a public health practitioner might develop a programme to reduce a specific health hazard like smoking. Health-promoting schools are a classic example of the settings approach, in which all aspects of health are considered, but only as far as they are relevant to the setting of the school.

Beattie's model of health promotion, published in 1991, is perhaps the most relevant to health promotion practice today because it is comprehensive (see Fig. 5.22). It covers four areas involving different levels of individual and collective action, and both 'top down' and 'bottom up' approaches: health persuasion, legislative action, personal counselling and community development. It encompasses the creative tension present in public health and health promotion practice between, on the one hand, empowering and supporting individuals to have an impact on their communities and societies and to develop the skills to maintain their own health and wellbeing; and, on the other hand, coercing or manipulating people so that they behave in healthy ways. The belief that 'the end justifies the means' has been prevalent in public health practice in past eras, but in the longer term coercion is often counterproductive. Sometimes it is essential (for example in laying food handlers with gastro-intestinal infections off work until they are recovered, or closing down catering outlets that are a health hazard); sometimes it is highly effective (seat belt and drink-driving legislation); and sometimes it is a step too far (forcing parents to have their children immunized before attending school). Like the subtle manipulation of information which can be present in health campaigns it is, however, always disempowering, giving people the feeling that they are not responsible for their own health and that 'the government will do what is necessary' on their behalf.

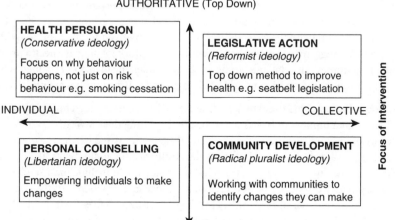

Fig. 5.22 Beattie's model of health promotion.
Source: Reproduced with permission from Beattie, A. (1991) Knowledge and control in health promotion: a test case for social policy and social theory. In J. Gabe, M. Calnan and M. Bury (eds) (1991). The sociology of the health service, London, Routledge.

Health education

According to Ewles and Simnett, health education

> comprises planned interventions or programmes for people to learn about health, and to undertake voluntary changes in their behaviour.

Knowledge about health and its determinants is important for the maintenance of health; ignorance, on the other hand, is disempowering. But as well as providing information, health education has a role in transferring skills and building self esteem. Nutbeam describes the outcome of health education in terms of an improvement in *health literacy*

> cognitive and social skills which determine the motivation and ability of individuals to gain access to, and understand and use information in ways that promote health.

Although it may be delivered at a group, community, or even population level, health education aims to improve the knowledge and skills of individuals, and thus represents the individual end of the health promotion activity spectrum. For example, personal, social and health education (PSHE) in settings such as schools and young offenders institutions has the potential to improve young people's knowledge about the impact of health-related behaviours such as substance misuse or (for a younger age group) road safety.

The relationship between acquisition of knowledge and skills and changes in health-enhancing behaviour is not straightforward, however. Many factors are involved in making decisions about and then achieving behaviour change, and there is wide recognition that didactic teaching is insufficient on its own to alter behaviour. For example, self-awareness and readiness to change are important mediating factors – which are in turn closely related to emotional wellbeing. Various models have been proposed to elucidate the process and the factors involved in effecting individual behaviour change, thus providing a theoretical framework for effective health promotion programmes. They include the health belief model, the theory of reasoned action, social learning theory, and the stages of change model. Brief outlines are given below.

Health belief model (Rosenstock and Becker) This relies on the concept that individuals hold a number of beliefs about health, including their own susceptibility, the severity of the condition being targeted, and the benefits of and barriers to the recommended preventive actions. All these beliefs influence the individual's likelihood of taking action. Cues to action or strategies to activate might include mass media campaigns, advice from health professionals and others, and experience of the condition in a friend or member of the family. Health-promoting activities are framed as influencing these belief systems. You are more likely to act if you think you are likely to get the disease and that it is serious, and if you believe that the benefits of taking action outweigh the costs (time, pain, money, inconvenience).

Theory of reasoned action (Azjen and Fishbein) This model holds that your behaviour depends on your intentions, which in turn depend on your attitude (influenced by beliefs about the consequences of the behaviour and the value that you ascribe to these outcomes) and subjective norms (your feelings about other people's perception of the behaviour and how much you care about this). Health promotion interventions are aimed at altering beliefs about the behaviour or perception of the peer group's views. This model recognizes that individuals rarely act alone and are influenced by norms set by those around them. Perceived behavioural control makes it easier or harder for a particular individual to act on their intentions based on what power or control each choice gives them.

Social learning theory (Rotter) The key concepts in this model are based on an ecological approach: reciprocal determinism (behaviour change results from interaction between the individual and the environment), behavioural capability (knowledge and skills to influence behaviour), expectations (beliefs about likely results of action), and self-efficacy (confidence in ability to take action and persist with it). The main premise is that behavioural change in individuals comes about by change in the social environment.

Stages of change (Prochaska and Di Clemente) This approach is based on understanding that people are at different levels of readiness to take action or change their behaviour at different times in their lives. Health promotion interventions must be appropriate to the stage that the person is at. Five stages are described – precontemplation, contemplation, preparation, action, and maintenance. Health-promoting interventions focus on either the thinking stages (e.g. conciousness raising, environmental re-evaluation e.g. non-smoking areas, self re-evaluation) or the doing stages (e.g. facilitating social support, reinforcement management, building up personal rewards for desirable actions), and have been found to be more effective if they match the stage the individual has reached in terms of altering their behaviour.

Pulling it all together

As the reader may have spotted from this overview of concepts and definitions, public health is full of paradoxes: between the promotion of health and wellbeing and the prevention of disease; between protecting and caring for the sick and vulnerable and enabling and encouraging people to look after themselves; between requiring or coercing people to behave in certain ways and empowering them to take charge of their own lives. Sometimes these paradoxes make uncomfortable bedfellows – statistical concepts and spiritual insights seem hard to reconcile – yet at the same time they are an important source of creative tension, demanding that public health changes and develops to suit current needs and that it is practised with an open mind.

Further reading

Public health

Bradshaw, J. (1990) *Poverty and child health*. National Children's Bureau, London.

Detels, R., Holland, W., McKewan, J., and Omenn, G.S. (ed.) (1997) *Oxford textbook of public health*. Oxford University Press, Oxford.

Donaldson, L.J. and Donaldson, R.J. (2000) *Essential public health*. Petroc Press, Newbury.

MacFarlane, A., Dunkley, R., and Wright, J. (1988) *Child public health training: a European perspective* (*see end of section for details). Public Health Resources Unit, Institute of Health Sciences, Oxford.

Epidemiology

Hill, A.B. (1965) The environment and disease: association or causation? *Proceedings of the Royal Society of Medicine;* **58**: 295–300.

Howick, J., Glasziou, P., and Aronson, J. (2009) The evolution of evidence hierarchies: what can Bradford Hill's guidelines for causation contribute? *Journal of the Royal Society of Medicine;* **102**: 186–194.

Last, J.M. (ed.) (1988) *A dictionary of epidemiology.* Oxford University Press, Oxford.

Mausner, J.S. and Kramer, S. (1985) *Epidemiology – an introductory text.* W.B. Saunders, Philadelphia.

Rose, G. (1992) *The strategy of preventive medicine.* Oxford University Press, Oxford.

Rothman, K.J. (1986) *Modern epidemiology.* Little Brown, Boston.

Health and well-being

Blaxter, M. and Paterson, E. (1982) *Mothers and daughters: a three generational study of health attitutes and behaviour.* Heinemann, London.

Chida, Y. and Steptoes, A. (2008) Positive psychological well-being and mortality: A quantitative review of prospective observational studies. *Psychosomatic Medicine;* **70**: 471–765.

Huppert, F.A. (2000*) Psychological well-being: Evidence regarding its causes and its consequences. Review commissioned by the Government's Foresight Mental Capital and Well-being Project www.foresight.gov.uk

Huppert, F.A., Bayliss, N., and Keverne, B. (2005) *The Science of Wellbeing.* Oxford University Press, Oxford.

Pennington, J. (2002) Feeling happy and healthy, having fun and friends. Thesis submitted for degree of Doctor of Clinical Psychology. British Psychological Society.

Ravens-Sieberer, U. and the Kidscreen Group. (2007) The KIDSCREEN – 27 quality of life measure of children and adolescents: psychometric results from a cross cultural survey in 13 European countries. *Quality of Life Research;* **16**: 1347–1356.

SF-36 Health Status Questionnaire User's Manual (1989) Quality Quest, Mineapolis.

Steptoe, A., Wardle, J., and Marmot, M. (2005) Positive affect and health realted neuro-endocrine cardiovascular and inflammatory processes. *Proceedings of the National Academy of Sciences;* **102**: 65089–12.

Tennant, R., Hiller, L., Fishwick, R., et al. (2007) The Warwick-Edinburgh Mental Well-being Scale (WEMWBS): development and UK validation. *Health and Quality of Life Outcomes;* **5**: 63 doi:10.1186/1477-7525-5-63

Varni, J.W. (1998) *Pediatric quality of life inventory version 4.0* www.pedsql.org/pedsql13.html

Health promotion

Downie, R.S., Tannahill, C., and Tannahill, A. (1996) *Health promotion: models and values.* Oxford University Press, Oxford.

Earp, J.E. and Ennett, S.T. (1991) Conceptual models for health education research and practice. *Health Education Research;* **6**: 163–71.

Naidoo, J. and Wills, J. (1994) *Health promotion: disciplines and diversity.* Routledge, London.

Nutbeam, D. and Harris, E. (1999) *Theory in a nutshell: a guide to health promotion theory.* McGraw-Hill, Sydney.

Ottawa Charter for Health Promotion (1986) World Health Organisation, Geneva.

Prochaska, J.O., DiClemente, C.C., Velicer, W.F., and Rossi, J.S. (1993) Standardised, individualised, interactive and personalised self-help programs for smoking cessation. *Health Psychology*; **12**: 399–405.

Quah, S. (1985) The health belief model and preventive health behaviour in Singapore. *Social Science and Medicine*; **21**: 351–63.

Research Unit for Health and Behavioural Change (1989) *Changing the public health*. John Wiley, Chichester.

Social capital and inequalities

Coleman, J.S. (1990) *The foundations of social theory*. Harvard University Press, Cambridge MA.

Cooper, H., Arber, S., Fee, L., and Ginn, J. (1999) The influence of social support and social capital on health. *A review and analysis of British data. Surrey Institute of Social Research*. Health Education Authority, London.

Earls, F. and Carlson, M. (2001) The social ecology of child health and well-being. *Annual Review of Public Health*; **22**: 143–66.

Helliwell, J. How's Life? Combining Individual and National Variables to Explain Subjective Well-Being. "http://www.nber.org/papers/w9065"NBER Working "papers/w9065.pdf" Paper No. 9065 (Cambridge: National Bureau of Economic Research). July 2002. (subsequently published in "papers/Helliwell-EM2003.pdf"Economic Modelling **20(2)**: 331–60. 2003).

Jarman, B. (1983) Identification of underprivileged areas. *BMJ*; **286**: 1705–9.

Kawachi, I. and Berman, L. (2000) Social cohesion, social capital and health. In *Social epidemiology* (ed. Berkman, L. and Kawachi, I). Oxford University Press, Oxford.

Kawachi, I., Kennedy, B.P., Lochner, K., Prothrow–Stith, D. (1997) Social capital, income inequality and mortality. *American Journal of Public Health*; **879**: 1491–8.

Putnam, R. (2000) *Bowling alone*. Simon and Schuster, New York.

Putnam, R. (1993) *Making democracy work: civic traditions in modern Italy*. Princeton University Press, Princeton.

Rifkin, S. (1990) *Community participation in maternal and child health/family planning programmes*. World Health Organisation, Geneva.

Runyan, D.K., Hunter, W.M., and Amaya Jackson, L. (1998) Children who prosper in unfavorable environments: the relationship to social capital. *Pediatrics*; **101**: 12–18.

Sampson, R., Raudenbush, S., and Earls, F. (1997) Neighborhoods and violent crime: a multilevel study of collective efficacy. *Science*; **277**: 918–24.

Townsend, P., Philmore, P., and Beattie, A. (1998) *Health and deprivation: Inequality and the North*. Routledge, London.

Waterston, T., Alperstein, G., and Stewart Brown, S. (2004) Social capital: a key factor in child health inequalities. *Arch Dis Child*, **89**: 456–459.

Risk

Edwards, A.G.K. and Elwyn, G. (ed.) (2001) *Evidence based patient choice – inevitable or impossible?*, pp. 3–18. Oxford University Press, Oxford.

O'Connor, A., Fiset, V., Rosto, A. et al. (2002) *Decision aids for people facing health treatment or screening decisions. Cochrane Library Issue 1*. Update Software, Oxford.

Screening

Current UK health promotion programme – http://www.health-for-all-children.co.uk

First, second, and third reports of the National Screening Committee. Available at www.nelh.
org/screening

Hall, D. and Elliman, D. (2003) *Health for all children* (4th edition). Oxford University Press,
Oxford.

Chapter 6

Child health and adult health

History revisited

The belief that health in childhood is an important determinant of health in adulthood was widely held a century ago, and the particular vulnerability of infants and fetuses was well recognized. This belief contributed to the development of a number of the public health programmes described in Chapter 4, which aimed to enhance maternal, infant, and child health and welfare. The dramatic improvement in child, and then infant, mortality rates that occurred during the last half of the nineteenth and first half of the twentieth century, together with the more static adult mortality rates (see Chapter 4), fuelled the belief that child health was no longer a problem. The focus of public health interest shifted to the newly emerging 'epidemics' of adult cardiovascular diseases and cancer. Recent research on the early care of infants and the biological underpinning of socio-emotional development, together with the identification of a growing number of childhood risk factors for adult disease, has rekindled the interest of academics and policy makers in the health and care of children. Interventions to improve child health are once again coming to be seen as important to the improvement of public health in general.

Different research paradigms

This recent research draws on the work of the small number of academics from different disciplines who maintained an interest in the links between child and adult health throughout the period when such ideas were not fashionable. They include the biologists and nutritionists interested in growth, development, and in the long term sequelae of infectious diseases; social scientists interested in the impact of poverty and social deprivation across generations; and child psychologists, psychiatrists, and psychotherapists interested in the impact of childhood experience on adult personality and mental health. These groups used different methodologies and focused on different aspects of childhood; each has favoured different explanations for the way in which the factors they identified impact on adult health.

During the last decade, when research into the childhood origins of adult health has blossomed again, various different disciplines have started to work collaboratively on child-adult health links and the boundaries between the different approaches have softened. Now biologists are undertaking research to elucidate the neural, endocrine, and other mechanisms through which early care influences adult health, and the social scientists are incorporating psychosocial variables into their models of child-adult health links, alongside those related to the more traditional variables of poverty, housing and education.

More holistic models are appearing in which a wide variety of modifiable factors are seen to be important both individually and in interaction with each other, as depicted in the Mandala on page 48. Bronfenbrenner's ecological model was an important early prototype. She described the influence of micro (family environment) meso (school environment) exo (digital environment TV/games) and macro (economic environment) systems on human development, together with the way in which these systems are interconnected and also influenced by the individual child. Her model thus included the influence of 'nature' as well as 'nurture' and presaged the work of the research groups now beginning to demonstrate the interplay at a biological level between the modifiable childhood risk factors for adult disease and genetic determinants of health and wellbeing (see chapter 3, p. 47).

The picture is thus becoming increasingly complex, but whilst recognizing the potential for oversimplification, there is merit in starting the story of child-adult health links with a description of the three different research paradigms from which our current understanding has emerged, and the principal concepts and ideas that they have contributed.

Biological programming

The belief that insults to health early in life can have an irreversible impact on health throughout life is well supported by observation, as is the idea that these insults may only matter during critical periods of human development. The impact of rubella infection on the fetus in the first trimester of pregnancy is a good example. This infection, which is relatively innocuous to human health at other times of life, can have a devastating and irreversible effect on the development of the cardiovascular and nervous systems of the fetus. Rubella immunization, first in teenage girls, later in one year olds in the combined MMR vaccine and now in infants, is one of the many public health successes attributable to the biological sciences. It has led to the virtual elimination of disability caused by rubella infection. The studies of Nobel prize winners Hubert and Wiesel, demonstrating that the development of vision is dependent on the stimulus of light rays entering the eye during a critical period in the life of the kitten, is another good example, and one which has also had an important impact on clinical practice in child health. The concept of stimulus and response is now recognized to be fundamental to many aspects of neural development.

These are all examples of what has come to be known as biological programming. Observation of the development of other functions without a clear cut 'critical period' – where there is an optimum time for development but some level of development can take place outside this period – has given rise the concept of 'sensitive periods', sometimes referred to as 'prime times'. The development of speech and language provides an example of a neurological function with a sensitive period in which the stimulus of hearing the spoken word is optimum to the development of language during the preschool period, but in which some function can be developed after this time.

> Biological programming—a biological stimulus (such as an infection or the lack of a key nutrient) at a critical period of development causes a lasting positive or negative effect on health.

Socio-economic effects across the life course

Social scientists have focused on the explanatory paradigm of socio-economic circumstances, demonstrating that poverty and social deprivation in childhood have an impact on the risk of disease, not just in childhood, as we saw in Chapter 3, but throughout life. This group have coined the term 'life course approach'. As well as demonstrating a wide variety of persisting effects of childhood social circumstances on adult health, they have developed theoretical models to help understand childhood effects on adult health. Some of these build on those of the biologists, recognizing that biological programming during a critical or sensitive period may be compounded or minimized by later 'effect modifiers'. The Western child whose language development is impaired by deafness may develop good language because he/she is given hearing aids at an early age, whereas the poor child in the developing world who is not offered aids does not. Country of birth and poverty are 'effect modifiers' in this model.

Two basic models underpin all life course studies of the impact of childhood social circumstances on health in adulthood. In the first, childhood poverty directly predisposes children to certain diseases and health problems, which persist into adult life; long term disability related to accidental injury is a good example of this mechanism. In the second, childhood poverty predisposes children to poverty in their adult lives, which brings risks to adult health and influences adult health without intervening child health problems.

Most studies suggest more complex mechanisms, recognizing the accumulation of risk over the life course. Such risks may be independent of each other, but are more commonly clustered. As we saw in Chapter 3 'risk clustering' is common in families living in poverty, as poverty increases the chances of a wide range of risks to health including poor educational opportunities, road traffic accidents, inadequate diet, and exposure to passive smoke. Many social resources and opportunities are constrained by social stratification, like social class, and by social institutions, creating 'social patterning'.

Risks may also occur in 'chains' or 'pathways' where each exposure increases the risk of a subsequent exposure; for example damp housing increases the risk of glue ear, which increases the risk of poor language development, which increases the risk of educational failure and behaviour problems, all of which reduce the risk of employability in adulthood, which brings with it its own health risks.

Finally, some childhood experiences may be detrimental, not because they have a direct impact on health, but because they reduce the individual's resilience to other negative experiences. Examples of this include schools which undermine rather than enhance children's self esteem, leaving children less able to compete for jobs, and more vulnerable to depression in the face of negative life events like unemployment or marital breakdown.

Together, these childhood risk factors interfere with the development of what has been called 'health capital'— health protective factors such as healthy lifestyles, robust self esteem and educational achievement – leaving individuals vulnerable to a wide range of diseases throughout the course of their lives.

Life course studies show that socio-economic circumstances in childhood, particularly poverty, impact on health in adulthood (a) because these predispose to health problems in childhood which track through into adult life, and (b) because poverty also tracks through into adult life, leaving the adults vulnerable to adult diseases related to poverty and social deprivation.

Many socio-economic risks to health occur in clusters, and others in chains or pathways.

All can reduce health capital and thus resilience to future health risks.

Early care and nurture

Psychologists, psychiatrists, and psychotherapists interested in the development of mental health and social wellbeing have demonstrated that the quality of the relationship between babies and their carers impacts on social and emotional devolopment, skills in interaction with others and the capacity to manage or regulate emotions. In their early studies, they defined relationship quality according to observable infant behaviours and identified different levels of 'attachment' security to 'carers' (almost always mothers). In these studies roughly 70% of infants were identified as securely attached with 30% insecurely attached in different ways. Emotional regulation and positive social and emotional interaction are critical for the development of mental health in the positive sense. They are important for psychological resilience to stressful life events and they influence access to social support in adulthood. The individual without social support is more vulnerable to health problems, as described in Chapter 5, under the heading of 'social capital'. These attributes are also important for cognitive development, because the insecurely attached, poorly regulated child has problems with learning.

Researchers working in this paradigm have shown that children are particularly vulnerable to lack of nurture in the first three years of life. It is now possible to demonstrate anatomical and physiological differences in the brains of children who have not been appropriately nurtured in early life. The brain scans below (Fig. 6.1) illustrate this starkly, showing differences in brain structure as a result of extreme neglect in the early years.

The effects of parenting on development continue into adolescence; an example of a 'sensitive period' in life course terminology.

Fig. 6.1 MRI Brain scans. Source: Reproduced from Perry B. (2002) Childhood Experience and the Expression of Genetic Potential: What childhood neglect tells us about nature and nurture, *Brain and Mind*, 3: 79–100, with permission.

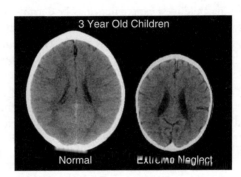

Early care and nurture—the relationship between babies and their carers – has a decisive and long-lasting impact on mental health, relationships, and the ability to learn. The 'sensitive period' for social and emotional development is in the first three years of life. Emotional trauma, lack of sensitive attuned parenting and/or the absence of appropriate stimulation at this time are more likely to have sustained and serious effects, but detrimental relationships later in childhood can also be damaging. Some of these effects can be reversed later in life.

Classic studies

The different paradigms are each associated with classic studies which address different determinants and health outcomes.

Cardiovascular disease and birth weight

A strong and consistent relationship has been demonstrated between birth weight and cardiovascular disease risk in later life (Table 6.1). The original UK based studies were carried out by Barker, who believed that this was an example of biological programming, with nutritional insults to the fetus during pregnancy determining vulnerability to cardiovascular disease in later life. His early studies were based on the archived records of health visitors in Hertfordshire and Sheffield in the early part of the twentieth century, and the linking of birth and early life records to death certificates. Many other studies in the UK, US, Scandinavia, and developing countries have confirmed the association between birth weight and coronary heart disease mortality risk.

Together, these studies show a doubling of risk for babies weighing less than 5.5 lbs compared to those weighing 9.5 lbs, and a dose–response relationship. A body of evidence (not quite as strong as that for coronary heart disease) also links birth weight to stroke in later life. As stroke shares many risk factors with heart disease, this is not altogether surprising.

Table 6.1 Death rates from coronary heart disease among 15,726 men and women according to birth weight

Birth weight in lbs (kg)	Standardized mortality ratio	Deaths (no.)
≤5.5 (2.50)	100	57
Up to 6.5 (2.95)	81	137
Up to 7.5 (3.41)	80	298
Up to 8.5 (3.86)	74	289
Up to 9.5 (4.31)	55	103
≥9.5 (4.31)	65	57
Total	74	941

Source: Reproduced from Osmond, C., Barker, D.J.P., Winter, P.D. et al. (1993) BMJ 307:1519–24, with permission from BMJ Publishing Group Ltd.

Barker's hypothesis that the mechanism is nutritional derives support from animal experiments. These show that under-nutrition *in utero* can lead to persisting changes in blood pressure, cholesterol metabolism, insulin response to glucose, and a range of other metabolic and immune processes known to be important in the development of cardiovascular disease in humans. There have, however, been a number of criticisms of this hypothesis.

Criticisms of the Barker hypothesis

Growth in childhood, as opposed to growth *in utero* or in infancy, has also been shown to be strongly associated with coronary heart disease risk, suggesting that the impact is not confined to a critical period in pregnancy or the first year of life. However, a small number of studies have examined birth weight data, child height data, and final adult height data together, using regression analyses to adjust statistically for the potential confounding effects of adult health-related lifestyles and adult socio-economic status. These studies have shown that the birth weight/cardiovascular disease relationship remains significant, if attenuated, even when all these other factors have been taken into account, thus supporting Barker's belief in the importance of biological programming *in utero*.

Studies supporting the Barker hypothesis have been criticized on the grounds of publication bias—that is, only studies in which a relationship has been found have been written up and submitted for publication. A meta-analysis carried out by Huxley of studies of the relationship between birth weight and blood pressure has demonstrated that larger studies show smaller effects and that some very large studies from other research groups have not been able to corroborate Barker's findings.

While these studies have suggested that the impact of birth weight on cardiovascular disease risk may be smaller than previously supposed, it nonetheless seems likely that there is an epidemiological relationship between the two. The mechanisms involved in this relationship, however, are not well established. Studies set up by the Barker group to identify the specific nutritional deficiencies in pregnancy which might lead to low birth weight and cardiovascular disease risk in humans have failed to produce clear-cut findings. Randomized controlled trials of nutritional supplementation in pregnancy have likewise failed to produce positive findings on birth weight.

Alternative, non-nutritional hypotheses to explain the relationship between birth weight and cardiovascular disease in adulthood suggest that birth weight may be acting as a marker of family socio-economic conditions, and that it is these, rather than the specific nutritional insults, which are responsible for adult disease risk. There is also a possibility that nurture plays an aetiological role in this process. Studies (see, for example, Lou et al., Rahman et al., Bailey et al., Barreau et al., and O'Connor et al.) have suggested that maternal stress and/or depression in pregnancy and early life are linked to low birth weight, poor growth and a number of pathophysiological processes, such as raised cortisol levels and impaired immune and gastrointestinal function, which have the potential to interfere with health in later life. Poverty and social deprivation are potent causes of maternal stress and depression. Alternatively, maternal distress (for example in the form of post-natal depression) interferes with the development of attachment security, emotional regulation, and their sequelae. Maternal distress is therefore a further potential confounding factor between poor socio-economic conditions, fetal and childhood growth, and adult cardiovascular disease. These different mechanisms are of course not mutually exclusive and all three may be acting together.

Summary: birth weight and cardiovascular disease

- ◆ Multiple studies have linked birth weight with later cardiovascular disease risk.
- ◆ These studies were important in rekindling interest in child-adult health links.

Whilst biological programming, in the form of nutritional insults in pregnancy, was proposed as the likely explanation, this now seems unlikely to be the sole mechanism.

Socio-economic circumstances in childhood and adult health

Social scientists have taken advantage of the data gathered in birth cohort studies, which were once unique to the UK, to demonstrate that socio-economic conditions in childhood have an influence on health in adult life through both the main mechanisms outlined on page 187. These studies have been gathered together by Diana Kuh in her now classic book, *A Life Course Approach to Chronic Disease Epidemiology*.

Figure 6.2 illustrates the key pathways through which, research suggests, socio-economic circumstances in childhood affect health in later life.

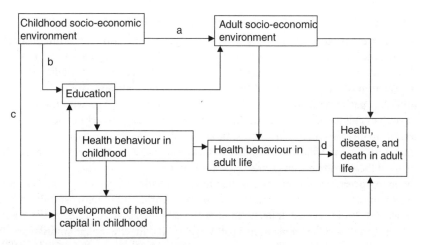

Fig. 6.2 Pathways between childhood and adult health: a simplified framework. Source: Reproduced from Kuh D, Ben-Shlomo Y, *A life course approach to chronic disease epidemiology*. Oxford University Press, 2004, with permission.

Social inequality in childhood tracks through to adulthood

Pathway (a) in Fig. 6.2 illustrates the fact that an adverse social environment in childhood predisposes to an adverse social environment in adulthood. There are a very large number of studies showing that such circumstances in adulthood—poverty, unemployment, and poor work environment in particular—increase the risk of ill health. The 1946 and 1958 birth cohort studies both demonstrate that those born into poor social backgrounds were more likely to be poor themselves in adulthood.

This pathway is illustrated in many studies; for example having an unemployed father at the age of 16 doubles the risk of a man experiencing unemployment in adulthood, and long-term unemployment of the father at age 16 increases the risk five-fold. In this way, cycles of social disadvantage are created, with each generation at increased risk of being exposed to the same detrimental social circumstances as the previous generation.

One of the intervening factors accounting for this social continuity may be educational achievement (pathway b). Family background has an influence on educational attainment, with low socio-economic status predicting educational failure. Educational attainment has an influence on adult income and occupation. Poor educational attainment earlier in school life is also predictive of health outcomes which presage poor health in adulthood – smoking and drug and alcohol misuse. School drop out is strongly associated with substance misuse, unsafe sex, and violence. The chances of a teenager starting to smoke are also influenced directly by family socio-economic circumstances; children are much more likely to start smoking if their parents smoke, and parental smoking is much more common in lower social groups. All these effects, of course, track through into adulthood (pathway d) creating adult health risks. Qualifications on leaving school can be shown to predict adult mortality, blood pressure, and self-rated health.

Poor health in childhood tracks through to adulthood

Studies have tried to unravel the separate effects of education, and other aspects of social deprivation in childhood, on health in adulthood. They have failed to show that educational under-achievement can account for the full effect of childhood social deprivation on adult health and this means that other pathways are involved. The other key pathway identified in these studies is that which starts with the effect of poverty in childhood on child health, and the development (or lack) of health capital leading to increased prevalence of disease and disability in adulthood (pathway c). The numerous ways in which poverty affects child health were reviewed in Chapter 3, and many of these health effects clearly track through into adulthood. The diets of children living in poverty are less nutritious than those of children from other social groups, increasing the risk of obesity in the developed world and of short stature in the developing world. The adult health impact of disability related to accidental injury in childhood is a good example of this pathway, leading directly though to disability in adulthood.

Child health also has an effect on socio-economic outcomes in adulthood. Congenital disability and infectious diseases are both more common among children in families living with poverty, and both, partly through their impact on schooling, increase the chance of adult unemployment. Growth at all stages of childhood is associated with socio-economic position, with children from more affluent backgrounds being taller. Childhood height predicts adult height, and adult height is an important predictor of social position. Men who are tall have a greater chance of upward social mobility. For women, it is the influence of low socio-economic status on obesity that has a greater influence. Obese women have a reduced chance of marrying up the social scale and thus increasing their life chances, and obesity itself is an important risk factor for disease.

Relative influence of social inequality in childhood and adulthood

This wide range of studies together provide unequivocal evidence that socio-economic factors operating in childhood have an influence on health in adulthood. However, they also give rise to questions, important in determining strategies for prevention, as to whether it is the experience of adverse social circumstances in adulthood or childhood that matter most. Studies which have tried to tease this out have demonstrated an independent impact of both, suggesting an ongoing vulnerability attributable to poor social circumstances in childhood, coupled with increased risks attributable to exposure in adulthood. Those living in poor socio-economic circumstances throughout life have the poorest health, at least as measured by coronary heart disease risk.

Summary: socio-economic circumstances

- There is robust evidence to show that socio-economic circumstances in childhood have an effect on health in adulthood.

- Children brought up in poverty accumulate health and social risks, and those living in poor socio-economic circumstances throughout life have the poorest health in adulthood.

Attachment, parenting, and family relationships

Contributions to the literature showing that early care and nurture have an impact on health in adulthood have been made from several different academic groups. One group with a psychotherapeutic orientation takes its lead from John Bowlby, who developed attachment theory. He studied children in care, documenting the progression to profoundly disturbed mental health and interpersonal relationships in adulthood of those who were deprived of a caring relationship with an adult during the early period of their lives. Bowlby's research was seized on in the post-war period by policy makers concerned about unemployment amongst men being decommissioned from the armed forces. They used his findings to make the case that mothers should stay at home to care for their children rather than participating in the labour force, thus freeing up jobs for ex-soldiers.

This distortion of Bowlby's recommendations brought his theories into disrepute. In spite of this, his writings have had an enduring impact on paediatric practice, leading to changes in hospital policies which formerly separated children from their parents. They have also influenced child psychiatrists, who, during the last fifty years, have continued to research the importance for mental health and relationships of the parent–child relationship, and the phenomenon of attachment or bonding of mother and baby.

Donald Winnicott and many others have built on and developed Bowlby's work, making careful observations of mother–infant relationships, following children up over time and demonstrating the ways in which attachment is important for normal human development. They have shown that children who develop mental health problems and difficulties with peer relationships as a consequence of not experiencing attuned, sensitive parenting in infancy are at high risk of growing up to be adults with mental illness, personality disorder, drug and alcohol misuse, and problems with relationships. Up to half of all babies can be shown in some recent studies to have less than optimal attachment patterns.

Psychologists such as Paterson, Baumrind, and others have made a different but important contribution to this field, demonstrating that the quality of parenting (including warmth, supervision, and positive discipline) remains important throughout childhood. They have focused respectively on the outcomes of antisocial behaviour and educational achievement. Family conflict and domestic violence also interfere with normal emotional and social development, as described in Chapter 3. The long-term impact of child abuse, particularly sexual abuse, on mental health has been most studied in women, where it has been shown to be an important risk factor for depression and drug misuse in adulthood. The development of post-traumatic stress disorder in childhood as a consequence of abuse represents one possible biological mechanism.

As described in Chapter 3, studies have shown, both with regard to the outcome of antisocial behaviour and with regard to abuse and depression, that parenting interacts with genetic endowment, making more impact on children with particular genotypes. Collectively, studies in this field show that adverse parenting, both very early in life and throughout early and mid childhood, increases the risk of:

- criminality and imprisonment
- delinquency, violence, and antisocial behaviour
- depression and anxiety
- drug and alcohol misuse
- forming destructive relationships and experiencing marital breakdown.

Figure 6.3 illustrates the risk of one of these psychosocial effects in the context of the socio-economic factors outlined in the previous section. The data come from a Swedish panel study with long term follow up. They show that three important childhood socio-economic factors—poverty, large family size, and family breakdown—all independently increase the odds of mental health problems in adulthood, after taking age, sex, and adult social class into account. But they also suggest that family conflict is a more important predictor of adult mental health than any of these three socio-economic indicators. This study also illustrates the impact of childhood psychosocial factors on physical health in adulthood, as discussed below.

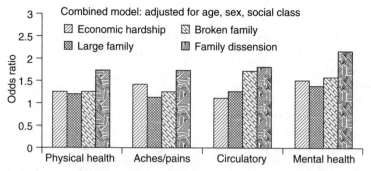
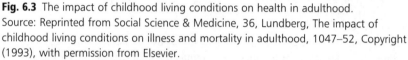

Fig. 6.3 The impact of childhood living conditions on health in adulthood.
Source: Reprinted from Social Science & Medicine, 36, Lundberg, The impact of childhood living conditions on illness and mortality in adulthood, 1047–52, Copyright (1993), with permission from Elsevier.

By increasing the number of children who develop antisocial behaviour, criminal activity and violent relationships, poor early care and nurture has an additional diffuse effect on adult health, reducing the level of 'social capital' of communities in which these children end up living. One of the features of communities with high social capital is that they show norms of social trust, a commodity that is scarce in places with high crime rates. As we have seen in Chapter 5, social capital is an important determinant of adult health. Through this link, therefore, poor parenting experienced by some children can have important detrimental effects, when both reach adulthood, on the health of other children.

Summary: attachment, parenting, and family relationships

♦ The social and emotional development of children is dependent on the care they receive in childhood.

♦ Those whose parents are not sensitive to their needs are at increased risk of mental illness, personality disorder, drug and alchohol misuse and problems with relationships.

♦ Lack of supervision, neglect, and negative approaches to discipline predispose children to antisocial behaviour.

Broadening the research base: other child-adult health effects

These classic studies from the different disciplines have been built on by others, some of whom have worked in a more interdisciplinary way, broadening our knowledge of child-adult health links and increasing our understanding of possible mechanisms. They have increased the range of diseases and health problems now recognized to have, at least in part, a childhood origin.

Respiratory disease

Respiratory diseases are caused by a complex interaction of infection, allergy, mucous secretion, and airways obstruction. Pollutants such as tobacco smoke also play an important role.

Historical cohort studies have provided evidence to link both infection and allergy development in childhood to respiratory health in adulthood. For example, there is growing, but incomplete, evidence that allergic sensitization (atopy), which is important in the development and prognosis of asthma, may be influenced by events during critical periods in infancy. This hypothesis centres on the belief that early exposure to infectious agents *protects* against the development of atopy. There may be a switching to alternative immunological pathways which is triggered by *non-exposure* to infectious agents.

The hypothesis is supported by the observation that children from large families and those from less affluent families are at reduced risk of developing atopic diseases such as hay fever and eczema. The evidence is less clear when it comes to determining the length and stage of the critical period, if indeed such a mechanism does exist.

Whilst exposure to infectious agents in general early in childhood has been proposed to be protective against some chest disease, chest infections in childhood have been shown to increase the risk of productive cough, wheeze, and impaired ventilatory function in adulthood. This relationship does not seem to be confined, as was first suggested, to a particular period of childhood, in the way that would be expected if biological programming was operating.

The detrimental impact on the respiratory system of exposure to tobacco smoke seems to operate throughout childhood, starting with the impact of exposure to 'passive smoke' *in utero*. This increases the risk of chest infection in childhood. Passive smoking in childhood also increases the risk of chest infections and plays a role in the aetiology of childhood asthma. Through the link between childhood chest infection and adult respiratory disease, this exposure has an influence on health in adulthood. As yet, the evidence suggesting that respiratory health in adulthood may be programmed by infections or other exposure in infancy is circumstantial and does not propose any obvious interventions. In contrast, the evidence suggesting that the inhalation of tobacco smoke at any time in pregnancy and childhood leads to respiratory problems in both childhood and adulthood is strong, and has much clearer implications for intervention.

Food allergies

Early exposure to microbes also plays a part in the development of food allergies, which are much less common amongst children born into disadvantaged conditions and in rural areas. Food allergies occur because of breakdown of immunological tolerance and their prevalence has increased dramatically in the past two decades. Allergies to cow's milk, soy, egg, wheat, and peanuts are the most common, and both acute and chronic reactions affecting the skin, respiratory and gastrointestinal systems occur. Colonization of the gut immediately after birth had been shown to be different in allergic and non-allergic infants, and colonization is now recognized to play a key role in allergy development. Colonization is likely to be affected by the use of broad spectrum antibiotics in the neonatal period.

Whilst most of the studies on food allergy relate to children, it is clear that some of these effects track through into adult life. Animal studies also identify intriguing links with other pathophysiological processes, including those involved in stress. Microbial colonization of the gut in infancy has been show to affect the physiological response to stress in rats, and maternal deprivation early in life promotes long term alterations in colonization and the functioning of the colonic epithelial barrier. (see Sudo, Barreau, and Bailey, for example)

Obesity, diabetes, hypertension

Obesity is an increasingly important determinant of health, and the new epidemic of childhood obesity is attracting widespread attention partly because of the implications for adult health. Whilst the relationship is not uncomplicated, childhood obesity does increase the risk of adult obesity and also of type 2 diabetes and the insulin resistance syndrome.

Links with birth weight are also complex. Higher birth weight is predictive of adult obesity, a relationship which is partly confounded by maternal obesity (as measured by Body Mass Index). Low birth weight, on the other hand, is predictive of central adiposity, which is an independent risk factor for cardiovascular disease. Low birth weight also increases the risk of type 2 diabetes, hypertension, and the insulin resistance syndrome independently of obesity. The relationship between birth weight and blood pressure is held to be particularly strong.

Both bottle feeding and over-controlling parenting also increase the chances of obesity in childhood and later life.

Ageing

A range of animal models suggest that food restriction in early life leads to premature ageing, and both intrauterine and infant growth have been linked to a number of physiological processes associated with premature ageing, including muscular strength, bone mass, and osteoarthritis. Obesity in adulthood is a potential confounder of this relationship, but most studies have shown an independent effect of growth in utero and early childhood.

Cognitive development

Preterm delivery increases the chance of poor cognitive development. Early nutritional intervention in preterm babies, using breast milk as opposed to artificial alternatives, results in significant improvements in the cognitive development of such children at eight years. The fact that the relationship between preterm delivery and cognitive development can be reversed by breast milk provides evidence that nutritional inadequacy very early in life can influence mental performance in later years. Longer term follow-up studies will be needed to demonstrate that this effect is carried

through to adulthood, but there are many studies showing that educational performance at eight years predicts educational achievement in late adolescence, and that this
in turn predicts employment prospects in adulthood.

Physical health in general

A series of intriguing studies have begun to show links between early care and family
relationships, and a wide range of physical health problems in later life. One such study
has already been referred to above (Fig. 6.3); another involved Harvard University
students in the USA in the 1950's. Those who did not feel close to and respect their
parents were shown to be at greatly increased risk of poor health, including heart
disease and musculoskeletal disease 40 years later (Fig. 6.4).

Data from the British birth cohort studies also shows physical health effects relating
to parent-child relationships (see Stewart-Brown). The results of very long term studies such as these are impressive but relatively rare. They are often subject to methodological problems because of the expense and logistics of conducting cohort studies.
A much larger number of studies with fewer methodological problems confirm that a
short term relationship exists: poor quality parent-child relationships and adverse
parenting increase the risk of a wide range of physical health problems in childhood.
(see Repetti, Waylen, Belsky, Bell)

These intriguing studies beg questions about possible mechanisms, and a number
of these have been proposed, some operating through socio-economic influences,
some psychological and some biological. For example, as described above, adverse
parenting increases the chance of educational failure, increasing the chance of poverty
and unhealthy lifestyles in adulthood with their attendant health risks. Adverse parenting is also a cause of impaired social and emotional functioning, reducing access to

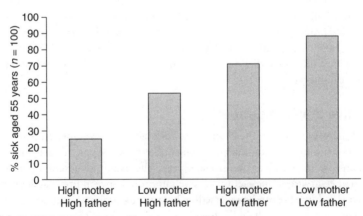

Fig. 6.4 Parental caring and health status in midlife.
Source: Reproduced from Russek and Schwartz (1997). *Psychosomatic Medicine*; 59:
144–9, with permission.

social support in adulthood, which protects against health problems like cardiovascular diseases. These two mechanisms relate more to long term health effects, whereas the third proposed mechanism potentially explains both long and short term effects. The latter relates to the neuro-humoral effects of adverse parenting as outlined in the next two sections.

> Life course studies now show at least a partial childhood origin for respiratory disease, obesity, diabctes, hypertension, food allergies, cognitive development, ageing, and 'physical' health problems more generally.

The development of the emotional brain

Recent developments in brain imaging—functional magnetic resonance imaging (MRI), positron emission topography, and non-invasive electro-encephalographic (EEG) recording—have enabled neuroscientists to study brain development in the human infant. These techniques, together with animal studies, have revolutionised our understanding of brain development. Brain growth is at is its peak in the first three years of life, but is dependent on optimum environmental conditions. At three years of age, the infant brain has twice the number of synapses of the adult brain. Subsequent brain development is use-dependent. Pathways that are well used become protected, whereas those that are not used are pruned. Rats raised in enriched environments have 25% more synaptic connections as adults than those raised in sparse environments. The growth of the brain and the pattern of neural pathways that develops in childhood is thus hugely dependent on experience. Many functions are termed 'experience expectant'; that is, in the absence of experience they do not develop at all.

Studies in animals and in humans show that pathways relating to social and emotional functioning are critically dependent on nurturing care in the very early years. The prefrontal cortex, hippocampus and amygdala are poorly developed in babies who have not received such care. Observation of the behaviour of animals who have been deprived of sensitive nurturing care in early life and of infants who have lived in fear of abandonment, humiliation, or physical attack suggest that they are 'hard wired' in later life to anticipate threatening relationships with others. The dominance of such pathways puts people at risk of mental illness, makes learning difficult and creates the expectation that relationships with others will be harmful. In contrast, infants who have received nurturing care are more likely to anticipate supportive, encouraging relationships and to behave accordingly.

Studies on different aspects of brain development—cognitive, sensory, and emotional—suggest that, whilst there are no critical periods, there are sensitive periods for optimal development. For example, the optimal time for language development is in the preschool period. They also suggest that brain development is remarkably plastic and that it is possible for functions which have not developed at the sensitive period to develop later. It is, however, more difficult for them to do so, and optimum conditions are required. The sensitive period for the development of the parts of the brain involved in emotion appears to be the first three years of life. The potential for neural development or learning to continue throughout life, and the ability of one part of the brain to support deficient functioning in another (neural plasticity), means that some damaging neural pathways developed during childhood can be reversed later in life. Long-term follow-up studies of damaged children suggest, however, that in the absence of intervention this does not normally happen, and that children who grow up with parents who cannot provide supportive care are at increased risk of problems in a wide range of aspects of adult functioning. These include memory, interpersonal relationships and the management of stress. One of the key skills which is poorly developed in these children is the capacity to self-soothe. This trait seems to be learnt from parental soothing of the infant and child. In adulthood, inability to self-soothe results in poor emotional regulation.

> Recent developments in neuroscience have revolutionized our understanding of the development of the brain and shown the vital role that early nurture and care play in this process.

Neurohumoral mechanisms

Sensitive attuned care also appears to be necessary for the development of a normal hypothalamic–pituitary response to stress. This finding has been critically important in understanding child-adult health links because it provides a conceptual mechanism through which the somewhat 'soft' subjective risk factors like adverse parenting, family stress, conflict, and abuse could have a wide ranging influence on adult health (Fig. 6.5).

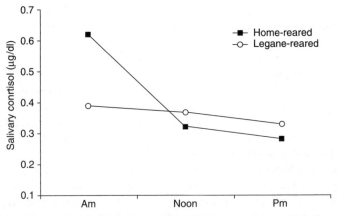

Fig. 6.5 Loss of normal circadian salivary cortisol measurements in chronically stressed children in Romanian orphanages (Leganes).
Source: Reproduced from Carlson, M. and Farls, F. (1997). Psychological and neuroendocrinological sequelae of early social deprivation in institutionalised children in Romania. *Annals of New York Academy of Sciences*; 807: 419–28.

It now seems clear that babies receiving warm nurturing care are less inclined to respond to stress by producing cortisol, and they can more rapidly and efficiently turn off this response. In children who are not so fortunate, each stressful life event results in greater cortisol concentrations, for longer periods. These individuals are described as suffering a high allostatic load. Cortisol interferes with the optimum functioning of many physiological processes including the immune response, cardiovascular functioning and the development of healthy bones and joints. Over time, increased levels of circulating cortisol take their toll on many aspects of physical and mental health. High corticotrophin releasing hormone (CRH) levels are associated with increased neuronal cell death, and this may be of particular significance in the young and rapidly developing infant brain. Children with chronically high levels of cortisol are more likely to show developmental delay. Studies of children in Romanian orphanages and others who have been subjected to chronic stress and maltreatment have shown blunting of the normal cortisol biorhythm. This early 'resetting' of the hypothalamic–pituitary–adrenal system represents a possible mechanism through which chronic hypocortisolism of adulthood develops. The latter has been linked to increased risk of psychological and physical morbidity.

> Nurturing care appears necessary for a normal hypothalamic–pituitary response to stress. The resetting of this response in children who live with chronic stress represents a possible mechanism for deleterious effects on physical and mental health.

Bringing it all together

The evidence base in support of the early care and nurture school of thought is strong and diverse, including both epidemiological and intervention studies published over a long time span. It is interesting, therefore, to consider why this school has, until recently, had such a minor influence on clinical, public health, academic, and political thinking. One of the problems may be that understanding of the mechanisms which underpin this theory has depended on a knowledge of the psychology and psychotherapy literature with which few clinicians, public health practitioners, epidemiologists, or policy makers are familiar. The studies of the psychoneuroimmunologists and developmental neuroscientists are important in this respect, demonstrating the biological mechanisms that underpin the conclusions psychologists and psychotherapists have drawn from their observational studies.

Combining the knowledge bases of all three approaches, and putting in place interventions and social policy which take account of all three, could have an important effect on public health. Many of the interventions which could reduce the burden of adult health attributable to childhood influences are also indicated for other reasons, and many are already evident in public policy. These include interventions to reduce childhood obesity, smoking, and teenage pregnancy (see chapter 8 for further details). A range of interventions have been developed to promote maternal sensitivity and attunement, and to increase parents' confidence and parenting skills. These are described in more detail in Chapters 3 and 8. These interventions are effective in improving emotional and social development and peer interaction, and in reducing delinquency and violence in later life. Many are now being implemented in the UK, Europe, USA, and Australia. In the UK, the health sector is systematically trialling interventions to improve very early relationships through nurse-led home visiting, and the education sector is providing support for parenting in families with children of school age. Support for parenting is a key initiative of the new Children's Centres (see chapter 4) serving 0–4 year olds.

The prevention and elimination of childhood poverty is an important strand of public policy in Scandinavian countries and an aspiration in others, including the UK. Effective anti-poverty strategies include the provision of high quality day care from child minders, and nursery education for older pre-schoolers. They offer children stimulating experiences and, if of high quality, also compensate for unhelpful parenting. Sadly, little available day care provision in this country is of high quality, and there are now significant doubts that institutional daycare can be expected to provide the attachment relationships babies need. There have been studies in the US showing long term positive effects from very high quality day care, usually coupled with parenting support in disadvantaged children, and some studies suggest that they can deliver improvement in the health of parents as well as that of their children. The development of social policy which makes the job of parenting easier and abolishes the stresses created by parenting in poverty would have an important effect on child and adult health.

Although life course studies have pointed to the potential importance of early life nutrition, they have failed to deliver convincing evidence relating to specific nutrients. Whilst it seems intrinsically likely that good nutrition for pregnant women, infants, and children will have a beneficial impact on children's development, the policy implications of research findings are not clear. Research in this area continues and the impact of some specific deficiencies – for example Vitamin D – are becoming clearer.

Further reading

(See also Chapters 1,3,7 and 8 for further reading on issues mentioned here but covered in more detail in these chapters.)

Anisman, H., Zaharia, M.D., Meaney, M.J., and Merali, Z. (1998) Do early-life events permanently alter behavioral and hormonal responses to stressors? *International Journal of Developmental Neuroscience*; **16**(3/4): 149–64.

Bailey, M.T., Lubaj, G.R., and Coe, C.L. (2004) Prenatal stress alters bacterial colonization of the gut in infant monkeys. *Journal of Padiatric Gastroenterology and Nutrition*; **38**: 414–421.

Barker, D.J.P. (1998) *Mothers, babies and health in later life*. Churchill Livingstone, Edinburgh.

Barreau, F., Ferrier, L., Fioramonti, J., et al. (2004) Neonatal maternal deprivation triggers long term alternations in colonic epithelial barrier and mucosal immunity in rats. *Gut*; **53**: 501–506.

Baumrind, D. (1991) Parenting styles and adolescent development. In *The encyclopaedia on adolescence* (R. Learner, A.C. Peteresen, J. Brooks-Gunn, eds.), pp. 746–58. Garland, New York.

Belsky, J., Bell, B., Bradley, R., and Stewart-Brown, S. (2007) Socio-economic risk, parenting during the preschool years and child health age 6 years. *European Journal of Public Health*; **17**: 508–13.

Bell, B. and Blesky, J. (2008) Parenting and children's cardiovascular functioning. *Child Care health and Development*; **34**: 191–203.

Bowlby, J. (1957) *Childcare and the growth of love*. Pelican Books, Middlesex. (Also Penguin, 1980).

Boyce, W.T. and Keating, D.P. (2004) Should we intervene to improve childhood socio-economic circumstances? In Kuh, D. and Ben-Schlomo, Y. *A Life Course Approach to Chronic Disease Epidemiology*. Oxford University Press, Oxford.

British Medical Association (1999) (1) Emotional and behavioural problems. (2) Fetal origins of adult diseases. (3) Inequalities in child health. In *Growing up in Britain: ensuring a healthy future for our children. A study of 0–5 year olds*. British Medical Association, London.

Bronfenbrenner, U. (1979) *The ecology of human development*. Harvard University Press, Cambridge Mass.

Caspi, A., McClay, J., Moffitt, T.E., Mill, J., et al. (2002) Role of genotype in the cycle of ciolene in maltreated children. *Science*; **297**: 851–854.

Committee on Integrating the Science of Early Childhood Development (2000) (1) Nurturing Relationships. (2) Inequalities in child health. In *From neurons to neighborhoods: the science of early childhood development*. National Academy Press, Washington, DC.

Forouhi, N., Hall, E., McKeigue, P., and Gillman, M.W. (2004) A life course approach to diabetes. In *A Life Course Approach to Chronic Disease Epidemiology* (eds. Kuh, D. and Ben-Schlomo, Y.) Oxford University Press, Oxford.

Gerhardt, S. (2004) *Why Love Matters: How affection shapes a baby's brain*. Brunner Routledge, London.

Gillman, M.W. (2004) A life course approach to obesity. In *A life Course Approach to Chronic Disease Epidemiology* (eds. Kuh, D. Ben-Schlomo, Y.) Oxford University Press, Oxford.

Gunnar, M.R. (1996) *Quality of care and buffering of stress physiology. Its potential in protecting the developing human brain*. University of Minnesota Institute of Child Development.

Heim, C., Ehlert, U., and Hellhammer, D.H. (2000) The potential role of hypocortisolism in the pathophysiology of stress-related bodily disorders. *Psychoneuro-endocrinology*; **25**: 1–35.

Hollick, M. (2007) Vitamin D deficiency. *New England Journal of Medicine*; **357**: 266–81.

Huxley, R., Neil, A., and Collins, R. (2002) Unravelling the 'fetal origins' hypothesis: is there really an inverse association between birth weight and blood pressure? *Lancet*; **360**: 659–65.

Kuh, D., Ben-Schlomo, Y. (2004) Introduction. In *A Life Course Approach to Chronic Disease Epidemiology* 2nd edition (ed. Kuh, D. and Ben-Schlomo, Y.) Oxford University Press, Oxford.

Kuh, D., Power, C., Blane, D., and Bartley, M. (2004) Social pathways between childhood and adult health. In *A Life Course Approach to Chronic Disease Epidemiology* 2nd edition (ed. Kuh, D. and Ben-Schlomo, Y.) Oxford University Press, Oxford.

Ladd, C.O., Owens, M.J., and Nemeroff, C.B. (1996) Persistent changes in corticotropin-releasing factor neuronal systems induced by maternal deprivation. *Endocrinology*; **137**: 1212–18.

Leucken, L.J., and Lemery, K.S. (2004) Early care giving and physiological response to stress. *Clinical Psychology Review*; **24**: 171–191.

Lou, H.C., Hansen, D., Nordentoft, M., et al. (1994) Prenatal stressors of human life affect fetal brain development. *Developmental Medicine and Child Neurology*; **6**: 826–32.

Lucas, A., Morley, R., Cole, T.J., Lister, G., and Leeson–Payne, C. (1992) Breast milk and subsequent intelligence quotient in children born preterm. *Lancet*; **339**: 261–4.

Murch, S. (2000) The immunologic basis for intestinal food allergy. *Current opinion in gastroenterology*; **16**: 552–557.

O'Connor, T.G., Ben-Schlomo,Y., Heron, J, Golding, J., Adams, D., and Glover, V. (2005) Prenatal anxiety predicts individual difference in cortisol in pre-adolescent children. *Biological Psychiatry;* **58**: 211–217.

Patterson, G.R. (1989) A developmental perspective on antisocial behaviour. *American Psychologist*; **44**: 329–35.

Perry, B.D. (1994) Neurobiological sequelae of childhood trauma: PTSD in children. In *Catecholamine function in PTSD* (ed. Murberg, M.) American Psychiatric Press, Washington DC.

Perry, I.J. and Luney, L.H. (2004) Fetal growth and development: the role of nutrition and other factors. In *A Life Course Approach to Chronic Disease Epidemiology* 2nd edition (ed. Kuh, D. and Ben-Schlomo, Y.) Oxford University Press, Oxford.

Plotsky, P.M. and Meaney, M.J. (1993) Early postnatal experience alters hypothalamic corticotropin-releasing factor (CRF) mRNA, median eminence CRF content and stress-induced release in adult rats. *Molecular Brain Research*; **18**: 195–200.

Rahman, A., Iqbal, Z., Bunn, J., Lovel, H., and Harington, R. (2004) Impact of maternal depression on infant nutritional status and illness. *Archives of General Psychology*; **61**: 946–952.

Repetti, R.I., Taylor, S.E., Seeman, T.E. (2002) Risky Families: Family Social Environment and mental and physical health of offspring. *Psychological Review*; **128**: 330–336.

Sayer, A.A., Cooper, C. (2004) A life course approach to biological aging. In *A Life Course Approach to Chronic Disease Epidemiology* 2nd edition (ed. Kuh, D. and Ben-Schlomo, Y.) Oxford University Press, Oxford.

Sroufe, A. (1996) *Emotional development*. Cambridge University Press, New York.

Stewart-Brown, S.L., Fletcher, L., Wadsworth M.E.J. (2005) Parent child relationships and health problems in adulthood in three national birth cohort studies. *European Journal of Public Health*; **15**: 640–6.

Stewart-Brown, S., and Shaw, R. (2004) The roots of social capital: relationships in the home during childhood and health in later life. In *Social Capital for Health: issues of definition, measurement and links to health.* (eds Morgan, A., Swann, C), Health Development Agency, London http://www.nice.org.uk/nicemedia/documents/socialcapital_issues.pdf

Strachan, D.P., and Sheikh, A. (2004) A life course approach to respiratory and allergic disease. In *A Life Course Approach to Chronic Disease Epidemiology* 2nd edition (ed. Kuh, D. and Ben-Schlomo, Y.) Oxford University Press, Oxford.

Suomi, S.J. (1997) Early determinants of behaviour: evidence from primate studies. *British Medical Bulletin*; **53**: 170–84.

Sudi, N.M., Chida, Y., Aida, Y., et al. (2004) Postnatal microbial colonisation programs: the hypothalamic-pituitary-adrenal system for stress response in mice. *The Journal of Physiology;* **558**: 263–275.

Waylen, A., Stallard, N., and Stewart Brown, S. (2008) Parenting and social inequalities in health in mid-childhood: a longitudinal study. *European Journal of Public Health*; **18**(3): 300–305; doi:10.1093/eurpub/ckm131

Weich, S., Patterson, J., Shaw, R., Stewart-Brown, S. (2009) Family Relationships in Childhood and Common Psychiatric Disorders in Later Life: Systematic Review of Prospective Studies. *British Journal of Psychiatry;* **194**: 392–398.

Whincup, P.H., Cook, D.G., Geleijnse, M. (2004) A life course approach to blood pressure. In *A Life Course Approach to Chronic Disease Epidemiology.* 2nd edition (ed. Kuh, D. and Ben-Schlomo, Y.) Oxford University Press, Oxford.

Winnicot, D.W. (1965) *The family and individual development.* Tavistock Publications: London.

Chapter 7

Techniques and resources for child public health practice

The practice of public health involves a focus on populations rather than individuals. The size and type of population can vary enormously: public health professionals can and do operate at international, national, regional, district, and local community level, with homogeneous and heterogeneous populations whose health, lives, and socio-economic circumstances span a wide range. There are clearly practical differences between projects focused at national and local level, and between work in countries with very different infrastructure and health problems, but the principles of public health practice are similar whatever the size and nature of the population, and certain tools and techniques are fundamental to everyone working in the field. Although much of this book assumes a focus at the level of a primary care organization in a developed country such as the UK, the approaches described can be generalized to any setting.

Public health involves a focus on populations rather than individuals, but—just as in clinical practice—the first step is to identify the problems to be addressed by defining and assessing health needs.

This chapter describes some of the tools used in child public health practice which enable a community diagnosis (also known as a health needs assessment) to be formulated.

Community diagnosis and needs assessment

The term community diagnosis is used for the process of assessing health needs within a community. To make a community diagnosis is to identify the problems, needs, and resources of a community in order to develop appropriate solutions to these problems. Community diagnosis should include both priorities identified by professionals via epidemiological methods, and locally determined (psychosociological) priorities. These are not necessarily the same. For example, professionals might identify smoking, alcohol abuse, and poor diet as the basis for a community's health problems, while local families might identify poor housing, safety concerns, lack of play space or child care, and inadequate local shops as the main health issues for them. (See Chapter 8 for a fuller discussion.)

The diagnostic process has many parallels in clinical and public health practice. The triad of history taking, physical examination, and investigations make up the cornerstone of clinical activity in response to a patient presenting with a 'problem'. In making a 'community diagnosis', we are applying similar processes of listening to the population, observing the population, and carrying out special investigations with a view to better understanding of the issues or problems presented (see Table 7.1).

The analogy can be taken further. At both the individual and the population level, there are frequently multiple, often inter-related problems to be found rather than a single diagnosis, and the clinician or public health professional may need to prioritize in deciding which are important, and which to tackle first. The views of the patient/population are vital in reaching such a decision, and imposing the paternalistic judgement of a professional about 'what needs treating' may be inappropriate in both cases. Perhaps most importantly, the purpose of making a diagnosis in either situation is to move on to action, with a view to resolving or alleviating the problem which has been presented, and the patient or population should wherever possible be an equal partner in that process.

> In public health practice, as in clinical practice, there are often several problems rather than a single diagnosis. Public health professionals, in conjunction with other professionals and local communities, need to decide which are priorities for action.

Some types of 'therapeutic activity' which are undertaken by public health practitioners have already been touched on in earlier chapters (for example, health promotion, disease prevention and screening) others (community development and advocacy) are discussed later in this chapter, and yet others (the development and implementation of health policy and strategies) will be explored in the final chapter. These are often less clear-cut than the clinical equivalents of treatment by medication, surgical intervention, or reassurance, and they invariably involve more players even than the modern multidisciplinary clinical team. However, there are still many similarities. At both the individual patient and community level trust, mutual respect, and fairness are crucial, together with a focus on producing a solution to the presenting 'problem'.

Table 7.1 Clinical and community diagnosis

	Clinical diagnosis	**Community diagnosis**
History	Symptoms, concerns, systems review, family and social, medications, allergy, etc	Concerns of local people and professionals Press reports of health issues Rapid appraisal needs assessment
Examination	Looking, feeling, listening	Examination of local and national statistics, local government reports, annual report of the director of public health, condition-based registers
Investigation	X-rays, blood tests, case conference	Surveys, case control or cross-sectional studies, geographical mapping

Finally, just as a good clinician will follow up his or her patient to assess the outcome of their treatment and the success of the therapeutic encounter as a whole—and to identify early the development of further complications or new problems—so the public health practitioner should always evaluate the outcome of any public health intervention or programme, and continue to reassess the situation to ensure that improvements have been maintained and any input continues to be appropriate and useful. The audit cycle is relevant to both situations, as are the principles of clinical governance and professional responsibility for the quality of the service provided.

One of the public health 'interventions' which may follow health needs assessment is the development or reconfiguration of local health (or social care) services to ensure that service provision reflects local need as far as possible. As in clinical practice, deciding what to do with the 'diagnosis' is often not a straightforward matter. It usually involves a stage of reflection and prioritization, balancing the relative significance of different problems—and different perspectives.

Consider, for example, the kind of problem lists which may emerge from the diagnostic process for a child with multiple disabilities on the one hand and a primary care organization's assessment of children's needs in its patch on the other. For the individual child, the list might include the improvement of mobility, the management of feeding, deteriorating control of epileptic fits, the development of contractures, and the fact that his parents are having increasing difficulty in coping physically as he grows. The child's dearest wish might be for a better wheelchair which would allow him to move around the school playground more easily and therefore integrate better with his peers. For the parents, overnight respite care a couple of nights a week might be the top priority. From the perspective of the medical team, referral to a surgeon for assessment of his contractures might be on the action list. His teachers might be pressing for adjustment of his anti-epileptic medication because they are having difficulty coping with fits in school. The social worker might be most concerned about behaviour problems in a younger sibling who has been receiving less attention lately and tensions in the parents' marriage, and might feel referral to a family centre is the most urgent need.

For the primary care organization, the problem list may include a shortage of nursing staff on the acute wards which means beds are currently closed; an increasing number of children with complex needs being placed (expensively) out of the area because of difficulty arranging appropriate educational provision for them locally; long waiting lists for child psychiatric assessment; a rising tide of substance misuse in local schools; the lack of community speech and language therapists; and a crisis of morale among health visitors due to reorganization of the service and conflicting priorities for their limited time. National targets, pressure points in services, and changes in demography and morbidity will all have to be taken into account. Again, different individuals and organizations may have a very different view of what matters most. It is clear that acute and community staff, parents and young people, teachers, social workers, community nurses, and therapists will have strong and probably conflicting opinions.

In both cases, many of the possible interventions will require additional resources, often from different budgets which are likely to be overstretched already and to have many competing claims on them. Others are simply a question of time, communication, and interdisciplinary working to improve the integration of care. In some cases, a small investment now might potentially mean less expenditure in the future. Needs assessment is one of the tools used to ensure that the health service uses its resources to improve the health of the population in the most efficient and effective way. The question of how best to employ limited resources, and the political and ethical debate about rationing of health care, is beyond the scope of this book. It is important to recognize, however, that needs assessment starts from the perspective of the population and its health status rather than from the perspective of the balance sheet, and that it does not shy away from identifying needs which may be difficult or expensive to meet—but nor does it shy away from identifying existing services that, for one reason or another, do not meet local need and may be inappropriate or superfluous.

Need, supply, and demand

We have assumed so far that the concept of 'health needs' is conceptually simple and readily understood, and that needs are easily identifiable in practice. Alas, this is not the case and, as with other apparently straightforward terms encountered in this book, it is important to be clear about definition and meaning. Several different kinds of health needs can be identified:

♦ *felt needs* are an individual's (or community's) subjective perception of poor health, which may or may not be articulated

♦ *expressed needs* are felt needs which have been articulated by individuals (or communities), usually in order to seek help to overcome their perceived poor health

♦ *normative needs* are those defined in relation to an objective norm of health, often by a professional who identifies interventions appropriate for the expressed need

♦ *comparative need* reflects a judgement about how one set of (individual or community) needs measures up to another, for example on the basis of severity, extent, and the range of interventions available or provided.

Simple examples are set out in Table 7.2.

There is also a distinction to be made between *health* needs and *health care* needs — essentially a need for health as opposed to a need for health care. Examples of health needs could include certain learning or behaviour difficulties, neglect, or anything else which compromises a child's wellbeing but may not be straightforwardly 'treatable' by health services. Health care needs are specific health problems, such as a fracture or bacterial infection, that can benefit from direct health services interventions. Some health needs may, however, be met by providing services, but they may also require or benefit from action on a wider scale to tackle determinants of health such as poverty, pollution, nutrition, housing, transport policy, employment opportunities, income inequality, or social capital.

Needs can be classified as *felt, expressed, normative,* or *comparative*—and can also be divided into *health care needs* and *health needs*. Health care needs are met by health services, whereas health needs may benefit from wider social, environmental, and economic action.

Table 7.2 Examples of different types of needs

Type of need	Individual patient examples	Community example
Felt	A child with abdominal pain which he or she is aware of but does not complain of	Members of a community who are concerned about the speed of traffic in their road
Expressed	A child with abdominal pain which he or she has reported and sought help from a health care professional	A community which has voiced its concern about traffic safety to the local council
Normative	A child with abdominal pain which has been deemed to require treatment or further investigation	A community whose road is recognized by the council to need traffic calming after accident statistics and traffic use have been examined
Comparative	A child whose abdominal pain has been assessed by a health care professional as more serious than the conditions of others waiting (e.g. in A&E)	A community whose road has been judged a priority for installation of speed bumps after comparison of local data with other potential sites

In reality, the distinction between the two is sometimes not so clear-cut. Both health needs and health care needs can be influenced by socio-economic status, the physical and social environment, and cultural and religious beliefs. Some health care needs would disappear if wider social and environmental action was taken; and in the absence of such wider action, some health needs can be mitigated by providing health care services. Does the rising tide of childhood obesity, for example, represent a health need or a health care need? What about deteriorating asthma in a child living in damp and mouldy accommodation? Is it appropriate to consider anaemia in a late-weaned baby as a health care need?

Another categorization which is helpful in needs assessment is the triad of need, supply, and demand, which is often illustrated diagrammatically by three overlapping circles, as in Fig. 7.1.

Here, *need* (usually assumed here to be a normative, objectively defined need for health care) is compared to the population's *demand* for health care (not dissimilar to expressed need in the set of definitions above) and to the health care which is currently provided or *supplied*. Certain conditions or interventions may fall into one, two, or

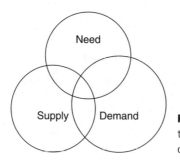

Fig. 7.1 The interrelated triad of need, supply, and demand.

three of the circles. For example, antibiotic treatment for acute ear infections may be demanded and supplied, but may not be needed since most cases will resolve without it. Similarly, child protection services for abused children may be needed and supplied but not demanded; appropriate adolescent health services may be needed and demanded but not supplied. Neonatal intensive care falls into the centre of the diagram where all three categories overlap, but a vaccination programme for an eradicated disease falls outside it altogether since it is neither needed, supplied, nor demanded.

Some authors impose a further qualification on needs which it is worth examining explicitly at this stage: that is, that health *care* needs exist only if an effective treatment is available for the condition in question. It follows that needs may change as research uncovers more therapies, or indeed exposes the ineffectiveness of established therapies. Thus a child with enlarged tonsils and troublesome but relatively infrequent tonsillitis would have been considered twenty years ago to have a need for tonsillectomy, but present evidence suggests that, in the absence of complications such as sleep apnoea, he does not need any surgical intervention. (Sometimes practice in one country differs from that in another because of a different attitude to research on effectiveness or a different assessment of needs—for example, lead screening in children is regularly undertaken in the US but not in the UK.) On the other hand, a child with a rare malignancy may be deemed to have no *health care* need in respect of active treatment, since no effective treatment has been identified for her condition, although she will have *health* needs for palliative care and support. However, that situation may change overnight with the publication of results from a research trial or a judgement by the National Institute for Clinical Effectiveness (NICE) that a new treatment merits general usage in the NHS.

Although it may seem logical to concentrate on those health needs that we have the means to address and to address with treatments of proven efficacy, it may also seem counterintuitive to define needs in such a conditional way. It is important to understand, however, how the niceties of definitions may affect policy decisions. Limiting health needs to conditions for which interventions of proven efficacy exist may exclude conditions and therapies for which adequate research has not yet been conducted. If this is so, then it is vital to re-evaluate the situation regularly in the light of new information—and to ensure that needs assessment feeds into the research and development agenda by identifying key areas in which research is needed to guide the provision of health care.

This is a complex and potentially confusing area, and it may seem that detailed consideration of what constitutes a health or health care need is of limited value in terms of day-to-day practice. It is important, however, that those working in the field of child public health are aware of these issues and explore their own understanding, definitions, and value systems before venturing forth into the field.

Approaches to needs assessment

There are many approaches to health needs assessment, some of which are listed below:

♦ Epidemiological
♦ Comparative

- Corporate
- Participatory
- Rapid appraisal

Needs assessment may focus on a particular condition (e.g. childhood diabetes), service (e.g. neonatal intensive care), or client group (e.g. children with learning difficulties), or it may be more open-ended, starting with a community and exploring its needs and problems to identify priority areas for more formal needs assessment.

Stevens and Raftery have described a tripartite framework for needs assessment which has been influential:

- **Epidemiological needs assessment** compares the demography and health (or more commonly the disease) status of the target population, the effectiveness of interventions for the problem(s) in question, and the local availability of services (see Fig. 7.2). It implicitly assumes, as described above, that needs only exist if effective treatment is available, and seeks to identify gaps in services for which there is a need and a remedy. Epidemiological needs assessment requires the collection of a considerable amount of information if it is to be conducted properly: the availability of data from different sources is explored later in the chapter.

- **Comparative needs assessment** contrasts services available locally with those available to similar populations in other areas.

- **Corporate needs assessment** gathers the views, desires, and knowledge of a range of stakeholders with different perspectives and experience.

It is often useful to combine all three approaches—epidemiological, corporate, and comparative—in order to develop as full a picture as possible of the health status and health needs of the population in question. For example, consider a needs assessment for a local population of asylum seekers, focusing particularly on unaccompanied minors. *Epidemiological* information may be limited, but it would be important to find out as much as possible about the population (how many unaccompanied minors there are; their age, sex, and nationality; the main health problems affecting them), the current availability of services for them (e.g. the number registered with local GPs and any special provision such as a dedicated health visitor), and any evidence that could be found about effective means of providing health care for this group (e.g. models of

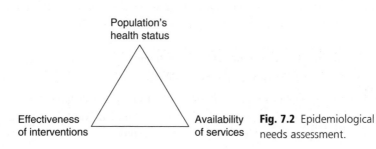

Fig. 7.2 Epidemiological needs assessment.

care which had been piloted and evaluated elsewhere). The *comparative* approach would involve finding out what neighbouring districts had done or planned to do in order to meet the needs of a similar population. The *corporate* approach would mean seeking the views of these young people themselves, and those working with them (including health and social care professionals, and voluntary and community workers) as to how their health needs could most appropriately be met. Sometimes information from these different sources forms a coherent picture; sometimes conflicting priorities or views emerge which have to be explored and resolved. However, a combined approach generally provides a more comprehensive view and is more likely to yield appropriate solutions which meet with general agreement.

Epidemiological needs assessment is based on information about the population's health status and the availability and effectiveness of health care. **Comparative** needs assessment assesses need and provision relative to other similar populations. **Corporate** needs assessment reflects the views of a range of stakeholders. **Joint strategic needs assessment** is the process whereby the health service and the local authority work together to identify problems which require action by both agencies, and **Commissioning** is the provision or establishment of services which will meet the health needs identified.

Other techniques have been developed which reflect the basic approaches to needs assessment set out above, but which have particular characteristics that make them especially appropriate for certain situations. **Rapid appraisal** needs assessment suits the need for expeditious responses to the child public health agenda in the twenty-first century; and **participatory** needs assessment, which builds on the theme of community approaches to health promotion described in Chapter 5, focuses on the target community and helps it to appraise its own needs.

Rapid appraisal

Rapid appraisal aims to gather a variety of information and perspectives on local health and social needs swiftly, and to translate these findings equally swiftly into proposals for action. It is a technique which is particularly well suited to investigating the health needs of a well-defined neighbourhood or population, or to any situation where a speedy overview is more important than an exhaustive survey—an approach sometimes referred to in the trade as 'quick and dirty'. It can be used to provide a starting point for a local community development project, or a more in-depth assessment of a specific issue or problem. Data are collected from three main sources:

◆ Interviews with a wide range of local informants

◆ Existing written records about the neighbourhood

◆ Observations made in the neighbourhood or in the homes of the interviewees.

From these sources a 'pyramid' of data is assembled (see Fig. 7.3) describing the neighbourhood's problems and priorities. Data from one source are validated

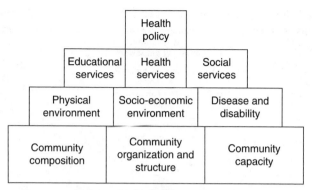

Fig. 7.3 Information pyramid for rapid appraisal.
Source: Reproduced from Murray, S. (1999), BMJ 318: 440–444 with permission from BMJ Publishing Group Ltd.

or rejected by checking with data from at least two other data sources or methods of data collection—a technique known as 'triangulation'. Informants are selected 'purposefully'—they are neither a comprehensive group nor a random sample, but have been identified by others as being in a good position to speak for the community on the issues involved. Professional views are often incorporated, as well as data collected from primary and secondary care.

Rapid appraisal needs assessment had its origins in work in developing countries, although it has subsequently been applied very effectively in the UK and other developed countries. An example of a suitable topic for rapid appraisal in child public health might be exploring the needs of a rapidly-growing town with a burgeoning community of families with young children, where services (health, social care, education, transport) have not kept pace with population growth.

Participatory needs assessment

Participatory needs assessment also addresses action to deal with the issues it raises. It aims to do this early in the process and requires needs assessment to be done *by* rather than *to* a community. Its basic philosophy emphasizes the importance of encouraging communities to tackle for themselves the problems that they consider important. It is intimately related to the concept of community development and often aims to improve health through improving quality of life at a more general level for the community (see Fig. 7.4). The 'community' here, as in rapid appraisal needs assessment, may be people who live in the same area (such as an inner-city housing estate or remote rural community) or who have something else in common (for example, children with disabilities).

Health impact assessment

Health impact assessment is a related but different technique which is growing in importance as a public health tool. It has emerged from the more established process of environmental impact assessment, and is used to assess the likely impact on health

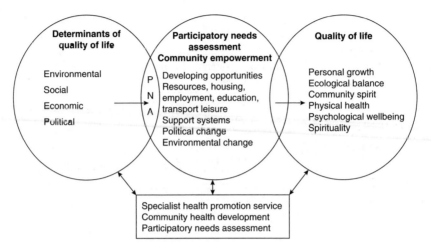

Fig. 7.4 The role of participatory needs assessment in improving quality of life. Source: Reproduced from Participatory Needs Assessment: a practical approach in partnerships between local residents and professionals', Rowley J & Bhuhi J, *Public Health Medicine* 1999, 1: 27–30. By Kind permission of Rila Publications Ltd, London.

of a planned development. It may be triggered by a community's concerns about, for example, a new traffic system or the closure of a school, or may be part of the planning process for larger developments such as the construction of a bypass or a new airport runway. It typically takes a broad view, examining both the positive and negative, and direct and indirect health effects of the proposed scheme (including perhaps pollution, noise, accident risk, employment, social disruption) and looking at ways of minimizing or mitigating its impact. This may involve proposals to build a new playground or to redevelop an access road to take traffic away from a local village. Health impact assessment requires the gathering of qualitative and quantitative data, and incorporates both lay and expert perspectives, engaging the local community and a wide variety of professionals and interest groups.

Community participation

Participatory needs assessment is one way of gaining community participation, which is a general term for the process of working with a community to improve its social wellbeing (and usually also the health and wellbeing of community members). Much of the experience of community participation comes from developing countries, but it has also been used in disadvantaged communities in the UK and other developed countries since the nineteenth century. Rifkin suggests four reasons why community participation in health is desirable:

1. Interventions to change behaviour and lifestyle—and thereby to improve health—can only succeed through individuals' conscious participation.

2. Participation of users in the planning and running of services should improve the appropriateness of those services for the population.

3 Communities have untapped resources which may be directed towards promoting health concerns, through the involvement of community members in the financing, building, and running of health facilities.

4 It is the right and duty of people to participate in activities affecting their daily lives.

Bringing needs assessments together – the Joint Strategic Needs Assessment

Joint Strategic Needs Assessment (JSNA) is the current process which brings together health services and local authorities to describe both the health care needs and the broader needs for health and wellbeing of local populations, and to consider the strategic direction for delivery of services to meet those needs. JSNAs play an important part in the local implementation of national policy – for example, Every Child Matters (see chapter 5) and the National Service Framework (NSF) for Children, which sets out standards of care to ensure that children's services are fit for purpose. JSNAs identify issues requiring future investment, informed by both national policy and the identification of local priorities for improving the health and welfare of children and young people. The JSNA process leads to the agreement of local Children and Young Persons Strategic Partnership Plans.

Developing a JSNA profile for a district – an example

This example looks at needs for perinatal health promotion to improve the health of babies in Plymouth. It aims to give a quick idea of the kind of data that might be used and the process that might be followed to weigh up local priorities. Fig. 7.5 maps the prevalence of smoking among mothers at birth in different localities in the city.

There is clearly a need to focus on smoking cessation interventions in the most disadvantaged areas, and those with the highest prevalence of maternal smoking. However, adverse risk factors cluster, and the mapping of mental illness and depression in parents across the city reveals a similar geographical pattern with higher prevalences in the south-west and north-west areas (Table 7.3).

This sort of clustering of risk might inform discussions between providers competing for limited resources in terms of recommendations how the programmes for smoking cessation and mental health promotion might need to be prioritized, commissioned, and delivered in different areas.

Commissioning

Joint Strategic Needs Assessment is closely related to the process of service commissioning (Table 7.4). A number of different individuals working with a variety of organizations are responsible for commissioning, which involves agreeing and defining the services which provider organizations will supply, and the financial arrangements for them. Figure 7.6 illustrates the relationship between needs assessment and commissioning.

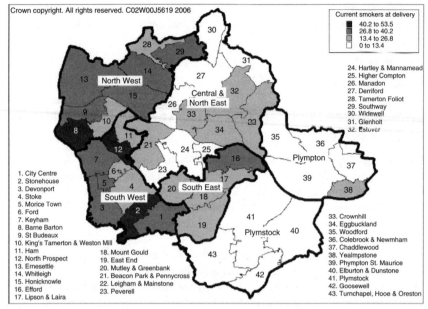

Fig. 7.5 Percentage mothers smoking at birth 2005/6 Plymouth.
Source: Reproduced from An atlas of child health and its determinants at neighbourhood level within Plymouth, Public Health Development Unit, November 2006, with permission.

A number of principles have been agreed by the Faculty of Public Health, Royal College of Paediatrics and Child Health, Association of Directors of Children's Services and the Child Public Health Special Interest group (CPHIG) UK, in order to align commissioning to a common strategy to support children's health and wellbeing.

Table 7.3 Parental mental illness, deprivation and locality in Plymouth

Deprivation group	Number	Percent
Most deprived	417	35.1
Middle group	182	19.0
Least deprived	82	11.3
Sub-locality	**Number**	**Percent**
Central/North East	87	14.9
North West	208	32.7
Plympton	33	10.3
Plymstock	24	10.2
South East	107	24.0
South West	222	33.9
Plymouth total	681	27.7

Source: Reproduced from An atlas of child health and its determinants at neighbourhood level within Plymouth, Public Health Development Unit, November 2006, with permission.

Table 7.4 Principles for successful joint commissioning

- Services should be commissioned with due respect for the philosophy of the *UN Convention on the Rights of the Child*, and on **principles of equity**
- Successful joint commissioning requires **secure inter-agency governance arrangements** to be in place, and an agreement over the scope of the service areas to be addressed in the joint commissioning process. The local **Children's Trust** should be the vehicle for this
- The **organisational accountability arrangements** should place the joint commissioning function at **an appropriately senior level** within the PCT and the local authority, ideally as a joint appointment
- Commissioning should be based on **a whole system approach,** which takes a holistic view of children and young people, and families' wellbeing, and which pools budgets where appropriate to commission and provide services
- There needs to be effective and appropriately resourced **specialist public health input** to the commissioning process, driven by the JSNA. One mechanism for this could be the appointment of a jointly funded consultant in public health to oversee this work
- A clearly agreed **commissioning framework** is needed, where local partners understand the process of reviewing, designing and improving services. The commissioning process should ensure that **expert practitioners and clinicians** from provider organisations, as well as other stakeholders, are able to work alongside commissioners to identify needs and inform service design and improvement
- The JSNA should be informed by **accurate and relevant data of high quality.** Indicators used should build on those used in the National Indicator Set, be well constructed and follow good scientific practice
- **Information sharing protocols** should be developed between agencies to allow for the sharing of certain detailed health information which would not normally be placed in the public domain, in order to inform the JSNA
- There needs to be meaningful public involvement and sophisticated tools to assess local need. Local areas should agree a **Statement of Good Practice** on ways of ensuring that the views of local children, young people and their families are ascertained as part of the JSNA process
- The commissioning process should be based on children's and families' all round needs, in biological, social and psychological terms, and should be **driven by an understanding of how these factors impact on health and wellbeing at various points in the lifecourse**, so that commissioners can invest wisely in services at different ages and transition points
- The commissioning process needs to ensure all elements of any child, young person and family pathway through services are in place and working well to achieve the desired outcomes. Key measures along the pathway should be used to drive a **culture of continuous improvement and learning**
- As resources become scarce, it is important not to weaken universal services in favour of a solely targeted approach to service commissioning for vulnerable groups. **Strong evidence-based universal services are a necessary foundation for more targeted services**

Source: Reproduced from Joint commissioning of children's services across local authorities and primary care trusts An Overview Faculty of Public Health. ISBN: 1-900273-30-6, April 2008, with permission.

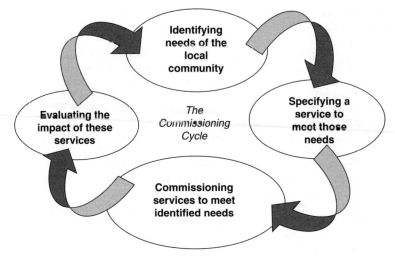

Fig. 7.6 The commissioning cycle.
Source: Adapted from Henschen, L., Lindfield, T. 2007. *Scoping Westminsters' Joint Strategic Needs Assessment*, with permission.

Community development

In fragmented communities with high social needs and/or high levels of disaffection and cynicism, community development may be necessary to engage communities sufficiently to enable their participation in needs assessment. Skilled practitioners from a variety of professional backgrounds who usually do not live in the community work alongside members of the community to establish a sufficient level of social trust and cohesion to start a discussion about common needs or issues. It is important that children and young people are involved in this process as well as their parents, where issues to do with their wellbeing are at stake. The role of the practitioner is to assist the organizational process while remaining in the background him or herself. The approach is also used to empower communities to take action about issues or needs that are important for the community, but are not priorities for the local authority or health service. When it is successful, this approach is very powerful in transforming communities and the lives of the individuals who live in them. However, if the approach fails and the community's needs are not met, cynicism and disengagement may escalate. Communities are collections of individuals with all the strengths and weaknesses of human kind, and community development projects can 'go wrong' because they are hijacked by powerful members of the community who have their own interests at heart rather than those of the community at large. These projects therefore need very skilled steering.

Some 'top down' initiatives, such as 'Healthy Schools' schemes, have been built on the principles of community development. The scheme incorporates a wide range of health initiatives but schools select those areas that are relevant to their needs. With support and advice from a local healthy school practitioner, teachers decide how they will tackle the health issues they are concerned about. Children and young people are involved sometimes through participation in a school council and sometimes through other mechanisms. They are offered the chance to take control of and improve aspects of school life, addressing what they perceive to be important problems. Proposed action might include starting a breakfast club or sports activities at lunchtime, altering the layout of the playground or the management of break times to tackle bullying, running a healthy snacks stall, or raising funds for new play equipment. As schools are given a very free hand in deciding which aspects of health to tackle and in what way, Healthy Schools schemes vary in the extent to which the principles of community development are employed.

Advocacy

According to the *Oxford Dictionary*, to be an advocate is 'to plead or raise one's voice in favour of [a cause or person]; to defend or recommend publicly'. In other words, advocacy is 'to stand beside', not 'to do for'. In public health terms, advocacy and lobbying ('seeking to influence legislators') are often directed at the highest level of health promotion, seeking to encourage healthy public policy—that is, policies that favour health rather than putting obstacles in the way of it. Examples of healthy public policy include the provision of cycle paths and safe routes to school at a local level, and the banning of tobacco advertising at national level. Health professionals with a concern for public health have an important role to play in raising health policy issues and putting pressure on governments and others to make changes in policy.

Advocacy can operate at an individual level as well as a population level. At the individual level, advocacy means making a commitment to support the child and family beyond the immediate issues related to their medical condition. It is integral to the work of many professionals involved with children—paediatricians, social workers, community nurses, GPs—and reflects a wish to meet all of a child's health-related and social needs within the context of his or her family and community. Factors outside the realm of direct health care provision (including family, educational, social, cultural, spiritual, economic, environmental, and political factors) often inhibit children's ability to achieve their full potential—particularly among children from disadvantaged families. Advocacy can also be part of community development; for example, young people can be taught the principles of advocacy and encouraged to use them to promote their health needs.

> Advocacy can operate at the individual level, supporting and arguing the case for a child or family, or at the population level to promote healthy public policy.

Advocacy for child health often begins with an individual patient, and may grow from there into local, regional, or national work in a public health capacity. Sometimes it follows through the same issues on a more general level—perhaps lobbying for certain services to be provided for the local population, rather than just for a particular child or children, or opposing cuts in services which will affect both known and unknown children.

Examples of opportunities for advocacy on an *individual* level include supporting an application for rehousing for a child with chronic serous otitis media and recurrent respiratory infections who lives in an overcrowded, damp house; writing to the school about the emotional consequences for a child with a disability who is in a mainstream school but falling behind, being bullied, and receiving inadequate teaching support; or helping teachers to feel more confident in dealing with a child with asthma in the classroom when they are reluctant to provide medication within the school setting.

Examples of opportunities for advocacy affecting a specific *population* include supporting a school campaign to improve safety in the streets nearby, promoting the emotional and social needs of local teenagers by lobbying local government for better youth facilities in the locality, or lobbying government to change outdated legislation which allows parents to use corporal punishment on their children.

Effective advocacy has a number of important elements and requires particular skills which those trained to deliver services (health, social care, education, etc.) may or may not possess, but can certainly learn and practice. The boxes below set out what advocacy involves and what skills professionals need in order to be effective advocates.

Essential components of advocacy for child health

- ◆ A problem within the system which is obstructing children's care, or a policy issue which is adverse to children's health
- ◆ The potential for individual or group intervention (such as lobbying) to bring about change
- ◆ Will and determination to make things better and to improve the system for children
- ◆ Presenting a good, succinct case and being prepared to see it through

Skills needed for advocacy

- ◆ Understanding of political system
- ◆ Lack of political bias
- ◆ Ability to manage change
- ◆ Assertiveness
- ◆ Media skills
- ◆ Holistic approach to health and health care
- ◆ Good team working and networking
- ◆ Ability to prioritize
- ◆ Persistence, patience, and tolerance of long time-scales

Social marketing

Advocacy is a mechanism for influencing health from 'bottom up'. Social marketing is an important 'top down' approach, in which the content of programmes is decided by professionals and policy makers and the general public are passive recipients.

Social marketing is being used increasingly as a means to change the behaviour of individuals and groups. It can be defined as the systematic application of marketing techniques to achieve specific behavioural goals for a social or public good. The core principles of social marketing (see Fig. 7.7) are derived from the commercial marketing of products which are by no means always 'health promoting', and it is a powerful approach with the potential (like tobacco advertising, for example) to be highly manipulative. So decisions about what is and what is not a 'social or public good' need to be taken with care.

The aim of social marketing is to achieve a measurable impact on a specific behavioural goal, such as healthy eating, smoking cessation, or physical activity. It requires an understanding of the target audience based on careful consumer research. That research will also help to define interventions which are likely to support the behavioural goals being targeted.

Social marketing interventions draw on theories derived from different disciplines and professions. The 'insight' segment of the social marketing triangle refers to the need to move beyond traditional public health information (such as demographic or epidemiological data) and look much more closely at why people behave as they do. What people think, feel, and believe is important, as well as what they do. The 'exchange' segment reflects the notion that the target audience will be trading off short-term and long-term benefits for any possible behavioural change. These might include money, time, effort, and some possible social consequences. Finally, social marketing uses the concept of 'competition' to consider all the different factors that can affect people's willingness or ability to adopt the desired behaviour. This includes external competition from those promoting negative behaviours, and also from those promoting other positive messages to the same audience. Internal competition includes the power of pleasure, enjoyment, risk-taking, habit, and addiction that can affect a person's behaviour.

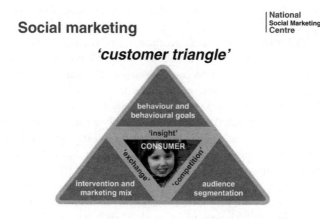

A device for highlighting a number of social marketing's key features

Fig. 7.7 Customer triangle diagram.
Source: Reproduced from *Social Marketing Big Pocket Guide*, National Social Marketing Centre, 2007, with permission.

Social marketing interventions need to be tailored to a particular target audience, and this is what 'segmentation targeting' aims to do. It looks at different ways in which people can be grouped and profiled, as a basis for choosing appropriate interventions. Programmes that include a number of different strands are more likely to be effective than a single intervention. The 'marketing mix' describes the balance between different approaches in the same programme (Fig. 7.8).

Evidence and evaluation

Meeting the health needs identified in needs assessment exercises and designing social marketing initiatives requires evidence of different kinds: for example, evidence about the determinants of health and about interventions, their effectiveness and their cost. Evidence and effectiveness are issues which have been touched on earlier, but it is helpful to explore a little further their usefulness, implications, and limitations for public health practice. These are huge topics in their own right, and we do not propose to cover them in detail here: the further reading list at the end of the chapter includes references where the interested reader can find all they wish to know about evidence-based medicine and the design of randomized controlled trials and epidemiological studies (such as cohort and case-control studies) which are used to generate evidence of effectiveness. The list includes books about health economics, an increasingly important component of evidence and evaluation which we do not deal with in any depth here.

The challenges of evidence-based practice in public health

As we saw in Chapter 4, the development of public health progammes in the past was often driven by belief and conviction, without the support of any research showing that the proposed interventions would be effective. While some of these interventions have been highly effective, others have failed or have had unintended consequences. Developing an evidence base for public health is therefore important, but this is a more complicated business than developing an evidence base in clinical practice. The complex interventions necessary to change behaviour are not well suited to randomized controlled trials, and it is rarely practical to trial changes in social policy. The World Health Organisation believes that randomized controlled trials are often 'unhelpful, inappropriate and unnecessarily expensive' in the evaluation of health promotion interventions. In its most recent advice on evaluation of complex interventions the UK Medical Research Council has also recognized that, whilst experimental approaches are to be preferred, they may not always be practical. Many interventions (such as car seat belts and 'pedestrian friendly' fronts to cars to promote road safety, developed on the basis of engineering design calculations and tested in laboratory trials) have been introduced to great effect without controlled trials.

Some areas of public health practice pose particularly difficult problems. Due to the logistics and expense of the very long-term follow-up necessary, studies showing a direct impact of child health interventions on adult health are rare. There are, however, other approaches to evaluation which can and have been employed by those trying to establish the effectiveness of childhood interventions that might be expected to affect adult health. The evidence base in this area therefore relies on the findings from a range of studies employing a variety of methodologies.

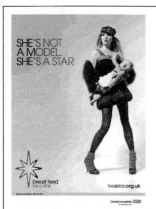

The Hub

Be A Star—Breastfeeding initiation case study

Originally commissioned by Central Lancashire PCT, 'Be A Star' is a social marketing intervention designed to increase breastfeeding initiation within deprived communities. Since launch, the programme has been developed into a model that can be applied in similar socio-economic contexts, regardless of location and with minimal supplementary research. As such, Be A Star is currently being implemented by PCTs throughout the UK.

Be A Star takes a holistic approach to health improvement based on social marketing principles and established behavioural theory. The programme incorporates service development, co-creation, peer-to-peer mobilisation, stakeholder engagement, group identity formation and a groundbreaking, through-the-line communications campaign.

12 months after launch, evaluation of the programme within the Central Lancashire PCT boundary reported the following impressive results:

- 13% increase in breastfeeding initiation over first 6 months against a 2% target
- 9% increase over first 12 months against a 2% target
- National and regional government targets exceeded 4 times over
- Peer support service extended to 27,000 young mothers
- Significant cost savings on service development through the co-creation of peer-driven support provision
- Establishment of a position of authority and a reputation for innovation from which to influence regional and national agendas
- Increased efficiencies and cohesion in delivery of breastfeeding services
- Mobilisation of internal staff through increased morale and aspiration
- Wider acceptance of social marketing approaches due to compelling evidence base

Fig. 7.8 An example of social marketing: the Be A Star campaign www.nsmcentre. org.uk

Source: An example of Social Marketing: the Be A Star campaign from the National Social Marketing Centre's ShowCase database: http://www.nsms.org.uk/public/ CSHome.aspx. © 2009 Hub Marketing Ltd, reproduced with permission.

There is a balance to be struck here between rigour and pragmatism—between the need to operate today within the realities of the messy everyday world where information, evidence, and certainty may all be lacking, and the ideal of a clear theoretical framework and strong evidence base on which to base public health action. It is important to remember that the lack of research evidence to guide clinical or public health interventions to meet certain individual or population health needs does not invalidate those needs, nor mean that no attempt should be made to address them. Indeed, it is sometimes necessary to act without full information about effectiveness, either in the clinical or public health spheres—for example, in extreme cases where life is at risk or when something needs to be done for reasons of precaution, humanity, or commonsense.

The introduction of non-evidence-based policies continues today: UK governments have tried to improve children's diets in the past by providing free school milk and school meals to children whose families are on income support, and currently by providing fresh fruit to all school children, with the aim of improving growth and development and reducing adult disease risk. While these interventions seem like a good idea from a commonsense point of view, no studies have ever been undertaken to demonstrate that free provision is followed by a sustained increase in consumption leading to better health outcomes.

> Developing an evidence base for public health is important, but is more complicated than in clinical practice. Randomized controlled trials may be neither feasible nor helpful. Many successful public health interventions have been introduced without prior evidence of effectiveness—but it is vital that such interventions are properly evaluated, so lessons can be learned for the future.

The importance of evaluation

Where interventions are introduced on the basis that it seems very likely that they will improve health rather than on the basis of unequivocal scientific evidence that this will happen, it is vital that they are properly evaluated in order that lessons can be learned about their effectiveness and operation, and future action can draw on the evidence yielded by past experience. Even in the case of evidence-based interventions, it is important that their implementation is monitored. Public health interventions are more complex than clinical interventions, such as the administration of a drug, and much more can go wrong. Benefits demonstrated in well-funded research studies cannot always be replicated in practice, and research reports rarely provide the pragmatic details about the delivery of the intervention that can make the difference between success and failure.

There is an extensive literature on health promotion evaluation, to which the 'Further reading' section again signposts those interested in this area, but a brief summary may be useful here. Health care evaluation has been defined as:

> The critical assessment, on as objective a basis as possible, of the degree to which entire services or their component parts... fulfil stated goals.
>
> (St Leger)

Cochrane first stressed the importance of evaluation and defined *effectiveness* and *efficiency* as key elements of performance to be assessed. Maxwell described six dimensions of quality which it is often helpful to consider when designing an evaluation: access, relevance, effectiveness, equity, acceptability, and efficiency. Holland has emphasized that acceptability can apply to professionals as well as the public.

Donabedian's influential model divides the system or intervention being studied into three elements to be examined during the evaluation:

- *Structure*: fixed resources and how they are organized
- *Process*: what is done (and how much); how activities and individuals interact
- *Outcome*: impact and end results

Evaluations of pilot or ongoing interventions may draw on the classical study designs, but as we have already seen these methods may be inappropriate and a more flexible approach may be needed. It is always important to include the perspective of users and the public; it is also vital to be clear what the intervention hopes to achieve, and to evaluate against specified targets and objectives wherever possible. In many cases, however, it is difficult or impractical to assess changes in the ultimate outcome—such as lower rates of premature death from coronary heart disease or cancer in the case of the school fruit scheme. Intermediate or proxy outcomes (such as changes in fruit consumption, population blood cholesterol levels, or childhood obesity) may have to be assessed, or it may be more appropriate to look at the process level in Donabedian's model (the number of children receiving free fruit in school as a result of the scheme being implemented).

> Evaluating health promotion interventions presents a challenge. It is often necessary to look at intermediate outcomes rather than focusing on endpoints (e.g. mortality and morbidity), or to assess process measures or changes in knowledge, attitude, or behaviour.

Several authors have proposed ways of studying the effectiveness of health promotion interventions. Tannahill suggests examining their impact at several points on a hierarchy of change:

- Change in knowledge
- Change in attitude
- Change in behaviour
- Change in morbidity or mortality

Nutbeam suggests four levels for evaluation which build on Donabedian's model:

1. *Process* – unravelling the reasons for the success or failure of an intervention
2. *Impact* – evaluation against the programme's objectives, such as improved community participation or individual health literacy
3. *Intermediate outcomes* – the development of healthy lifestyles, healthy environments, or effective health services

4 *Health and social outcomes* – improvements in quality of life, reductions in morbidity, disability, or avoidable mortality

Some of the particular methodological challenges in developing an evidence base in public health include:

◆ Studies of interventions delivered through a school or community require very large, expensive trials in which the communities or schools are randomized to intervention and control group (cluster randomized controlled trials).

◆ Many public health interventions depend for their success on the implementation of several different approaches at the same time. Most trials aim to isolate the impact of individual approaches and these trials can miss synergistic or enabling effects.

◆ Public health interventions often depend on interpersonal skills, which are not measured or reported in most trials. In many interventions it is the quality of relationships and communication between practitioner and client that count most in effecting change, and these skills are rarely measured.

◆ Public health interventions are often holistic. For example, the effectiveness of domiciliary health visiting is difficult to measure because good health visitors address the issues of greatest relevance and importance for individual families. Those undertaking randomized controlled trials are required to nominate a 'primary outcome measure' against which the success of the trial is measured. Unless this outcome is selected carefully and is holistic in nature, health visitors may not have addressed the primary outcome in a significant proportion of families

◆ Trials of public health interventions give priority to documenting the impact on health outcomes, and critical details about the process of implementation are often not gathered or reported. Such reports help practitioners know that something was or was not effective, but can leave doubts about what exactly the 'something' was.

◆ Studies of interventions to promote health have been limited by the lack of well-validated measures of wellbeing. As discussed in chapter 5, this situation is now beginning to change, but reliance on measures of disease or ill health is still common. This is often inappropriate in evaluating interventions which take a population approach, and 'ceiling' or 'floor' effects (when many participants score maximum at the beginning of the study) can mean that important improvements in health are missed.

Evaluating costs and benefits

Establishing the costs of interventions is now an important and sometimes complex part of evaluation. Costs can be viewed from various different angles: – costs to the NHS, costs to the public purse more generally, and costs to society (which include for example the cost of time off work to take part in an intervention). Health economists set these costs against the benefits of the intervention and their analyses now play an important and explicit role in decision making about whether a new intervention or programme should be provided. Several different types of analysis are undertaken of which two are key: cost effectiveness analysis measures the cost of achieving a specific outcome (e.g. reduction in time off school for asthma); and cost benefit analysis measures the cost of achieving impact on a generic outcome for example quality of life. The latter aims to allow the benefits of very different interventions (e.g. insulin for diabetes, smoking cessation progammes in pregnancy, or a wheel chair for a child with cerebral palsy) to be compared and policy makers to invest in those which offer the best value for money. One generic outcome favoured by health economists is the QALY or quality adjusted life year. QALY scores range from 1 which is perfect health to 0 which is death; a year of life wheel chair bound might be valued as 0.7. The DALY (disability adjusted life year) is another generic measure used in international comparisons to estimate the burden of disease from a specific condition. It is calculated from the number of years of life lost through premature death added to the number of years of life lived with disability. One DALY is equal to one year in good health; a year with conduct disorder might rate as 0.6 DALY. Health economic analysis of childhood interventions is still in an early phase of development.

Data sources

Robust, reliable data is essential for most of the techniques and processes described in this chapter. There are a number of sources of routinely collected data which can be used to build up a picture of the health needs of the population. These broadly divide into data which describes:

+ populations (demographic data)
+ health (often 'ill health') event data, such as mortality, hospital admissions, and consultations
+ lifestyle and health status.

Below are listed some important routine sources of data on children and families in each category: some examples of data available from these sources were given in Chapter 1.

Population data

Census data

Population censuses have been carried out in England and Wales since 1841, when the population was 15.9 million, with 46% aged under 20 and only 4% over the age of 65. They are carried out at ten-yearly intervals and provide key data for service planning and epidemiological studies. The population aged under 20 almost doubled between 1841 and 1911, from 7.3 million in 1841 to 14.4 million in 1911. Although the size of the overall population has continued to grow, the child population has shrunk since this time, to 11.0 million in 2001. This dramatically affects the structure of the population and the balance between different age groups within it. Census data also includes details of ethnic origin, occupation, and life-limiting illnesses.

Birth and death registration

Registration of births and deaths has been a statutory requirement in England and Wales since 1837. All births need to be registered by the parent within six weeks of delivery. There is no time limit after death for registration. NHS numbers, which give

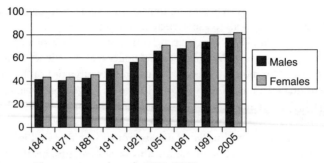

Fig. 7.9 Average life expectancy (years), 1841–2005.
Source: Data from Office for National Statistics.

the child rights of access to health services, are now generated at birth: this is a useful advance for information systems, enabling linkage of data on infants and mothers to improve care and research into early determinants of child morbidity.

Death registration data (Fig. 7.9) shows that life expectancy for men improved from 42 years to 75 years between 1841 and 2005. Currently there is a five-year gap in life expectancy between males and females, with women living longer. A gender difference in mortality exists throughout childhood and is reflected in differential morbidity patterns.

Population data sources include the decennial census and birth and death registrations.

Health events

Information about illness and disability is less comprehensive than information about deaths. Data sources include hospital episode statistics and GP consultation data (Royal College of General Practitioners, Birmingham Research Unit Weekly returns). These sources describe the common reasons why children and young people seek routine health care services (see Table 7.5). They are event-based rather than child-based, so they do not distinguish multiple events in a single child from single events in several children.

Table 7.5 Children consulting general practitioners (annual rate per 100,000 children) by type of condition, 2007, England and Wales

Disease group	Age group (years)		
	<1	1–4	5–14
Infectious and parasitic diseases	605	403	192
Neoplasms	11	4	12
Endocrine, nutritional, and metabolic disease, and immunity disorders	14	3	4
Disease of the blood and blood forming organs	5	5	3

(continued)

Table 7.5 (continued) Children consulting general practitioners (annual rate per 100,000 children) by type of condition, 2007, England and Wales

Disease group	Age group (years)		
Mental disorders	10	10	15
Diseases of the nervous system and sense organs	782	555	214
Diseases of the circulatory system	4	1	2
Diseases of the respiratory system	1837	1043	386
Diseases of the digestive system	240	66	30
Diseases of the genitourinary system	40	57	50
Complications of pregnancy, childbirth, and the puerperium	2	0	0
Diseases of the skin and subcutaneous tissue	715	351	206
Diseases of the musculoskeletal system and connective tissue	14	27	74
Congenital anomalies	67	7	4
Certain conditions originating in the perinatal period	114	1	0
Symptoms, signs, all ill-defined conditions	483	254	137
Injury and poisoning	58	81	81
Supplementary classification of factors influencing health status and contact with health services			

Source: Data from RCGP 2007 Weekly Returns Service.

Hospital episode statistics (HES)

Hospital episode statistics (HES) contain the following information:

- Hospital name
- Health authority of residence
- Demographic details (NHS number, sex, birth date, postcode of usual address)
- Admission details (referring GP, admission/discharge details, method/source of admission)
- Consultant episode details (consultant code, specialty)
- Clinical diagnoses, operations, and procedures undertaken.

With the growth in community services and day cases, children are admitted to hospital less often as Table 7.6 illustrates.

Most health care episode data is coded according to the health problem(s) triggering the event. Several different coding systems exist, the most common being the International Classification of Diseases (ICD), READ codes, SNOMED, and Healthcare Resource Groups (HRGs). The ICD coding manual, used for coding hospital data, is regularly updated and is now in its tenth edition. READ codes are used for general practice data.

Preventive care

Each UK area now has a computerized database of all children living in the area. This is used to manage preventive care services like immunization and surveillance episodes.

Table 7.6 Number of ordinary vs day case paediatric in-patient admissions and outpatient consultations in Scotland 1997–2001

	1997	1998	1999	2000	2001
Inpatient episodes					
Total	55,058	56,147	55,218	53,799	53,506
Medical Paediatrics	45,880	46,693	46,231	45,881	45,805
Surgical Paediatrics	9,178	9,454	8,987	7,918	7,701
Day cases					
Medical Paediatrics	2,054	3,303	4,047	3,378	4,256
Surgical Paediatrics	4,566	4,409	4,339	3,826	3,706
Total	6,620	7,712	8,386	7,204	7,962
Outpatient attendances					
Total	135,324	137,416	138,479	137,499	135,208
Medical Paediatrics	111,250	114,073	115,399	116,214	115,684
Surgical Paediatrics	24,074	23,343	23,080	21,285	20,524

Source: Data from ISD Scotland Child Health Statistics website.

It contains data about immunization and screening, together with some data on disability. The quality of data in these systems is very variable and depends on investment both in software development and staff, together with the degree of interest taken by health professionals. Their usefulness for epidemiological studies varies from one area to another.

Chronic disease

Information about the incidence and prevalence of a small number of diseases—including congenital malformations, cancer, cerebral palsy, cystic fibrosis, and diabetes—is recorded in disease registers. Disease registers have four principal uses:

1 *Service planning* e.g. determining the numbers of children with severe communication disability who require special educational provision
2 *Epidemiological research* e.g. the evaluation of a prenatal screening programme (such as that for Down's syndrome) or studying geographical variation in congenital anomalies
3 *Clinical audit* e.g. using the register as a sampling frame to identify children with continence problems or challenging behaviour, for whom the quality of care can be evaluated
4 *Individual patient care* e.g. to aid the co-ordination of multidisciplinary and interagency case reviews and planning meetings.

Some of the characteristics of a disease register are:

♦ it identifies individuals
♦ the individuals have certain characteristics in common

- ◆ it is longitudinal (a record kept over a period of time) and in some cases is systematically updated

- ◆ it records individuals within a geographically defined population.

The usefulness of a register can be compromised by poor initial planning, conflicting priorities for its use, incomplete or inaccurate data (case ascertainment), difficulties in maintaining staff interest and continuing managerial commitment, and failure to safeguard confidentiality and access arrangements.

> Other sources of information on health and health care include child health databases (covering all children in an area) and disease registers for children with conditions such as cancer and diabetes.

Population-based survey data

General Household Survey

The General Household Survey (GHS) commenced in 1971 and is a continuous survey of approximately 12,000 representative private households in Great Britain. Interviews are conducted with the adults in the household; a limited number of questions are included about children under the age of 16 years living in the household. A number of government departments use the data, which includes questions on housing, economic activity, pensions, leisure activities, education, and the family.

The health aspects covered include acute illness in the past two weeks, health during the previous year, the presence of chronic illness, consultations with a doctor, outpatient and in-patient visits to hospital, wearing of glasses or contact lenses, as well as smoking and drinking habits. According to the findings of the GHS, chronic illness affects one in five children aged 5–15, but only 50% report that their illness limits their day-to-day activities. Respiratory disease is the most common illness, reported by 7% of child respondents. This data is consistent with routine data showing the high prevalence of respiratory disorders in the child population.

Lifestyle and risk factors

Other surveys, such as the Health Survey for England and the Health Education Population Survey in Scotland, now regularly collect data on the prevalence of other specific illnesses, disabilities, health related lifestyles, and risk factors for ill health. In recent years national surveys have also been carried out on the prevalence of disability and of mental illness in UK children. The WHO carries out an international survey on health behaviour of school children (HBSC) which includes data from the UK and allows international comparisons of trends in lifestyle factors (see Chapter 3).

Such data can help inform health promotion policy at several levels, from local (e.g. within a school) to national. The Schools Health Education Unit in Exeter also carries out surveys of health and health-related lifestyles in schools, providing data which help schools plan health promotion activities. As a very large number of schools have participated, the dataset is now large enough to be used to discern trends.

> Surveys can gather information on acute and chronic illness, disability, health-related lifestyles, and risk factors for ill health, from a sample of the population or a particular group such as a school. Surveys may be regular or ad hoc, local, national, or international.

Limitations of routine data for health needs assessment

Routine sources of data provide only a limited perspective on children's health. Increasingly, interest is being shown in measuring health needs from the perspective of children, young people, and their parents. There is a need to collect data on such indicators as health-related quality of life, functional health status, health-related educational capability, and family functioning.

Several groups in the US, the UK, the European Union, and Australia are attempting to enhance routine data collection so that these aspects of health can be measured more accurately and universally. However, as the Medical Officer of Health for Nottingham noted in his Annual Report over 50 years ago:

> the collection of reliable information regarding the ills—both minor and grave— to which man is subject is a very slow process.
>
> (W. Dodd, 1950)

> Data sources vary in terms of completeness and accuracy; their usefulness depends on many factors including the quality, appropriateness, and accessibility of their information, and commitment to their development and use.

Further reading

Evaluation

Craig, N., Dieppe, P., Macintryre, S., Michie, S., Nazareth, I., and Petticrew, M. (2008) Developing and evaluating complex interventions: the new Medical Research Council guidelines. *BMJ*; **337**: a1655

Cochrane, A. (1971) *Effectiveness and efficiency: random reflections on health services.* The 1971 Rock Carling Fellowship monograph. Nuffield Provincial Hospitals Trust.

Donabedian, A. (1988) The quality of care: how can it be assessed? *Journal of the American Medical Association*; **260**(12): 1743–8.

Holland, W.H. (ed.) (1983) *Evaluation of health care.* Oxford University Press, Oxford.

Maxwell, R.J. (1984) Perspectives in NHS management: quality assessment in health. *BMJ*; **288**: 1470–2.

Phillips, C. (2005) *Health Economics: an introduction for health professionals.* BMJ: London.

St Leger, A.S., Schnieden, H., and Walsworth–Bell, J.P. (1992) *Evaluating health services' effectiveness: a guide for health professionals, service managers and policy makers.* Open University Press, Buckingham.

Needs assessment and community diagnosis

Cook, J., Pechevis, M., and Waterston, T. (1995) Community diagnosis and participation. In *European Textbook of Social Paediatrics* (B. Lindstrom and N. Spencer (eds.)). Oxford University Press, Oxford.

Stevens, A. and Gillam, S. (1998) Needs assessment: from theory to practice. *BMJ*; **316**: 1448–52.

Stevens, A. and Raftery, J. (1994) *Healthcare needs assessment: the epidemiologically based needs assessment reviews.* Radcliffe Medical Press, Oxford.

Advocacy

Hodgkin, R. (2000) *Advocating for children,* RCPCH London e-version on http://www.rcpch. ac.uk/publications.

Schmidt, L., Garrat, A., and Fitzpatrick, R. (2002) Child/parent assessed health outcome measures: a structured review. *Childcare health and development,* **28**: 237.

Waterston, T. and Tonniges, T. (2001) Advocating for children's health: a US and UK perspective. *Archives of Disease in Childhood*; **85**: 180–2.

Waterston, T. and Haroon, S. (2008) *Advocacy and the paediatrician. Paediatrics and Child Health.*

Waterston, T. (2009) Teaching and learning about advocacy. *Archives of Disease in Childhood. Education and Practice Edition*; **94**: 24–28.

Evidence-based medicine

Nutbeam, D. (1999) Making the case for health promotion: the questions to be answered. In *The evidence of health promotion effectiveness: shaping public health in a new Europe* (D. Boddy, ed.). EU, Brussels.

Sackett, D.L., Scott Richardson, W., Rosenberg, W., and Brian Haynes, R. (1997) *Evidence based medicine.* Churchill Livingstone.

Thorogood, M. and Coombes, Y. (1999) *Evaluating health promotion: Practice and Methods.* Oxford University Press, Oxford.

Registers

Abra, A. and Woodroffe, C. (1991) A special conditions register. *Archives of Disease in Childhood*; **66**: 927–30.

Blair, M.E. and Hutchison, T. (1997) Special needs registers – dreams and nightmares. In *Progress in community child health* 2, (ed. Spencer, N.), pp. 57–67. Churchill Livingstone.

Sources of data on child health

Botting, B. (ed.) (1995) *The health of our children decennial supplement.* Office for National Statistics (ONS), London. ONS website: www.ons.gov.uk.

Woodroffe, C., Glickman, M., Barker, M., and Power, C. (1993) *Children, teenagers and health – the key data.* Open University, Buckingham.

Health Economics

Ceri J. Phillips (2005). *Health economics: an introduction for health professionals.* Blackwell Publishing BMJ Books, London.

Chapter 8

Child public health in practice – case scenarios

In this chapter we give a number of practical worked examples relating to key areas of child public health for health professionals and their colleagues. The first describes the general process, for a newly appointed community paediatrician, of making a community diagnosis; the rest address specific problems. For each, a case scenario is described and there is a short review of the epidemiology, a list of the stakeholders likely to be involved, a survey of the evidence, and a suggested practical approach to tackling the problem. The framework for action is based on the concepts and information presented in earlier chapters.

Scenario A: 'Walking the patch'–developing a public health approach to a locality

This example describes the route taken by a community paediatrician taking up a new post in a deprived area of a large city, and wishing to assess the health and social needs of the local child population with the help of local primary care teams and public health specialists. Health visitors and other professionals with a geographical base use the phrase 'walking the patch' to describe what they do when coming into post for the first time and getting to know their case load. The term reflects the fact that the local community is the locus of interaction (as opposed to a GP's case load, for example, which might span several different distinct communities). Similarly, a new community paediatrician will often be allocated a 'patch' or geographical locality within which to base their activities.

Case Study

Karen Blackford has been appointed as a paediatrician with an interest in public health in a former mill town in the North of England called Milton. It is well known for its high unemployment rate and relatively large child population. There have been a number of high-profile cases in the area including two child deaths from abuse in the past three years and an outbreak of measles for the first time in 20 years. Children and young people who misuse drugs are over-represented compared to the norms for the region, and vandalism and car crime is high.

Karen decides that she would like to take a systematic approach to finding out about the child health problems in the area and convenes a meeting with a range of local professionals to discuss this project. Those attending include representatives from local primary care teams, the public health lead for children within Milton's primary care organization (i.e. PCT in England), and the designated nurse for child protection. They agree that there has been little emphasis on child health locally, and that few recent initiatives have addressed children's needs. This is partly due to competing national targets and priorities in adult health which have preoccupied service planners, and partly to the lack of a clear and united voice advocating for children in Milton. Karen suggests that a more co-ordinated approach should begin with a needs assessment.

Discussion at the meeting is recorded on flip charts and is later typed up and circulated to participants as a series of agreed actions and points to consider. The notes read as follows:

- Public health department to obtain available child health data.
- Need list of key people delivering services in the patch for Karen to meet: informants to be identified by GPs, community nurses, and local community development officer.
- Need to include other agencies—social services, education, Sure Start Children's Centres, police, youth offending team, voluntary sector, community leaders.
- Need to map current provision and possibilities (e.g. potential for community development work in Beechlands housing estate—family centre there run by National Children's Home).
- Community-based mental health services for children a particular problem.
- Any new interventions must meet needs identified by local community, must be sustainable and evidence-based, and must be evaluated.

Further discussion with the public health lead for children's services helps Karen to frame her approach in terms of a formal needs assessment, combining elements of both corporate and epidemiological approaches and of community participation (as described in Chapter 7). They set out the following framework:

Corporate needs assessment

- Stakeholder views—including young people and families, professionals from different agencies, and voluntary sector—about key health problems and interventions needed.

Epidemiological needs assessment

- Routine and other data on demography, morbidity, mortality of local child population.
- Information on current local services—health, social care, voluntary sector.
- Evidence of effectiveness, especially in relation to possible new services or developments.

Community participation

- Encourage wide range of local people to be involved in identifying problems and suggesting solutions.
- Be prepared to support local community in developing its own initiatives.

Child health data from routine data sources/local surveys

The data presented to Karen by the public health department are somewhat limited. Although there are good data on mortality, information on morbidity is sparse and is suspected to be unreliable and incomplete. Karen is particularly interested in information about child accidents and behavioural problems which are not available from routine sources. The data available is illustrated in Table 8.1.

Local health visiting and school nursing 'profile' data helps to fill in some of the gaps, and useful information is also obtained from other sources. The social services department is able to provide detailed data on looked-after children from its 'Quality Protects' returns and on children on the child protection register. The youth offending team has information on young people's involvement in crime; and the education department provides details of school exclusions, truancy, and attendance at special schools, including those for children with emotional and behavioural difficulties. The police have data on road traffic accidents involving children. Some GP practices, which have been involved in a pilot project to promote recording and accessibility of information on their computer system, are able to provide details of consultations and referrals for patients under 16. Karen also accesses online data on neighbourhood statistics to help build up a profile of the local area, especially in relation to deprivation. The Index of Multiple Deprivation scores for the four wards in Milton place them between the 3000th and 7000th most deprived wards out of 8414 in England and Wales, and the Child Poverty Index scores tell a similar story.

Table 8.1 Child health data from routine sources

Size and breakdown of child population under 15s	49,500
Births	3400 births per year
Proportion birth weight below 2.5 kg	7.4%
Black and ethnic minority	5%
Neonatal mortality rate	6 in 1000
Infant mortality rate	7.3 in 1000
Breast-feeding rate at birth	55%
Coverage of six-week check	95%
Child mortality and causes of death	20 per yr.—mainly prematurity, accidents, cancer, infection, and one case of non-acccidental injury in the last year
Teenage pregnancies	63 in 1000 women aged 14–19
Hospital out-patient consultation/A&E attendance	16% (varies from 3%–34% depending on local authority ward deprivation indices)
Immunization rate (completion of primary course)	87%
Immunization rate (MMR)	85%

Lack of appropriate health data is a common problem, and one of the tasks of a public-health oriented paediatrician is to identify information that is needed, what is available routinely, and what must be collected specifically. It is increasingly important for all health professionals to become familiar with child health information systems and data collection so as to inform their future development and improvement.

Discussion with key health professionals and local people

Over the course of several weeks, Karen meets a wide variety of people from the health sector, the local authority, and local voluntary organizations. They are listed in the box below.

Stakeholders in child health in Milton

- Health visitor representative on primary care organization (PCT) board.
- Chief Executive of primary care organization (PCT).
- Lead school nurse.
- Senior social worker for safeguarding children.
- Senior educational psychologist.
- Psychologist from child and mental health service.
- Other community paediatricians.
- Heads of Sure Start Childrens Centres and Extended Schools.
- Local Authority children's services lead.
- Parents who attend the Childrens Centre.
- Local councillor.
- Youth workers.
- Educational social workers.
- Heads of local schools.
- Director of local NCH (National Children's Homes) programme.

Karen wanted to meet children and young people to find out what they think about local services, and what they perceive as the key health and social problems they face. She is told of a study that has recently been completed by school nurses in the area, involving a series of workshops facilitated by a youth worker, to ascertain the views of children and young people on health issues. Karen is able to attend a follow-up focus group meeting at which some of the findings are discussed.

Some of the information provided by stakeholders is described below.

Health visitor Health visitors are trained to collect information on populations and have developed expertise in community profiling, making them an important resource in community diagnosis. Mandy covers one of the most deprived estates in the patch (Beechlands). The information she has obtained through community profiling enables her to identify the main problems in children's health locally, the strengths of the community, and which families are particularly high-risk. She considers that the main problems are in child behaviour and nutrition including breast feeding (for which little support is available), pedestrian accidents, and delayed speech and language development.

School nurse Liz is the school nurse for the largest of the local secondary schools. She has to cover several other schools and is conscious that she has insufficient time to meet the needs of the pupils adequately. She is aware that stress levels are high among young people and that there are many unresolved emotional and behavioural problems. A recent survey of behaviour and attitudes in local schools revealed much high-risk behaviour especially in relation to sexual health and drug and alcohol misuse.

GP Rajiv is a partner in a five-doctor practice that covers the same estate as Mandy. He is conscious of a poor understanding of health and disease among his patients and feels that local health services are not always appropriately used. There are many call-outs at night for minor complaints such as high temperature, upper respiratory infection, or crying in a baby. He reports a high level of smoking locally, examples of inadequate care of young children, excessive use of junk foods, and high rates of teenage pregnancy.

Parents The parents attending the family centre describe a different set of problems. These include difficulty in getting appointments to see a doctor, difficulty in understanding what the doctors say, lack of local play facilities for children, little local availability of fresh fruit and vegetables, poor public transport, and fear of letting children play outside because of 'problem families' in the neighbourhood.

Children and young people Stress over school pressure, community safety, lack of any play areas such as a skateboard park, and concerns about the lack of shops are all important issues for young people locally. Lack of job prospects, conflict with parents and teachers, and a failure to have their point of view taken into account exacerbate the situation for them. They don't feel local health services are accessible or appropriate to their needs and are reluctant to go to see the local GP about 'private health problems'. Nor would they know whom to consult over 'mental health' issues (such as eating disorders, anxiety and stress, and relationship problems.)

Social worker Mavis has worked in Milton for ten years and is despondent about the impact of budget cuts and difficulties in recruiting new staff, which have put increasing pressure on her team. She feels the needs of families and children are increasing all the time and that there is less scope to intervene except in the most serious cases, so that problems often get out of hand before they can be addressed. She is particularly worried about the parenting skills of very young mothers and the difficulty in providing adequate support to care leavers.

Chief Executive of primary care organization Although sympathetic to the needs of children in Milton, Sean's main concern is to bring the PCT into financial balance and to meet the many 'must-do' targets the government has set for the next few years—few of which concern children. He is keen to support initiatives mentioned in the NHS Plan such as 'Sure Start', universal neonatal hearing screening, breast-feeding, and parenting programmes, and to ensure that community staff employed by the PCT are working effectively. However little additional funding is available owing to the rapid growth of hospital budgets.

Karen also maps existing services, including the current work of the child health team in her patch (including health visitors and school and community nurses) and considers their suggestions about reprioritization. It is agreed that this will be discussed collectively at a later stage in the light of the needs assessment findings and evidence base. The public health lead searches the literature for evidence of effectiveness in relation to certain interventions that have been proposed.

A follow-up meeting is convened to present and discuss findings from the needs assessment process. Despite differences in perspective, clear priorities for child health emerge from the discussions with local stakeholders. These include a focus on children in different age groups: preschool children, younger school-age children, and teenagers.

Milton community diagnosis – key problems in child health

- ◆ *All children*: poverty and inequalities in health, community safety, parenting education and support, mental health.
- ◆ *Preschool children*: behaviour problems, delayed development, poor nutrition and low breastfeeding rates, low coverage of immunizations, availability of child care and nursery provision.
- ◆ *Primary school children*: accidents, nutrition, dental health, antisocial behaviour.
- ◆ *Teenagers*: nutrition, high-risk behaviour (drugs, alcohol, sexual health, accidents), stress and anxiety, deliquency.

Next steps

It is clear that the 'community diagnosis' requires an inter-agency approach over a long period of time, a re-evaluation of current services and work practices, and a clarity about the evidence base for improvement. Karen is conscious of the fact that, whilst there is no time like the present for assessing problems and scoping possible solutions, as a newcomer to the area, she needs to tread carefully at first in terms of action. It will be essential for her to spend time building the relationships which will be vital to sustained success in tackling the problems identified and to get a better understanding of 'how things work' locally. A measured and appropriate response is likely to be more effective than an attempt to solve every problem at once. She is also aware that many of the problems such as poverty and environmental degradation are outside the scope of her service, though the local authority has a responsibility in this direction, and councillors are part of the decision-making group.

Together with the primary care and public health leads, an inter-agency child health improvement team is developed with a wide membership, under the aegis of the primary care organization's public health department. The team recognizes that concerted action and the involvement of local people and professionals working together will be vital, and that the first step is to agree priority areas to focus on initially. As well as the most pressing problems identified by local stakeholders, these might include a couple of projects identified as 'early winners' likely to yield fairly swift results, and areas in which national targets have been set or which can benefit from specific funding streams. The PCT may be able to find non-recurrent funding for some short-term projects. The local Children and Young Persons Strategic Partnership Board, which is led by the Childrens Lead for the Local Authority, are informed of the health priorities and contribute to interagency training and development of the Childrens Centres staff.

It is agreed that three workshops will be held in different localities within the patch to discuss possible projects and developments. There will also be two workshops for children and young people, facilitated by experienced youth workers. The team agrees that the criteria for taking forward any new initiative in child health will be:

- Perceived importance in the eyes of local people
- Possible to monitor outcome
- Some evidence of effectiveness of the proposed action and therefore likelihood of success
- Sustainability
- Tackles structural issues (e.g. not just provision of information)
- Includes some element of parent empowerment

The workshops are successful and many specific areas for action are raised that reflect the concerns of local people, including play areas for children, nursery and child care provision, shopping facilities, and the negative impact of recent service cuts, especially in social services. It is agreed that councillors will take these concerns to the relevant local authority planning groups. The child health team also volunteer to take on an advocacy role in supporting parents such as the group that has already formed to lobby the transport and housing departments to improve road safety and ensure windows and railings are repaired on the local estate. The police representatives at the workshops agree to feed back community safety concerns and to discuss these further with local residents.

The topics of greatest importance for the community in relation to health service provision are children's behaviour problems, accident prevention, and adolescent health issues. The latter include access to services; drug, tobacco, and alcohol use; stress; sexual health issues; and relative lack of physical fitness. Proposals for action include:

- a 'Sure Start' Children's Centre bid with health facilities incorporated in the plans
- developing a 'healthy living' centre in Beechlands
- providing evidence-based parenting programmes based in the Children's Centre and schools
- starting a community-run nursery
- a needle exchange designed to be accessible to young people
- developing a 'BodyZone' scheme (outreach health information and advice centre) and breakfast club in local schools
- 'Healthy Schools' projects and the development of after-school clubs particularly around physical activity and also a school based peer counselling programme for emotional concerns

- a loan scheme for home safety equipment
- funding of community worker to help with initiating specific local projects.

Several of these will require considerable development work, which the child health improvement team agrees to consider. Karen and the public health lead will explore the time-scale for Sure Start scheme bids. Other individuals are invited to submit brief proposals for smaller projects which might be started with the help of the PCT's short-term funding: these include the breakfast club, community nursery, and safety equipment loan scheme. Increasing awareness of alternative sources of out-of-hours health advice, such as NHS Direct, was also felt to be important, and Karen agrees to seek the help of her community team in promoting this.

In developing new initiatives, time-scale and sustainability are all-important. Change does not come quickly and it is depressing to find that funding has run out after two or three years just as the benefits of an intervention are becoming apparent. Before starting a new project, there needs to be agreement about how it will be continued within mainstream resources once any special funding has been used up.

The developments proposed in Milton are likely to be too extensive to introduce all at once: several involve many steps that will require careful consideration and planning and, of course, the identification of funding, and each will need to be managed by someone who is able to take a global view of their aims. A phased development over a number of years is likely to be more effective and feasible. Appropriate public accountability is also vital to ensure a long-term commitment to sustaining change. However, the process of needs assessment has been successful in identifying some key problems and possible solutions, and has also been of benefit in developing relationships between different agencies, and between professionals and the community. Engaging local people and encouraging them to participate in the process has already helped to empower them and to tap into the considerable resources of the community. It will be important, however, not to raise unreasonable expectations and to ensure that momentum is sustained in order that disillusion does not follow.

In practice, public health projects often come in smaller and less comprehensive packages than this example suggests, so that the action needed is not quite so daunting. The remaining scenarios focus more closely on a number of specific problems and interventions.

Further reading

Alperstein, G. and Nossar, V. (1998) Key interventions for the health improvement of children and youth: a population based approach. *Ambulatory Child Health*; 4: 295–306.

Blair, M. (2000) Public health: Taking a population perspective on child health. *Archives of Disease in Childhood*; 83: 7–9.

Children and Young People's Unit (2001) *Learning to listen: Core principles for the involvement of children and young people.* CYPU, London.

Cook, J., Pechevis, M. and Waterston, T. (1995) Community diagnosis and participation. In *European textbook of social paediatrics* (B. Lindstrom and N. Spencer, eds.). Oxford University Press, Oxford.

Edmunds, S., Garratt, A., Haines, L., and Blair, M. (2005) Child Health Assessment at School
Entry (CHASE) Project: evaluation in ten London primary schools Child:Care, *Health and
Development;* **31**(2): 143–154.

Eisenstadt, N. (2002) Sure Start: Key principles and ethos. *Child care, health and development;*
28: 3–4.

Every Child Matters http://www.everychildmatters.gov.uk/

National Evaluation of Sure Start http://www.ness.bbk.ac.uk/

Sure Start website http://www.surestart.gov.uk/

Waterston, T. (1995) How can child health services contribute to a reduction in health
inequalities in childhood? In *Progress in community child health* (ed.Spencer, N.),
pp. 11–29. Churchill Livingstone.

Scenario B: Infant mental health promotion

Case Study

Sue Bailey, a health visitor at Burnwood Primary Care Trust, has been delighted to find that
programmes to support parenting are mushrooming all over her patch. Muchester City Council
appointed a Parenting Commissioner two years ago who led a successful bid to establish the city
as a Parenting Early Intervention Pathfinder site. For the past year, primary schools across the
city have been able to offer high risk families advice from a Parent Support Adviser and a place
on the Incredible Years Parenting programme. Attendance at this programme is increasing rapidly. Local Children's Centres now offer a programme suitable for all parents that helps with
relationships as well as behaviour management. These new initiatives mean Sue feels more supported when she encounters a family experiencing problems with children's behaviour. She
knows the one to one support she offers is valuable, but cut backs in health visiting services have
increased her case load, and she rarely feels able to offer enough. Back up from formal parenting
programmes gives her confidence that the mental health of children in her patch is being supported. She hears that colleagues in Child and Adolescent Mental Health Services are also pleased
and that their workload is becoming more manageable.

When she first saw the new government policy 'Every Parent Matters', Sue realized that
Muchester was ahead of other local authorities in terms of parenting support, but she also realized that Burnwood PCT wasn't playing its full part. Other PCTs had bid to become pilot sites for
the Nurse-Family Partnership programme, but she hadn't heard mention of this in Burnwood.

At the CPHVA (Community Practitioners and Health Visitors Association) conference last
year, Sue had heard several presentations about infant mental health. She'd learnt how easily the
infant's social and emotional brain is molded by early relationships, how much impact this
molding has in later life, and how difficult it can be to reverse its effects later in childhood. She
decided that before she retired she'd try to get the PCT to play its part in supporting infant
mental health. She'd never done anything like this before, but this was something she felt pas-
sionately about and she was determined to have a go. She knew the PCT was under financial
pressure and that preventive services were easy targets for cuts. She also knew a change of government at the next election might mean further reduction in NHS spending, but she was
cheered when a colleague told her a conservative-party commission had just produced a report
called 'Breakthrough Britain: The Next Generation', which focused on the importance of infant
mental health.

As she read around the subject Sue realized that policy making in relation to parenting had focused on antisocial behaviour and its consequences – educational failure, criminality and violence – rather than the health aspects, but she knew the PCT would be more impressed by the potential for improving health. She also realized that she had a lot to learn when it came to presenting a case to the PCT: – about interpreting the epidemiological literature, understanding the evidence base for interventions, and making an argument on health economic grounds. Looking around for training that might help, she found a Masters course in Public Health at a nearby university which offered a module on parenting and infant mental health. She decided to enroll for two modules and see how she got on. Her manager told her there were no funds to help pay for the course, but agreed to give Sue time off for studying.

Background

Infant mental health has only recently surfaced as a topic of concern to public health and child health services. It has its roots in psychotherapeutic disciplines and careful observational studies of mother-infant interaction. Large scale, robust, epidemiological and intervention studies are relatively new. These show that 60–70% of infants are securely attached at one year of age (see chapter 3). Follow up studies of infants who lack secure attachment show increased risk of mental health problems, including anxiety and depression, as well as behavioural problems, delinquency, problems with peer relationships, and educational difficulties. In reality, the picture is less black and white than this suggests, but the more severe the 'attachment security', the greater the problems in later life. Some degree of insensitivity, intrusiveness, and/ or hostility is common, and babies do not need perfect parenting to learn to self-soothe and recover from distress. However, parent-child relationship problems that fall short of creating 'attachment security' can still interfere with the development of mental wellbeing. Adults with mental wellbeing (see chapter 5) have *agency* (the belief that they can influence the world around them to ensure their needs are met); they can self-soothe and modulate emotional arousal; they have positive social skills and make trusting reciprocal relationships easily; they are curious, interested in learning and able to act autonomously. Population norms for these attributes of wellbeing are not yet available, but collectively they are uncommon. They are, however, important determinants of health; to quote the World Health Organisation, 'there is no health without mental health'. Agency is critical in health promotion, since people with agency are better able to change to healthier lifestyles. Modulation of emotional arousal is important for preventing both chronic anxiety and violence. Positive social skills are a more important determinant of future employment than academic performance and are critical in establishing supportive relationships.

Most studies have focused on the mother-baby relationship and two key attributes– sensitivity and attunement – have been shown to be important. Mothers who can read cues and respond appropriately can give their infants a secure base from which to grow and develop. Maternal hostility, intrusiveness, or emotional withdrawal are all damaging. Emotional security becomes embedded in the developing brain in such a way that infants who lack it respond to threat with an exaggerated stress response (see chapter 6). This contributes to the development of cardiovascular disease and impaired immunity as well as mental health problems in later life. The full impact of parenting in infancy on public health is not yet known because most studies follow children for at most a few years. Enough is however known to make a very strong case for intervention.

Long term outcomes

Most follow up studies focus on social outcomes like peer relationships and antisocial behaviour, but others have shown that problems with mother-infant relationships increase the risk of depression and poor physical health (e.g. cardiovascular risk factors) in later childhood. Parent-child relationships in adolescence can also have an impact on adult health – both mental and physical (see chapter 6). Many studies link the quality of very early relationships with the quality of relationships in later childhood. The extent of risk is related to the extent of problems with parenting. Abusive relationships increase risk greatly (up to 20 fold in some studies) whereas odds ratios for sub-optimal parenting are in the range 1.5–2.5; because of the large numbers of children involved, the population attributable risk from sub-optimal parenting is large.

Risk factors

Risk factors for poor parent-infant interaction include teenage parenting, history of abuse, parental mental illness (especially antenatal and postnatal depression), and parental drug and alcohol misuse (see chapter 3). Intergenerational transmission is common, with a high correlation between insecure attachment as an adult and parenting that creates insecure attachment in the child. Postnatal depression interrupts parent-infant communication; mothers can be frankly hostile towards the baby or emotionally withdrawn and neglectful. The father-infant relationship is also important and fathers' mental health (both before and after birth) also predicts poor child outcomes.

Poverty and social deprivation are also risk factors, but here the story is more complicated and most evidence comes from studies of relationships in early and mid-childhood. Whilst parenting is socially patterned, there is more variation within social groups than between them, and path analyses suggest that poverty influences child outcomes mainly through its effect on parental mental health, parental relationship quality, and parenting. When good parenting can be maintained in the face of deprivation, children are protected from many of its damaging effects. One study showed maternal mental health to be a much more important determinant than poverty. In particular, parenting did not improve in families whose level of social deprivation reduced.

What works?

Several systematic reviews have recently been undertaken – one for the English Department of Health. These reviews collate and assess the available evidence from trials and reviews. They cover interventions ranging from intensive long-term parent-infant psychotherapeutic approaches to universal approaches such as distributing magazines and DVDs. The greater the problems with the parent-infant relationship, the more intense the intervention needs to be.

Universal services:

- The Brazelton Neonatal Behavioural Scale, administered by midwives or health visitors, helps parents recognize their infant's abilities and interpret cues
- DVDs, television programmes, books and newsletters like Baby Express and the Social Baby DVD are beneficial in informing parents about infant mental health matters
- Soft infant carriers and kangaroo care are low cost interventions for which the evidence base is reasonable – the latter has mostly been used in the developing world
- Infant massage supports the development of sensitivity in some mother-infant pairs
- Group based programmes like PIPPIN which develop parents' emotional literacy and sensitivity to babies' needs increase attunement and sensitivity in controlled trials.
- Some programmes have been trialled with fathers as well as mothers and can be offered antenatally as well as postnatally

High risk targeted programmes:

- Holistic home visiting programmes which aim to improve the parent-infant relationship (exemplified by The Family Nurse Partnership programme) improve outcomes for the infants of teenage parents. Programmes delivered by nurses work better than those delivered by paraprofessionals. Some programmes require weekly home visiting for up to two years.
- Mellow Parenting is an effective group based programme for families where abuse is an issue. One version of this programme is designed for parents of infants.
- Parent-infant psychotherapy is useful for severe relationship problems and may also need to be offered intensively and long term.
- Interaction guidance is effective and may be used in home visiting and psychotherapeutic sessions. Parents are videoed with their infants and later watch the video with a skilled psychotherapist, who reflects with the parent on the baby's interactions and the parents' affect and responses.
- Both cognitive therapy and psychotherapy reduce the severity of postnatal depression. However, improved maternal outcomes do not seem to change maternal-infant interaction or infant outcomes (though interaction guidance may be useful for depressed mothers).
- Social support programmes provided by volunteers can also be useful in subclinical post-natal depression but not in clinical depression.
- Parenting under Pressure is one of the few programmes which shows improved parenting in families where parents abuse drugs or alcohol.

Delivery

The literature is clear that practitioners need to focus on what the parent can do and build from there. Reflective approaches including video observation and role modelling are valuable. Home-based practice using achievable steps is empowering. Sensitivity and non-judgemental attitudes are essential, and building trust can take a long time where parents had a damaging childhood themselves. Training in these skills is offered by Infant Mental Health Masters courses, the Solihull Approach and the Family Nurse Partnership Programme.

Drop out from parenting programmes is not uncommon. Practical support (free transport and meals, crèche care) increases engagement in centre-based programmes.

Who are the stakeholders?

The PCT Board is the primary stakeholder. To convince the Board, Sue needs the Manager of the Health Visiting Service, the Director of Public Health and the Chief Executive on her side. Paediatricians, midwives and health visitors are potentially important allies, and Child and Adult Psychiatrists have a stake as key service providers when problems arise. The Mental Health Trust might be persuaded to offer financial support as a way of implementing Standard 1 of the Mental Health NSF or the New Horizons framework, which will supercede it. As the only organization with universal access to families with newborns, the PCT has to be the provider of infant mental health services. However, the County Council Social Services and Education Departments have a stake because of the childhood outcomes of infant mental health problems. The Parenting Commissioner is likely to be a staunch ally.

The support of these stakeholders could be engaged through the Joint Planning Process. National voluntary organizations like the Association for Infant Mental Health might provide resources and support in making the case. Local voluntary organizations offering infant mental health and parent support services in the area might also help.

An approach

Sue attends her Masters course modules and gains agreement that her written projects can focus on building the case for infant mental health services – thus enlisting the support of the academics teaching her. She writes a strong, well-referenced case which considers the relative importance of universal and targeted approaches. Most of the evidence she discovers favours providing both, because universal programmes reduce stigma and increase access to those with more severe needs. Sue realises that universal approaches will need to be low key in order to be affordable. She unearths a report on the health economics of parenting support, which shows that whilst these programmes are costly, the savings over the long term are likely to be substantial.

Sue proposes including two sessions on infant communication in routine antenatal classes providing all new parents with a DVD about parent-infant relationships and normal infant communication and starting an age-paced parenting newsletter for families with newborns. She also proposes home visiting for high risk families, including teenage mothers and parents who have been in care as children. She identifies several local health visitors trained in the Solihull Approach who might undertake further training in the Family Nurse Partnership Model. She makes the case for local psychologists and psychotherapists to receive training in interaction guidance as a resource for parents with clinical postnatal depression and others identified as needing this approach. The Director of Public Health helps her with costing these new services. Sue realises this plan leaves out much that could be done, but she knows resources are limited and feels this constitutes a very good start. Sue sends her proposal to her manager, who agrees to take it to the PCT Executive Board. The CEO puts the paper on the agenda for the Joint Strategy Group with the County Council.

Meanwhile the local Parenting Commissioner has been very supportive. She has put Sue in touch with a local charity which has had to withdraw its infant mental health services through lack of funding. The charity uses Sue's paper to lobby county councilors.

Sue has also met the Clinical Lead for Paediatrics and spoken to health visiting and midwifery colleagues. Much to her surprise she received a measure of support from both.

At the Joint Strategy meeting with the County Council Sue's paper was well received and councilors who had been lobbied spoke in its favour. However, there was passionate opposition from a Labour councilor who was angry that mothers were being blamed for what she described as the sins of society. How could mothers who were trying to make ends meet on a low income have time for such things? Their first priority was to put food on the table. It was much more important, she argued, to give these mothers access to good quality daycare, which had been shown to be a cost-effective way of making a difference.

Fortunately one of the councilors had been briefed by the charity, who had anticipated this argument. He cited research showing that daycare, especially in the first year of life, was almost always less good for the infant than parental care at home. He also quoted evidence that parental relationships were critically important even for children in daycare. Although the vote was close the council agreed to support the proposal and explore Joint Funding for the new service.

At the PCT board, antagonistic arguments were raised by a local GP whose three children had all been in daycare from the age of three months. Her arguments were so forceful that the plan was not approved at this meeting. However, by this stage the CEO was convinced of its benefits, and asked the Director of Public Health to look again at the evidence. Six months later the DPH's paper was accepted by the PCT and a five year plan was drawn up to develop and fund the services. The DPH also recommended setting aside a small sum for evaluation. Sue knew her course tutors might be interested in tendering for the evaluation.

All this had taken Sue two years of hard work and her retirement was creeping closer. She looked forward to that moment, feeling satisfied that what she had set in motion would make a real difference to the families her colleagues would be supporting in the future.

Further reading

Barlow, J., Schrader McMillan, A., Kirkpatrick, S., Ghate, D., Smith, M., and Barnes, J. (2008) Health-led parenting interventions in Pregnancy and Early Years Research report Department for Children, Schools and Families **RW** 070.

Department for Children, Schools and Families (2007) The Child Health Promotion Programme: Pregnancy and the first five years of life DH Publications. DfES Publications, Nottingham.

Centre for Social Justice. (2008) Breakthrough Britain, The Next Generation: a report from the Early Years Commission. Centre for Social Justice, London.

Cost Benefit Analysis of Interventions with Parents. (2008) Economics Research Report DCSF RW008. London.

HM Government (2007) Every Parent Matters DCSF.

Rees, C. (2007) Childhood Attachment. *British Journal of General Practice*; **57**(544): 920–922.

Repetti, R.I., Taylor, S.E., and Seeman, T.E. (2002) Risky Families: Family Social Environment and mental and physical health of offspring. *Psychological Review*; **128**: 330–336.

Sroufe, A. (1996) *Emotional development*. Cambridge University Press, New York.

Social Justice Policy Group (2007) Breakthrough Britain. http://www.centreforsocialjustice

Stewart-Brown, S., and Shaw, R. (2004) The roots of social capital: relationships in the home during childhood and health in later life. In *Social Capital for Health: issues of definition, measurement and links to health*. (Eds. Morgan, A. and Swann, C.) Health Development Agency, London http://www.nice.org.uk/nicemedia/documents/socialcapital_issues.pdf.

Waylen, A., Stallard, N. and. Stewart-Brown, S. (2008) Parenting and social inequalities in health in mid-childhood: a longitudinal study. *European Journal of Public Health*; **18**(3): 300–305. doi:10.1093/eurpub/ckm131

Waterston, T., Welsh, B., Keane, B., et al. (2009) Improving Early Relationships: A Randomized, Controlled Trial of an Age-Paced Parenting Newsletter. *Pediatrics;* **123**: 241–247.

Weich, S., Patterson, J., Shaw, R., and Stewart-Brown, S. (2009) Family Relationships in Childhood and Common Psychiatric Disorders in Later Life: Systematic Review of Prospective Studies. *British Journal of Psychiatry;* **194**: 392–398.

Van Doesum, KTM, et al. (2008) A randomised controlled trial of an home-visiting intervention aimed at preventing relationship problems in depressed mother and their infants. *Child Development*; **79**: 547–561.

Scenario C: Health promotion directed at reducing motor vehicle accidents involving school-age children

Case Study

Mr James, orthopaedic surgeon at St Stephen's Children's Hospital, is carrying out his ward round on a Monday morning following the weekend 'take'. On this occasion, he is accompanied by Stephen Charnley, the community paediatric trainee who has been attached to the firm. He notices that among the children on the ward who have fractures of the long bones, two live on the same street. On further enquiry, he establishes that this is one of the worst roads in the town for road traffic volume and speeding. He remembers reading in the local paper that there have been three deaths in the past year of young children crossing this road.

Background

Childhood accidents are the top cause of death in children and are highly amenable to prevention. The chief cause of death is collision between a motor vehicle and a child pedestrian or cyclist, where the degree of trauma to the child is very great. Motor traffic continues to increase in the UK, and there is insufficient protection for children.

What works?

There is considerable scope for prevention. The chief factors causing motor vehicle accidents (in which there is a large social class variation) are children playing on the streets, the lack of safe play areas – especially in areas of high social deprivation, high car speeds in residential neighbourhoods, lack of separation of cyclists, cars, and pedestrians, and the limited use of cycle helmets. Measures which can be taken to reduce risk are mainly outside the scope of the health sector. There is considerable evidence of the benefit of traffic calming, both in terms of injury reduction and in improving neighbourhood interaction (Fig. 8.1).

Other measures include promoting the use of cycle helmets, the introduction of more cycle paths, and traffic reduction policies. The latter would improve children's health in many ways, including the reduction of particulate emissions associated with respiratory infections and asthma. Evidence is building that as a result of increasing car transport of children, there is a reduction in physical fitness as a direct result of less walking or cycling opportunity.

This field is one of the most important for child health promotion, since accidents are such a high-ranking cause of death and disability, and the means of preventing them are well known. Other countries have demonstrated that success is possible. There is, however, a big question of political will – hence the important role of advocacy in this area. Paediatricians and public health practitioners were successful in lobbying for child-proof containers and need to be equally forceful in relation to leglislation on traffic reduction and the separation of cyclists from cars.

Evidence-based approaches to child injury prevention

Legislation and enforcement e.g. childcare products, building construction, health and safety in child care settings and schools.

Product modification e.g. child resistant containers for poisonous substances, redesign of wood-burning stoves.

Environmental modification e.g. road traffic calming schemes especially around schools and kindergartens, physical separation of different types of road user.

Supportive home visits focusing on hazard identification and avoidance.

Safety devices e.g. cycle helmets and smoke detectors.

Education, skills and behaviour – education programmes need to be combined with other strategies above to achieve behaviour change.

Emergency medical care improving prehospital and hospital care, e.g. staff training, standardized equipment.

(WHO 2008)

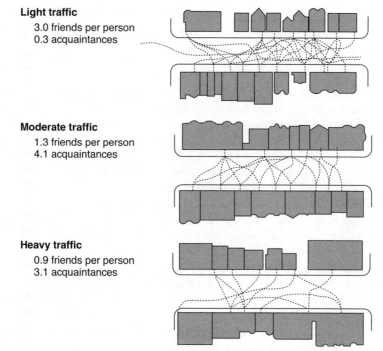

Light traffic
3.0 friends per person
0.3 acquaintances

Moderate traffic
1.3 friends per person
4.1 acquaintances

Heavy traffic
0.9 friends per person
3.1 acquaintances

Fig. 8.1 Diagram of the effects of road traffic density on social interaction. Source: Adapted from Appleyard D, Lintell M. The environmental quality of city streets: the residents' viewpoint. *American Inst of Planners Journal* 1972; 38: 84–101. Reprinted by permission of Taylor & Francis Group.

Health promotion is effective at both national and local levels. Nationally, measures might include: reduction of traffic speeds in built-up areas; greater encouragement of cycle lanes; legislation on wearing cycle helmets, and traffic reduction legislation. At regional or district level, measures might include promotion of 'Safe Routes to School', greater creation of home zones and 20 mph limits, local school and community schemes to promote cycle helmets, local council traffic calming schemes in all residential neighbourhoods, and local congestion charging.

Who are the stakeholders?

Those with an interest include paediatricians, A&E consultants, the public health department, school nurses, the health promotion unit; transport and road safety departments in the local authority, local councillors, and parents and school governors (especially in relation to Sustrans supported Safe Routes to School).

An approach

Stephen is aware that this can be a difficult issue to make progress on despite its importance. He talks first to the local child public health lead in the Primary Care Trust (Ms Dorothy Kenny, a former health visitor manager with a higher degree in public health) who has a special interest in this area. Dorothy is a strong supporter of Sustrans, an organization whose remit is sustainable transport and which is aiming to develop 'Safe Routes to School'. She is aware of other groups active in this area including the Campaign for Better Transport (working to reduce traffic and make roads more people friendly) and the National Children's Bureau initiative to support home zones. The local Child Accident Prevention Group has been dormant for some time, and Dorothy and Stephen decide that it would be useful to re-invigorate the group and use it as a focus for lobbying for safe routes to school, using the example of the two boys in hospital as the 'trigger'. The street the boys live on is part of a disadvantaged area that has already been targeted by the local Children and Young Persons Strategic Partnership (CYPSP) so that inter-agency networks have already been established locally and form the basis for the subsequent campaign.

The local school takes an active role by placing a highly visible black disc, 30 cm wide, on the nearest lamp post, for every serious accident which occurs within a half mile radius. The discs are a constant reminder to local people (and policy makers) of the dangers of traffic in the area. Using a small grant from the local authority, the school purchases high-quality cycle helmets in bulk to be sold to parents at cost. The home-school association become involved in developing a Safer Routes to School proposal and bidding for funding. The scheme is fronted by a local celebrity who has severe spinal injuries from a road traffic incident in her childhood and is wheelchair bound. The plan is to introduce cycle training and maintenance for senior pupils and build a new secure bike shed in the school grounds.

The Child Accident Prevention Group agree to meet regularly to review progress and to look at other injury prevention initiatives. It is agreed that Mr James will monitor injury rates using a monthly print-out of all fractures of the long bones and head injuries treated in the hospital. He agrees to display this in the A&E department as a map of accident 'hot spots' and to encourage hospital staff to take an active role in secondary prevention.

This is an example which originated in a hospital setting and was followed up as an active prevention outreach. Severe injuries are only the tip of the iceberg of morbidity associated with road traffic accidents but a useful place to start because of the heavy burden in terms of loss of function and time off school.

Further reading

Department of Health (2002) *Preventing accidental injury—priorities for action.* Stationery Office, London.

Duperrex, O., Roberts, I., and Bunn, F. (2002) *Safety education of pedestrians for injury prevention (Cochrane Review). The Cochrane Library, Issue* 4. Update Software, Oxford.

Towner, E., Dowswell, T., Mackereth, C., and Jarvis, S. (2001) *What works in preventing unintentional injuries in children and young adolescents? An updated systematic review.* Health Development Agency, London. http://www.sustrans.org.uk/

Safe Routes to school http://www.sustrans.org.uk/default.asp?sID=1094226578046

http://www.bettertransport.org.uk/ Accident Prevention Amongst Children and Young People A Priority Review DH, DT, DCSF. 2009.

Kendrick, D., Barlow, J., Hampshire, A., Polnay, L., Stewart-Brown, S., Parenting interventions for the prevention of unintentional injuries in childhood. *Cochrane Database of Systematic Reviews.* 2007, Issue **4**.

World Report on Child Injury Prevention Geneva, World Health Organisation, 2008.

Scenario D: Promotion of breast-feeding

Case study

Hilda Benson, a health visitor in a depressed Midlands town, in what was formerly a thriving coal-mining area, has a particular interest in breast-feeding. She has seen a recent government report which shows a modest increase in breast-feeding rates at birth nationally over the last few years, but with a more rapid falling-off over the first few weeks of life than in the past. She suspects from her own experience, and from talking to other health visitors in the area, that breast-feeding initiation rates locally are considerably lower than the national average of 69%. Hilda has recently been on a course which re-emphasized the value of breast-feeding and suggested ways in which health professionals can promote breast-feeding in their patch, and—fired with enthusiasm—she decides she wants to do something about this issue.

Background

Breast-feeding is known to confer substantial benefits on both mother and baby. Hilda's notes from her recent refresher course contain the following list:

Benefits of breast-feeding

Infant	Mother
Improved nutrition	Convenience and cost
Fewer gastrointestinal infections	No risk of errors in making up bottles
Fewer respiratory infections	Quicker weight loss after pregnancy
Less risk of atopic eczema, asthma, etc.	Decreased risk of breast and ovarian cancer
Lower rates of obesity, diabetes, and coronary heart disease in later life	
Possible decrease in risk of sudden infant death	
Possible increase in IQ	

Hilda knows that the World Health Organisation recommends exclusive breast-feeding for the first six months, and that the UK government supports this and wants local action to promote breast-feeding. She is aware that there is a large social class divide in breast-feeding prevalence (although the most recent government report shows a greater increase in lower social classes than higher, which is encouraging). She also knows that rates vary by ethnic group, with rates as high as 95% among mothers of African and Caribbean origin, and 87% among Asian mothers, with the white population trailing behind.

Hilda is aware that the La Leche League is active in neighbouring towns. This is a voluntary organization which supports breast-feeding by befriending new mothers and offering practical advice and emotional support. There are no La Leche groups operating in her town, and little promotion of breast-feeding in the local media. The reasons for low breast-feeding rates are thought to include cultural attitudes, lack of direct contact with breast-feeding mothers, limited knowledge of the benefits of breast-feeding, and heavy media promotion of bottle-feeding. She has been told of the evidence that certain measures to support breast-feeding—such as improving mother-infant contact immediately after birth and rooming-in mother and baby together in the post-natal ward—can be beneficial, and that NICE (the English National Institute for Health and Clinical Excellence) has recently published a review on the promotion of breastfeeding initiation. Hilda has heard of UNICEF's 'Baby friendly criteria', designed to encourage hospitals to develop policies which favour breast-feeding, but she doesn't think the local maternity unit has adopted them.

UNICEF's baby friendly hospital criteria: ten steps

1 Have a written policy that is routinely communicated to all health care staff

2 Train all health care staff in skills necessary to implement the policy

3 Inform all pregnant women about the benefits and management of breast-feeding

4 Help mothers to initiate breast-feeding within half an hour of birth

5 Show mothers how to breast-feed and how to maintain lactation even if they should be separated from their infants

6 Give newborn infants no food or drink other than breast milk, unless medically indicated

7 Practise rooming-in, allowing mothers and infants to remain together 24 hours a day

8 Encourage breast-feeding on demand

9 Give no artificial teats or pacifiers to breast-feeding infants

10 Foster the establishment of breast-feeding support groups and refer mothers to them on discharge from hospital

---

Who are the stakeholders?

Paediatricians, hospital and community midwives, health visitors, GPs, Director of Public Health and Director of Health Improvement in the PCT, hospital trust chief executives, Sure Start Children's Centres, voluntary and community groups.

An approach

Hilda writes a short paper setting out the benefits of promoting breast-feeding locally. She points out that there is a strong likelihood of health gain if more mothers breast-feed, particularly through the reduction of enteric and respiratory infections, which are known causes of mortality and morbidity in infancy. There will also be longer-term benefits for both mothers and babies, and there may be benefits to parent–child interaction. She includes what is known about the effectiveness of promoting breast-feeding, and sets out a few ideas for action locally.

Initially, Hilda takes the paper to the health visitors' professional forum, where there is widespread support for the idea of a local breast-feeding project. The health visitor representative on the Primary Care Trust Board agrees to take the paper to a board meeting and to pass it on to the Director of Health Improvement.

Some weeks later, Hilda hears that the PCT has agreed to make this a priority area for health promotion locally and has allocated a small amount of money for development work. Hilda agrees to chair the group, which is asked to submit a project plan. She initially recruits the following people to help her:

- a GP from the local practice who has an interest in maternal and child health
- a representative from the local branch of the National Childbirth Trust, whom she has discovered is very supportive of an initiative to increase breast-feeding. She will also liaise with La Leche League, which has no branch in the area.
- a community midwife
- a hospital children's health care assistant (HCA) who often supports infant feeding on the children's wards
- a specialist registrar in public health from the PCT.

At the first meeting of this group, it is agreed that the main difficulty in developing health promotion measures for breast-feeding is the large number of potential areas for action, and the limited evidence of effectiveness of any particular intervention. There is a clear need for more research, but little likelihood of progress in time to help this project. Evaluation of any interventions agreed by the task group will be important.

It turns out that the public health registrar has recently completed a local survey of breast-feeding, seeking information on breast-feeding prevalence at birth and six weeks, any advice which mothers were offered from different sources, and users' views about local services including the support available from midwives, health visitors, and others. The results showed that the local prevalence of breast-feeding is 60% at birth and 30% at six weeks, and that the main sources of advice cited were friends, female relatives, and the media, with midwives and health visitors rated much lower. A sizeable proportion of women felt local breast-feeding support services were inadequate and might have helped them continue breast-feeding for longer. However, another sizeable proportion said they had never considered breast-feeding. He also found out that there were on average, 6–8 admissions per month for dehydration and prolonged jaundice in infants who had failed to establish breastfeeding adequately in the area.

The group agrees that they should develop proposals both for health promotion interventions to increase the initial uptake of breast-feeding, and for improving support services to help breast-feeding mothers continue for longer. They agree to consider action at national, local, and individual level, since there is always scope for advocacy and lobbying to affect higher-level policy. After a brainstorming session, the group produces a long list of possibilities (see Table 8.2).

Table 8.2 Breast-feeding promotion initiatives

National level

- Strategic and policy support for breast-feeding
- Positive media advertising of breast-feeding and better information for parents on its benefits
- Control of advertising of bottle-feeding
- Longer statutory maternity leave
- Guidelines for training of health professionals
- Promotion of guidelines for 'Baby Friendly' hospitals and communities
- Legislation to protect mothers' rights to breast-feed in public places
- More routine data collection on prevalence

Local level

- Local media advertising in support of breast-feeding
- Encourage adoption of 'Baby Friendly' criteria
- Staff training for all midwives, health visitors, and GPs—breast-feeding lead for each patch?
- Breast-feeding support services, including drop-in clinics, outreach, possibly helpline
- Work closely with local voluntary organizations including NCT and La Leche League
- Develop peer support network / local breast-feeding champions
- Encourage facilities for breast-feeding locally, in restaurants, shops etc.—'Baby Friendly' awards for local businesses?
- Focus on hard-to-reach groups and those with low prevalence e.g. teenage mothers, lower socio-economic groups
- Link to Personal, Social and Health Education (PHSE) classes in local schools, youth clubs, etc. to educate young people about benefits of breast-feeding
- Work with fathers—believed to be a key influence
- Continuing/wider data collection on prevalence of breast-feeding

Individual level

- Advice and information on benefits of breast-feeding
- Support from professionals and peers for those initiating breast-feeding
- Support/equipment for those returning to work e.g. breast pumps

Programme of action

Following their discussions, the group agrees the following preliminary programme of action:

- Appointment of co-ordinator for the project, using development money
- District-wide audit of data collection and agreed standards for data collection at different ages
- Encouragement of maternity hospital to apply for 'Baby Friendly' status
- Organization of training workshops for health professionals (midwives, health visitors, GPs) on how to support breast-feeding
- Local advertising (e.g. on buses) on benefits of breast-feeding
- Introduction and evaluation of peer counselling schemes
- Links with NHS Direct to co-ordinate advice on breast-feeding support and management
- Work with PCTs on developing community 'Baby Friendly' initiative
- Link to 'Healthy Schools' scheme to explore possibility of including breast-feeding in the PHSE syllabus
- Link to teenage pregnancy task group to ensure support and advice to teenage mothers on breast-feeding
- Link to local Chamber of Commerce to explore 'Baby Friendly' businesses

This proposed work programme is submitted to the PCT and Director of Public Health for approval. Meanwhile, different members of the group agree to explore possible costs and resources for each proposal.

The task group may need to expand to include further representatives from this list, and will certainly need to keep them informed of action and progress. It is agreed that the group should produce a newsletter containing information on the benefits and prevalence of breast-feeding and updates on local action to promote it. This newsletter could be widely circulated to professionals and the public. Sponsorship for this will be sought from a local business. It is clear that there is a long way to go, but the group has made a good start in defining a framework for action.

Further reading

Cattaneo, A. and Buzzetti, R. (2001) Effects on rates of breast feeding of training for the Baby Friendly Hospital Initiative. *BMJ*; **323**: 1358–62.

Declercq, E., Labbok, M., Sakala, C., and O'Hara, M. (2009) Hospital Practices and Women's Likelihood of Fulfilling Their Intention to Exclusively Breastfeed. *American Journal of Public Health*; **99**: 929–935.

Dennis, C.L., Hodnett, E., Gallop, R., and Chalmers, B. (2002) The effect of peer support on breast-feeding duration among primiparous women: a randomized controlled trial. *Canadian Medical Association Journal*; **166**: 21–8.

Fairbank, L., O'Meara, S., Renfrew, M.J., Woolridge, M., Sowden, A.J., and Lister-Sharp, D. (2000) A systematic review to evaluate the effectiveness of interventions to promote breast feeding. *Health Technology Assessment*; **4**: (25).

Hamlyn, B., Brooker, S., Oleinikova, K., and Wands, S. (2002) *Infant feeding 2000*. The Stationery Office, London.

Hoddinot, P. and Pill, R. (1999) Qualitative study of decisions about infant feeding among mothers in the east end of London. *BMJ*; **318**: 30–4.

Nicoll, A. and Williams, A. (2002) Breast feeding. *Archives of Disease in Childhood*; **87**: 91–2.

National Institute for Clinical Excellence (NICE). (2006) Promotion of breastfeeding initiation and duration: Evidence into practice briefing.

Saadeh, R., and Akre, J. (1996) Ten steps to successful breastfeeding: a summary of the rationale and scientific evidence. *Birth*; **23**: 154–60.

Sikorski, J., and Renfrew, M.J. (2000) Support for breastfeeding mothers. *Cochrane Database of Systematic Reviews*. CD001141.http://www.babyfriendly.org.uk/

Scenario E: Child health surveillance programme – delay in diagnoses

Case Study

The District Child Health Promotion Co-ordinator (DHPC), Daniel Tan, has recently been involved in a medico-legal case involving a seven-year-old boy whose parents are suing the GP for late diagnosis of their son's testicular maldescent, resulting in the child having one testis much smaller than the other. This followed on closely from another medico-legal case where a child with phenylketonuria (PKU) had been diagnosed late, at the age of 18 months. These cases have occurred despite the fact that there is a district policy on early referral of undescended testes and PKU is a condition which is specifically screened for in the neonatal period. Daniel wants to look into these cases and explore the reasons for the late diagnoses.

Background

Most countries have developed preventive programmes for maternal and child health as a response to poor infant mortality figures or suboptimal child health status. To a greater or lesser extent these are published as national policies, albeit with regional variations. The basic elements are immunization, health education, and screening tests. Table 8.3 and 8.4 shows the current UK programme for screening and immunizations: the US equivalent is the Bright Futures programme. UK policy is based on a rigorous critical review of the international literature by a multiprofessional working group. In 2009, the programme was reviewed and published as the Healthy Child Programme (Fig 8.2).

In the UK, delivery of the programme is based in primary care, mainly in general practice and partly in community health clinics. The personnel involved often work in several different settings and are employed by different authorities.

Following the 1990 NHS reforms, preschool child health surveillance (CHS) was highlighted as an area for increased involvement of GPs. Targets were set for immuniza tion rates, with different payment rates conditional on reaching 70% or 90% coverage. In addition, a list of practices wishing to carry out CHS was established, which was held

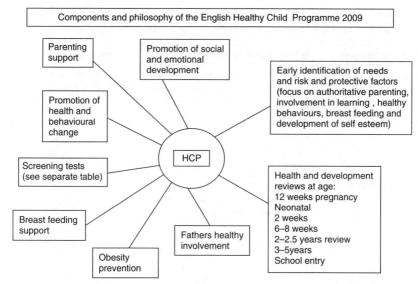

Fig. 8.2 Different components of the Health Child Programme philosophy.

Table 8.3 Summary of screening procedures in children under five recommended in the 2008 English Health Promotion Programme

Antenatal	Biochemical screening for Down syndrome Fetal anomaly ultrasonography
Birth	Full physical examination Newborn hearing screen by otoacoustic emissions (OAE)
72 hours	Cardiovascular screen, developmental dysplasia, risk babies to have ultrasonography Eyes Tests(boys) General examination and matters of parental concern
5–8 days	Bloodspot screening – hypothyroidism, phenylketonuria, cystic fibrosis, medium chain acyl-COa dehydrogenase deficiency, haemoglobinopathies
6–8 weeks	Physical examination cardiac, developmental dysplasia of the hips, eyes, testes (boys) general examination and matters of concern
By 5 years	Preschool hearing screen Visual impairment screen by orthoptist led service Height and weight as part of national growth public health surveillance programme
Growth monitoring carried out in response to parental or professional concers	

Table 8.4 Routine childhood immunisation programme UK as of 2009. Each vaccination is given as a single injection into the muscle of the thigh or upper arm

When to immunise	Diseases protected against	Vaccine given
Two months old	Diphtheria, tetanus, pertussis (whooping cough), polio and Haemophilus influenzae type b (Hib) Pneumococcal infection	DTaP/IPV/Hib and Pneumococcal conjugate vaccine (PCV)
Three months old	Diphtheria, tetanus, pertussis (whooping cough), polio and Haemophilus influenzae type b (Hib) Meningitis C (meningococcal group C)	DTaP/IPV/Hib and MenC
Four months old	Diphtheria, tetanus, pertussis (whooping cough), polio and Haemophilus influenzae type b (Hib) Meningitis C (meningococcal group C) Pneumococcal infection	DTaP/IPV/Hib and MenC and PCV
Around 12 months	*Haemophilus influenza* type b (Hib) and meningitis C	Hib/MenC
Around 13 months	Measles, mumps and rubella (German measles) Pneumococcal infection	MMR and PCV
Three years and four months or soon after	Diphtheria, tetanus, pertussis and polio Measles, mumps and rubella	DTaP/IPV or dTaP/IPV and MMR
Girls aged 12 to 13 years	Cervical cancer caused by human papillomavirus types 16 and 18	HPV*
13 to 18 years old	Tetanus, diphtheria and polio	Td/IPV

by the employing authority at the time (Family Health Services Association—FHSA). In order to be eligible for inclusion on the 'list', GPs had to establish they had sufficient competence either by holding appropriate postgraduate qualifications or by attendance at special training courses.

The professionals involved include:

◆ midwives (hospital and community)

◆ health visitors

◆ GPs

◆ community paediatricians

◆ school nurses

◆ clerical staff

◆ child health information system manager

Both PKU and undescended testes are relatively low prevalence conditions, as are the other key conditions for which screening is recommended: hypothyroidism, hip dysplasia, sensorineural hearing loss, and amblyopia. The performance of screening tests for these conditions have been shown, in a number of studies, to be very variable, especially for the physical and sensory impairment items. The Guthrie heel prick biochemical test (which involves taking a few drops of blood from babies on the seventh day of life, once feeding has been established, and sending it to a reference laboratory on a special piece of absorbent card to be tested for PKU and hypothyroidism) is effective. However, studies have shown that the programme as a whole can be problematic unless there is good flow of information between clinicians and laboratories. Simple things such as inadequate sampling technique, postal loss or delay, or mis-identification of infants through frequent name changes can lead to a potential catastrophe for the child and family. In the US, the identification of a new case of congenital hypothyroidism is considered a medical emergency.

Although primary care health professionals are the key target audience for delivery of this programme, there is good evidence demonstrating the effectiveness of parents in identifying a number of developmental and sensory impairments.

The District Child Health Promotion Co-ordinator (DCHPC) is responsible for setting up a multidisciplinary group to oversee the programme as a whole and monitor its quality as set out in the lastest guidance for commissioners of children's services. The functions of such a group are listed in the box below.

Functions of the District Child Health Promotion Co-ordinating (DCHPC) Group

1   To share ownership of the programme and to develop agreed written aims, objectives, referral guidelines, administrative processes, and training standards

2   To develop quality standards for provision of child health surveillance in primary care and schools and methods for monitoring these

3   To ensure equitable delivery of the programme and that 'hard to reach' children and those 'looked after' by the local authority are not missed by the universal programme.

4   To introduce and co-ordinate new programmes and alterations to the existing programme

5   To establish, develop, and maintain information systems

6   To facilitate consultation with parents, children, and voluntary groups in the planning and implementation of the programme

Who are the stakeholders?

Midwives and health visitors have a major involvement in ensuring that the screening tests are carried out, but feel that they receive little information about coverage and find out about 'abnormal' findings in an unreliable and often untimely manner. Other key individuals who are involved in the child health screening activities are the child health computer clerk and administrator of the child health system, the pathology laboratory staff, and clinic nurses.

At secondary (and tertiary) care level there are paediatricians with a special interest in endocrinology and metabolic conditions and paediatric surgeons.

Parents of young children nearly all receive a personal child health record (PCHR) which highlights the various components of the child health surveillance programme along with section for professionals to record their findings. The PCHR has helped to empower parents and demystify the process of preventive care. Increasingly, children of school age are being issued with their own records to keep along with the early years' pages. This record is thus the basis of the adult patient-held health record of the future.

An approach

There is a local evidence-based policy document, adapted from the national recommendations, which specifies referral pathways for key physical problems that the programme is aimed at detecting at an early stage. There have been a number of recent training updates organized by Daniel, with good attendance and an emphasis on clinical technique and referral pathways. Daniel is aware, however, that there is a certain scepticism locally about the value of the child health surveillance programme, especially among GPs who feel they are over-examining 'normal' children.

Daniel decides to look at each incident of delayed diagnosis as a 'critical learning exercise', with a view to sharing the findings more widely. These incidents are clinical governance and risk management issues and require a similar process of 'non-blame' enquiry. He consults members of the DCHP group, which includes representatives of most professional groups involved in the Child Health Promotion programme. The notes of the children in question are collated from primary care nursing, medical and hospital records, as well as regional laboratory data. It soon becomes apparent that there has been a deviation from the expected 'pathway' in each case. In the first case, the GP had made a prompt referral for maldescent of the testis at three months, but the surgeon and clerical staff failed to arrange further follow-up. In the second, there was an error at the point of neonatal blood sampling and testing (a midwife provided insufficient blood and the retesting was delayed).

A number of actions are agreed by the DCHP group:

- Training subcommittee to devise a staff educational session update on testicular maldescent, emphasizing the need for careful physical examination technique and prompt referral to surgical team
- Advice to parents in the PCHR to be reviewed, so that the threshold for self-referral is lowered
- Training and awareness-raising session for clerical staff who record Guthrie test results, stressing the importance of timely reporting of 'insufficient' samples (where too little blood has been collected from an individual child)
- An audit of age at orchidopexy to be carried out between the four surgeons in the hospital to help ensure concurrence with national policy recommendations and to reduce variance

Further reading

Blair, M. (2001) The need for and role of a coordinator of child surveillance/promotion. *Archives of Disease in Childhood*, **04.** 1 5.

Hall, D., and Elliman, D. (2003) *Health for all children (fourth edition)*. Oxford University Press, Oxford.

The Child Health Promotion programme – pregnancy and the first five years of life (2008) Department of Health, England.

Blair, M., and Hall, D.M.B. (2006) From child health surveillance to child health promotion. *Archives of Disease in Childhood;* **91**: 730–35.

Seymour, C., et al. (1997) Neonatal screening for inborn errors of metabolism: a systematic review. *Health Technology Assessment;* **1**(11).

Winter, M., Balledux, M., De Mare, J., and Burgmeijer, R. (1995) *Screening in child health care—report of the Dutch Working Party on Child Health Care.* Radcliffe Medical Press, Oxford.

Scenario F: Mitigating the health impact of social deprivation

Case Study

Max Sanderson, a community paediatrican in South Knowsley NHS Trust, has been asked by the Chief Executive for Oddington Park Primary Care Trust (PCT) whether he would attend a meeting to discuss the PCT's health improvement plan. The PCT has agreed that they should develop a plan to improve child health in Marton Estate, a community well known as an area of severe social deprivation. The practices in the PCT are particularly concerned about the high teenage pregnancy rates, high proportion of low birth weight babies, the high consultation rate for babies and children, and the low immunization rates.

Background

As Chapter 3 makes clear, social deprivation is an important risk factor for a range of child health problems, particularly injury, perinatal and infant mortality, preterm birth, low birth weight, congenital abnormalities, sudden infant death, child abuse, disability, and behaviour problems. Socially deprived communities suffer high levels of crime, and community members are more likely to be exposed to violence. Drugs are often a problem and teenagers are exposed to both drug taking and the opportunity to engage in illegal drug pushing. Social trust is usually low and community members are more likely to feel isolated and unsupported. Such communities often look depressing. However, deprived communities may differ from one another. Some have large populations of people from minority ethnic groups; in some, unemployment is the norm; and in some, single-parent families are very common.

There are many way of defining poverty (see Chapter 5). According to one commonly used measure—the proportion of the population living on less than half the average national income—over one in four children born in the UK are now brought up in poverty. Consistent definitions are important for measuring trends over time, but whatever measures are used it is possible to demonstrate that the proportion of children living in poverty doubled in most Western countries in the 1970s and 80s. At the beginning of the twenty-first century, the UK government has begun to tackle childhood poverty and rates have begun to fall slightly. There is a government target in England for the eradication of child poverty by 2020, but progress so far is slow.

What works?

Health promotion and disease prevention are part of Max Sanderson's job description, but in the five years since he took up his post, clinical commitments have prevented him from developing this aspect of his job—so he was pleased to be asked to the PCT's meeting, and decided that he should prepare himself by doing a little preliminary research. Searching through databases of systematic reviews in the library, he found several from well-respected sources that covered relevant interventions shown to have the potential to improve child health in deprived communities. These identified the following as being of potential benefit:

♦ *Injury prevention*: cycle helmet and seat belt use; smoke detectors; area-wide urban safety measures including traffic calming; pedestrian safety

♦ *Passive smoking*: nicotine replacement and behavioural self-help strategies for parents who smoke

♦ *Pregnancy and STD prevention*: sex education in schools delivered by teachers who feel at home with the subject matter and involving peer education; accessible, confidential family planning services both in GP surgeries and on an outreach basis in schools and youth centres

♦ *Breast feeding* : home visiting and social support, including peer counselling

♦ *Social and educational consequences of social deprivation* including delinquency and school dropout: support for parents including home visiting programmes, both professional and volunteer; group parenting programmes; drop-in centres; early years education programmes; health-promoting school initiatives that take a whole-school approach.

♦ *Infant mortality;* reducing maternal obesity, reducing smoking in pregnancy, reduction in sudden infant deaths by reducing bed sharing and prone sleeping position, as well as household overcrowding. Also reducing relative poverty by increasing income of routine and manual social classes.

Max was interested to read that it appeared to matter how health promotion interventions were delivered. Many seemingly valuable interventions had proved ineffective. He read that those that were developed with the community to meet needs they had identified, and where there was community involvement, were more likely to succeed. He also read that 'multifaceted' interventions (those which involved more than one approach) and multidisciplinary approaches were more effective. It appeared that the interpersonal skills and qualities of the person delivering the intervention mattered for effectiveness.

Max also decided that he should consult the local Trust's health promotion service. He thought he ought to know what was being done already. The Director told him about a range of initiatives which were happening in Marton's schools under the umbrella of the Healthy Schools Programme. The primary school had developed bullying and behaviour management policies, and the secondary school had a very strong and well-supported drug and smoking policy. He also learned that the school nurse in the secondary school was not keen on talking to teenagers about contraception.

Max mentioned what he had learned from his trip to the library and was surprised to find that the Director was not at all impressed. She told him that that sort of evidence was not usually helpful. Did he know that the World Health Organisation had just announced that randomized controlled trials were 'inappropriate, misleading and unnecessarily expensive' in evaluating health promoting interventions? She talked about disempowerment, explaining that it was very difficult for people with no long-term prospects to care much about their future health. She explained that Marton had been on the receiving end of a whole range of well-meaning projects. Many of these had been helpful in the short term, but invariably the project worker had got another job or the money had run out, leaving the community feeling let down and highly sceptical of 'projects'. She said she felt that the areas which were most important were skills development and employment initiatives. These were empowering and helped people out of poverty. She added that it mattered a great deal who was going to undertake the work and that their skills and experience were key. She also said that whatever the PCT did, they must do in conjunction with other agencies. She felt that a rapid appraisal might be a good starting point to gather information about the community's needs and concerns. She also mentioned that she had been part of a group that had put together an unsuccessful bid for a Healthy Living Centre in Marton.

After the meeting Max reflected that although the Director had been so dismissive of the systematic review evidence, quite a lot of it seemed to concur with what she had told him.

Who are the stakeholders?

Everyone is a potential stakeholder in a community health improvement project, but many of those who could be expected to take an interest are likely to be too busy to get involved. The PCT is potentially a very important player, especially in home visiting, parenting support provision, and school health service provision, and they had already expressed an interest. Local authorities need to be involved in employment and skill development initiatives as well as in early years' provision and youth centre activities. Road traffic initiatives are also the responsibility of the local authority. Social services are likely to want to get involved in initiatives which might prevent child abuse or the need for children to be 'looked after'. The police and probation service may want to help in drug and crime prevention strategies. Voluntary organizations may be the only organizations with people trained to provide certain services. Sometimes it is possible to involve local businesses in such schemes. Local authorities should know the history of any of the large number of government initiatives to improve the wellbeing of deprived communities, and the likelihood of accessing additional monies to support any initiative in Marton.

An approach

Reflecting on all that he had learned, Max decided that he should go to the meeting and express an interest in being involved. He felt that the most important thing he could bring to the meeting was an air of realism. He wanted to ensure that the PCT was planning to develop a sustainable multidisciplinary, multifaceted approach.

He wondered whether people from the local authority and voluntary sector would also have been invited, and whether it would be possible to get some members of the community involved. He realized that the first step in any health improvement plan might be to identify sources of funding. Of one thing he was certain—if anything useful was going to come out of the PCT's health improvement plan, they were going to need to take a long-term approach.

Max reflected that he could see this initiative spanning the next ten years of his life, and that it would be novel and attractive to be part of an initiative for which he did not have to assume responsibility single-handedly. He was also aware that it was inappropriate for him to have a clear plan in mind at this stage. In this area of work, it seemed plans needed to be made jointly and his views should not be accorded priority. It might be that none of the things he thought should happen would be addressed in the first instance. However, he also felt sure that it was important for him to be there and to be seen to be supporting the initiative, and to be prepared to be a 'critical friend' of new plans suggested.

The meeting turned out to have been well set up, and most of those who Max had thought about seemed to be represented—although he drew attention to the lack of a community representative. Those present all agreed to support a health improvement project on Marton estate focusing on child health in particular. Much to Max's surprise, the financially hard-pressed PCT agreed to fund a short-term, part-time post to co-ordinate the project initially, and it was agreed that one of the local health visitors with community development training and skills should be approached to see if she would be willing to take on the post. The meeting agreed that the project would begin with a rapid appraisal. The health visitor manager agreed to manage the project and support the project worker. The group agreed to meet quarterly and to consider at their next meeting how they might go about recruiting community members onto the group.

At the suggestion of the community members, it was decided initially to focus on infant mortality reduction. Since there was a definite excess of infant mortality in the area compared to similar areas, this was seen as a whole area priority of political significance and could involve all sectors with long term benefits. Recognizing that infant deaths were a rare event, Max and the health visitor manager worked closely with the commissioners of services to highlight the upstream determinants of infant mortality. A campaign was established based on these determinants, which they entitled the NO Death IS BEST campaign:

N utrition – prevention of **O** besity, folate, vitamin and calcium supplementation

I mmunisation uptake maximise in first year

S moking cessation in pregnancy and postnatally

B reast feeding initiation and maintenance

E arly antenatal booking

S IDS prevention – Back to Sleep and reducing bed sharing

T eenage pregnancy prevention/ support

The campaign was shared with key stakeholders and the Childrens Centre lead arranged a meeting for Max to present the evidence and support along with the breast feeding coordinator and midwife. The following month, all Childrens' Centres in the area were supporting the campaign with materials from the health promotion department and signposting to pharmacies in the area that were offering smoking cessation programmes.

A score sheet was produced to allow the local planning team to keep track of changes in these key determinants and ensure sustained action over a long period.

Further reading

Acheson, D. (1998) Independent inquiry into inequalities in health report. The Stationery Office, London.

Arblaster, L., Lambert, M., Entwistle, V., et al. (1996) A systematic review of the effectiveness of health service interventions aimed at reducing inequalities in health. *Journal of Health Services Research and Policy*, 1: 93–103.

British Medical Association (1999) Inequalities in child health. In Growing up in Britain: ensuring a healthy future for our children. A study of 0–5 year olds. British Medical Association, London.

Implementation plan for reducing health inequalities in infant mortality: a good practice guide Dec 2007 Department of Health, England.

Scenario G: Promoting vaccine uptake

Case study

Jane Farray, local GP in Durnswood, has just notified her second confirmed case of measles in a week to the local health protection team. There has not been a case since 1987, and she is concerned that this might be the beginning of a trend related to poor uptake of primary immunization. This poor uptake resulting from recent adverse publicity about side-effects of the MMR (measles, mumps, and rubella) vaccine and its relationship to childhood autism.

A review of Jane's own practice records reveals a 76% uptake rate for MMR and a 97% uptake for other vaccines. She contacts the public health lead for communicable diseases, Sheila Tellworth, who obtains district-wide data on immunization from the local child health office, where the computerized register is held. This shows that there has been a decrease in uptake of MMR since late 1998 for the whole area and that coverage is now at critical levels for herd immunity. Nationally measles notification rates have also increased (Fig. 8.3).

Background

MMR (measles, mumps, and rubella) vaccine was introduced in the UK in 1988, and led to a dramatic reduction in the incidence of these diseases (see Fig. 8.4).

Vaccination rates are very dependent on public confidence in vaccines and the perceived threat of the diseases being immunized against. There is often a fine balance, easily tipped by perceptions of adverse effects related to specific vaccines. The research reports linking pertussis (whooping cough) immunization with encephalopathy ('brain damage') resulted in a sharp decline in the uptake of immunization in the UK in the 1970s, leading to a rise in the incidence of the disease and increased infant mortality

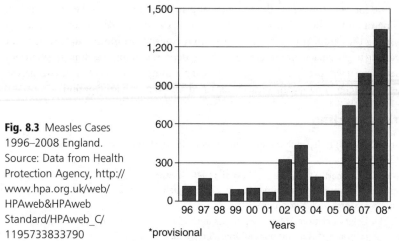

Fig. 8.3 Measles Cases 1996–2008 England. Source: Data from Health Protection Agency, http://www.hpa.org.uk/web/HPAweb&HPAwebStandard/HPAweb_C/1195733833790

*provisional

and childhood respiratory morbidity. It is estimated that it took 15 years for the effects of the 'scare' to subside and immunization rates to return to their previously high levels (see Fig. 8.5).

In that time, there were three major epidemics and many thousand children admitted to hospital with whooping cough and its complications. Dr Farray and her colleagues in Durnswood are not keen for a repeat of this trend to happen in their area.

Vaccine safety

Concerns about vaccine safety have been in existence as long as vaccines themselves. Indeed, following the Vaccine Act of 1853 (see Chapter 4), there were riots in Leicester by the anti-vaccine lobby and popular cartoons of the time depicted, as a side-effect, parts of cows growing out of humans! A clear description of the true side-effects of both immunization and the disease itself is important. Table 8.5 demonstrates these side by side.

There have been a number of scientific studies which have now excluded a causal link between MMR and autism both in terms of biological plausibility and on epidemiological grounds.

What works?

MMR vaccine is approximately 90–99% efficacious, with protection lasting between 14 and 27 years depending on the particular antigen used. Fig. 8.6 demonstrates the effect of having a reduced uptake in a school population of 1000 pupils.

A review of the evidence on increasing the uptake of immunization shows the following interventions work:

♦ Telephone reminders to parents

♦ Postal reminders (linked to the child's first birthday)

♦ Consistent and accurate advice from health professionals

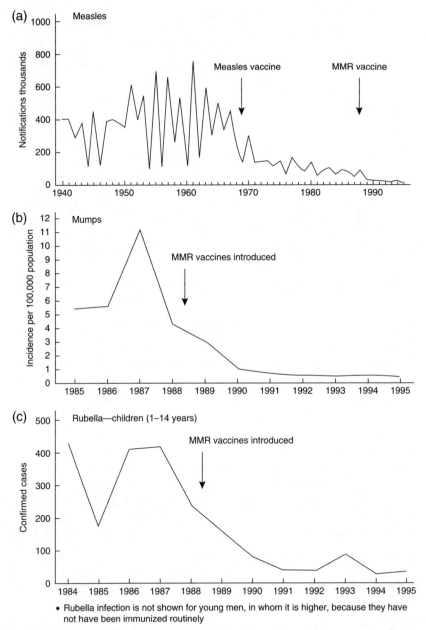

Fig. 8.4 Efficacy of vaccine introduction on the incidence of measles, mumps, and rubella.

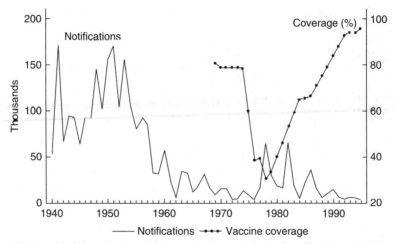

Fig. 8.5 Pertussis (whooping cough) immunization uptake and notifications of disease.

- Regular training and updating of health visitors and practice nurses on common immunization enquiries
- Written parent information which addresses common concerns
- Local immunization advisory clinic/telephone advice line
- Outreach immunization by health visitors for socially vulnerable groups (e.g. children of travelling families, those in temporary accommodation)
- Feedback of immunization uptake to practices, in a graphical form

Who are the stakeholders?

Stakeholders include parents, the district immunization co-ordinator, paediatricians, the anti-vaccine lobby, primary care team members, children, vaccine manufacturers, the Department of Health, and local health promotion departments.

The combination of an increasingly well-educated community, the availability of multiple sources of information (and misinformation) in the media (including the internet), and parents more willing to challenge medical authority, has resulted in the

Table 8.5 Adverse events following natural measles or vaccination with MMR

Condition	Rate after natural disease	Rate after first dose of MMR
Convulsions	1 in 200	1 in 1000
Meningitis/encephalitis	1 in 2000 to 1 in 5000	Less than 1 in 1,000,000
Conditions affecting blood clotting	1 in 3000	Less than 1 in 24,000
Severe allergic response (anaphylaxis)	–	1 in 100,000
Deaths	1 in 2500 to 1 in 5000	0

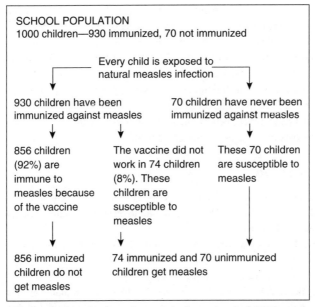

Fig. 8.6 The effects of suboptimal vaccine uptake in a school of 1000 pupils.

need for child public health professionals to become equally sophisticated in presenting the options available. A multi-dimensional approach is needed.

An approach

The district immunization co-ordinator, Dr Farray, and Dr Tellworth arrange to meet to discuss how best to tackle the problem in Durnswood. The Health Protection Agency (www.hpa.org.uk) has just produced an information pack on MMR for professionals with good-quality materials for parents too. The child health system manager is able to arrange for a special reminder to be sent to the parent of each child in the district at the time of their first birthday. It is agreed that this will be sent out together with a brief and well-designed information sheet taken from data given in the HPE pack, acknowledging the main concerns of the anti-vaccine lobby and local parents.

In addition, two of the health visitors in adjoining practices decide to set up a stall at the local supermarket, with the support of the local health promotion unit, to help raise the issue of declining immunization rates and how this might affect the local population. The radio station is invited to do a piece on a local health programme, and a press release is produced by Dr Tellworth for the local free newspaper. All practice nurses and health visitors are asked to attend a compulsory training session which features the use of parent 'scripts' and role play, so that negotiation skills can be improved in addition to acquiring clear and accurate factual information.

Outreach immunization is arranged for those children identified by the computerized child health system as being three months overdue for their MMR and where consent has been obtained already. Clear guidelines are produced for referral to the immunization clinic in the paediatric department for 'difficult' cases, but the emphasis is on empowering those responsible for vaccination to manage as much as possible in the community setting by raising the general level of expertise.

The effect of the programme is monitored on a quarterly basis, with all primary care practices receiving their immunization uptake figures in a ranked graphical display corrected for deprivation score.

Immunization is one of the most cost-effective preventive interventions available. During a period of loss in public confidence in the vaccination programme, it is especially important that concerted efforts are made by all those involved with child public health to restore the balance in favour of increased protection of the community as a whole.

Further reading

Barrett, G. and Ramsay, M. (1993) Improving uptake of immunisation. *BMJ*; **307**: 681–2.

Davies, G., Elliman, D., Hart, A., Nicoll, A., and Rudd, P. (1996) *Manual of childhood infections*. W.B. Saunders.

Department of Health, Welsh Office, Scottish Office Department of Health, DHSS (Northern Ireland) (1996) *Immunization against infectious disease*. HMSO, London.

Horton, R. (2004) The Lessons of MMR. *The Lancet*; **363**: 747–749.

Peckham, C., Bedford, H., Seturia, Y., and Ades, A. (1989). *The Peckham Report National Immunisation Study: factors influencing immunisation uptake in childhood*. Action for the Crippled Child, London.

Peltola, H., Jokinen, S., Paunio, M., Tapani, H. and Davidkin, I. (2008) Measles, mumps, and rubella in Finland: 25 years of a nationwide elimination programme. *The Lancet Infectious Diseases;* **8**: 796–803.

Scenario H: Reviewing the system for investigating suspected child deaths from abuse

Case Study

Anya Clegg is the newly appointed designated nurse for child protection for Sidborough North Primary Care Trust (PCT), which covers a population of 200,000 in the city centre and northern suburbs of a large town in East Anglia. She is concerned to discover that in the last 18 months, there have been two deaths of children on the child protection register within the PCT area. During her first few weeks in post, she obtains copies of the serious case review ('Part 8' review) reports for each of these children in order to find out more about these specific cases and about the workings of the local child protection system and the Safeguarding Children Board (SCB)

Details of cases

Case 1 was a baby aged six months whose mother was a known drug misuser. The baby had been subject to a pre-birth child protection case conference, and he and his two older siblings (aged two and four) were on the child protection register for actual neglect. One previous sibling had died on the special care baby unit after being born prematurely and being small for its date; a much older sibling, born when the mother was 15, had been long-term fostered and eventually adopted and was not in contact with the family. The mother had an abusive partner and the children had spent a good deal of time with their maternal grandparents, but this relationship had diminished since the new baby was born. The mother was in contact with a drug worker and had been on methadone, but admitted to having increased her heroin use again recently.

The baby died while co-sleeping with his mother on a sofa. At post-mortem he was found to be significantly underweight and to have a few superficial bruises which the mother attributed to rough treatment from his siblings, but there were no other findings suggestive of abuse, and the cause of death was found to be sudden infant death syndrome (SIDS). The pathologist was aware that the child had been on the child protection register but had been given no further details of the family circumstances. The social worker in charge of the case had visited two days before the baby's death and found the mother cheerful and the baby clean and apparently well-cared for, but he reported that the flat was 'in a tip as usual', that the older children were inadequately clothed, and that the mother's partner had behaved threateningly when he questioned the mother about the children's welfare. The health visitor had also seen the mother and baby recently when she brought him for his final primary immunizations; she had been quite concerned about his weight and a skin rash and had suggested the mother took him to the GP, but had not yet got in touch with the social worker because she was new in post and unclear about how to contact him. The police had attended the scene of death, but because of a mix-up over communication no sample had been obtained from the mother for a drug screen immediately after the baby's death.

The Part 8 review concluded that professional practice in this case had been appropriate and in line with agreed protocols, and that no acts or omissions by staff could have contributed to the baby's death. It made recommendations about record keeping, communication, staff training and supervision, and other issues, which had been followed up at six-monthly intervals by the SCB. The Coroner was satisfied with the post-mortem report and pronounced that death had been due to natural causes, without holding an inquest.

Anya was concerned that the possible role of neglect in this baby's death had not been adequately considered. She knew that co-sleeping with a parent on a sofa increased the risk of SIDS, especially if the parent smoked or had recently drunk alcohol or taken drugs. She felt the baby's physical condition was indicative of neglect, and that this too had increased his risk of SIDS. Overall, she was concerned about the level of communication between staff in different agencies, both before and after the baby's death.

Case 2 was a seven-year-old with epilepsy and learning difficulties. He had been entered on the child protection register as at risk of physical harm six months before, following an incident in which his father had pushed his mother down the stairs and the child also suffered extensive bruising. His father was, however, currently in prison on remand following a brawl in a pub in which a teenage boy had been stabbed. His mother had been diagnosed as depressed since this event and had been finding it increasingly difficult to manage her son alone. The week before, she had taken the child to the Emergency Department after he had apparently fallen off a chair, but his injuries were insignificant on that occasion and consistent with the story. The social worker had been informed and had visited soon after; her main concern was the mother's mental health, and she had been trying to arrange respite care for two nights a week. A review case conference was due to take place in four weeks' time and the social worker discussed with her supervisor the possibility of altering the category of registration, since physical harm no longer seemed the greatest risk to the child. She had written to the community paediatrician caring for the child and asked whether he would review the boy before the case conference. The special school he attended had noticed no change in his condition or behaviour: his epilepsy had been well controlled for the last year and he had had no fits in school for some time.

The child had apparently been found dead in his bed by his mother when she went to get him up one morning. She said he had shown no signs of ill health the evening before and she had not heard him wake in the night. She admitted, however, taking a double dose of the sleeping tablets recently prescribed by her GP. The physical and post-mortem findings indicated that the cause of death was acute asphyxia. The pathologist discussed the case with the community paediatrician. They agreed that the findings were consistent with accidental asphyxia during a seizure, and that this fitted in with the child's history, although it was impossible to distinguish this cause of death from asphyxia due to other causes, including deliberate smothering.

Again, the Part 8 review had found that no aspect of professional practice in this case had a bearing on the child's death, although it again made extensive recommendations, many of them along very similar lines to those from Case 1. An inquest was held in this case and an open verdict was recorded, but the Coroner was at pains to point out that this implied no criticism of the mother but simply reflected the fact that the post-mortem findings were not clear enough to be sure whether this death was accidental or from natural causes.

Anya was concerned about this case too. She knew that children with disabilities were at greater risk of abuse, and she felt the mother's mental health problems and the 'cry for help' the week before the child's death, when he was taken to casualty with a minor injury, had not been taken sufficiently seriously. Although the Part 8 review's recommendations did address these issues, Anya felt that the question of whether or not the mother had deliberately smothered the child—or indeed had not heard him fitting in the night because she had taken an excessive dose of sleeping pills—had not been faced squarely. She was also not clear that the recommendations from the Part 8 review had made any real difference to professional practice locally: the monitoring reports seemed to her to be a bureaucratic exercise.

Anya subsequently examined six further Part 8 reviews conducted within the SCB's area in the last five years. Many of them raised the same issues and concerns—and the recommendations were depressingly familiar in each. Anya talked to a few colleagues in health and social services who admitted that they were worried about how well child deaths were managed and reviewed locally, about whether lessons were appropriately learned from them, and about broader issues of inter-agency working. Several pointed to the existence of detailed and cumbersome protocols, and to concerns about confidentiality, to explain the reluctance of staff to share sensitive information. Some also said there had been other deaths and near misses locally which they felt should have been reviewed, but that they had no channel for proposing this.

Who are the stakeholders?

A wide variety of health professionals in both hospital and community settings, including health visitors, GPs, paediatricians, A&E staff, the local public health department, social workers and the social services department, teachers and the local education department, the police family protection unit, the probation service, the Coroner, the NSPCC, and paediatric pathologists. Many of these will be represented on the SCB.

An approach

+ At the next SCB meeting, there was an item on the agenda about a recent report from the NSPCC concerning child deaths from abuse and neglect. The NSPCC representative introduced this, pointing out that the NSPCC believes at least half of such deaths are never identified, and that lessons are not adequately learned from them. He reminded the committee about a high-profile case which had been in the news recently and suggested that there may be greater scrutiny of local practice in future. Anya took this opportunity tentatively to share her findings from looking at local Part 8 reviews, and there were many nods round the table and a general agreement that this was not an area which was well managed locally. Child Death Overview Panels (CDOPs) have recently been established in the UK and have specific terms of reference. Anya is asked to lead on the development of a death review panel locally and offered to look at the issues in more detail, and this suggestion was gratefully accepted.

The group included representatives from each of the SCB member agencies

- the community paediatrician, who is also designated doctor for child protection;
- the public health consultant responsible for child protection in the PCT;
- a senior education social worker;
- the social services lead for child protection;
- the Detective Inspector from the Police Family Protection Unit;
- a senior probation officer; and
- NSPCC representative.

They used the most recent report on the Confidential Enquiry of Sudden Deaths in Infancy (CESDI) and other national and international reports to highlight what lessons could be learned. The local death files were reviewed in detail with the paediatric pathologist and coroner to examine local themes.

Findings

Two months later, CDOP was convened to consider the findings from this project and agree recommendations for action. The main findings are:

- Around half of child deaths locally are referred to the coroner, and about two-thirds of these have an inquest. However, the findings are not routinely shared with other agencies.

- Only a tiny fraction of deaths have any multi-agency review, although in addition to the Part 8 review process, a Sudden Unexpected Death in Infancy Review Group had recently been established which looks at unexpected deaths under a year of age but there was a need to expand this for older children since approximately 40% of the deaths were in the later age group.

- Part 8 reviews locally are only conducted on children dying while on the child protection register or looked after by the local authority; 'near misses' are not included. The Department of Health guidance in *Working together to safeguard children* suggests a wider range of cases should be considered.

- Stakeholders expressed concern and confusion about a range of issues, including communication and joint working, the conduct of Part 8 reviews, suspicious deaths which are not reviewed, the impact of reviews on local practice, and the SCB's advocacy and leadership role.

- ◆ The literature review yielded a wealth of information on child death review systems, most of it from the USA and Australia—but few such systems have been formally evaluated, so there is little evidence about their effectiveness.

Next steps

A number of recommendations are agreed with the SCB and CDOP. These cover the following areas:

1 A thorough review of local practice in relation to the arrangements for and impact of Part 8 reviews.

2 Clarification of a protocol following the death of a child to ensure timely notification and action by key agencies

3 An emphasis on improving inter-agency communication, including training for all staff on confidentiality and the Children Act, and specific policies for communication in particular circumstances (e.g. ensuring the pathologist has adequate information before conducting a post-mortem, that all staff have a route for raising concerns about suspicious deaths with the SCB, and developing better links with the coroner).

4 Agreement that culture change is needed as well as practical change—that the SCB needs to develop a more proactive leadership and communication role; that all agencies need to re-establish a focus on child-centred, collaborative working; and that a balance needs to be struck between the safeguards offered by protocols and procedures, and the need to allow staff freedom to exercise their professional judgements in difficult situations.

There is a great deal of energy, enthusiasm, and commitment at this meeting, and Anya feels pleased to have made progress in clarifying the problems and engaging other stakeholders, and in having agreed actions with the SCB as a whole. She is aware, however, of the danger that other issues will emerge and divert attention from this work, and that she and others will have to work hard to maintain the momentum established at the outset.

Further reading

Department of Health, Home Office, Department for Education and Employment (1999) *Working together to safeguard children*. The Stationery Office, London.

Fleming, P. et al. (2000) *Sudden unexpected deaths in infancy: the CESDI SUDI Studies 1993–6*. The Stationery Office, London.

NSPCC (2001) *Out of sight: NSPCC report on child deaths from abuse 1973–2000* (2nd edition). NSPCC, London.

Reder, P. and Duncan, S. (1999) *Lost innocents: a follow-up study of fatal child abuse*. Routledge, London.

Sinclair, R. and Bullock, R. (2002) *Learning from past experience – a review of serious case reviews*. Department of Health, London Child Death Overview Panels CESDI report

Scenario I: Obesity: a public health strategy

Case Study

Julie Birchcroft has just been appointed as Minister of Public Health in the latest UK Government cabinet reshuffle. This is her first ministerial level appointment and she is keen to show that she can make a difference. On appointment to office, she has been given a clear brief to bring about a reversal of the upward trend in childhood obesity. She is aware that the Chief Medical Officers in all four countries of the UK: Scotland, Wales, Northern Ireland and England, have had obesity high on their agendas for the last five years and also that, in some respects, Scotland and Wales are further ahead than England. She is hazy on what has actually been done and what has been achieved. Like many others in the UK she has watched with fascination as a celebrity chef exposed, on prime time television, what has come to be known as the school meals scandal. She knows that like so many other public health issues any policy she produces will need to involve many government departments and embrace both public and private sectors at local, national and even international level. She is aware of the key role played by the food industry and also that this is a political 'hot potato'. She can see that the policy of increasing the number of mothers who are working outside the home may be playing a part in declining nutritional standards in the home. She also knows that many other governments throughout the developed world are working on this issue and that there might be lessons to be learnt from the USA and Australia, which both have major epidemics, as well as from continental Europe where the prevalence of obesity in children is much less than the UK.

She decides that the first step is to commission a briefing relating to the current situation and what has been implemented in which countries. Then she suspects that there will be a need an expert working party to update current activity and develop the next phase of strategy.

Background

In 2006, 17% of 2–15 year olds in England were estimated to be obese and a further 13% overweight. The picture in Europe is similar and the number of European Community children affected by overweight and obesity is estimated to be rising by 400,000 per year. Although the most rapid increases have been seen in the UK and USA, the problem is a global one with 75% of the world's overweight children living in low and middle income countries. There is some evidence that the rising trends may be leveling off in the UK and USA in the younger age groups, but these trends will only be confirmed if maintained for several more years.

Adiposity can be measured in a variety of ways including skin fold thickness, densitometry, scanning using dual energy X-rays, and bioelectrical impedance (BodPod). For practical purposes at population level, measurement is based on Body Mass Index (BMI) (Weight/Height2) plotted on a standard growth chart, with cut offs variously defined: eg 110% of ideal body weight = overweight and 120% = obesity; or BMI over the 85th, 90th, 95th, or 97th centiles.

In children, the main effects of obesity are psychosocial, including social isolation, bullying, and low self-esteem, with resultant lower levels of academic attainment;

whilst rare, Type 2 diabetes is now beginning to be seen in obese children. Childhood obesity is also associated with a range of adverse metabolic and cardiovascular traits including childhood hypertension and abnormal lipid profiles, exacerbation of asthma and, in the Western world at least, an increase in risk of obesity in adulthood. The adverse effects of obesity in adulthood are well known.

Health effects of obesity in adults

- Type 2 diabetes
- Cardiovascular disease and stroke
- Hypertension
- Cancers, particularly of the intestine and reproductive system
- Osteoarthritis and other joint disease
- Back pain
- Skin conditions
- Time off work
- Psychological effects

Risk factors for childhood obesity include genetic and epigenetic variation, intrauterine exposures, birth weight, bottle feeding, and parental adiposity. Children from manual social classes have marginally higher odds (OR 1.14, 95% CI 0.98 to 1.33) compared to children from higher income households, but the differences are small. Whilst of importance clinically these largely immutable risk factors are not of great relevance to solving the problem of the obesity epidemic, which has been caused by a change in the balance between energy input and output among children. Increasing portion sizes, together with snacks and drinks containing a high level of sugar and fat (particularly saturated and hydrogenated fats), reduction in nutritional standards of school meals, reduced outdoor play and independent travel due in part to parental fear of strangers, increased time spent in front of computer and TV screens, the dominance of the car, reduction in school sports facilities and time for games in the curriculum have all contributed. Although there is not a consensus on the relative importance of these various influences, in children the evidence points to the lack of physical activity as a key factor.

The International Obesity Task Force (IOTF) describes an obesogenic environment in Fig. 8.7.

What works?

Governments in several countries have now introduced mandatory measurement of BMI in the school populations. In 2006/7 80% of children in state schools in England were measured at two ages, and one in ten 4–5 year olds and 17.5% of 10–11 year olds were obese using the 95 th centile as a cut point. Legislation has been introduced to ensure that parents are given the results of these screening tests. The extent to which identification of the problem in the individual child effects outcome has not been

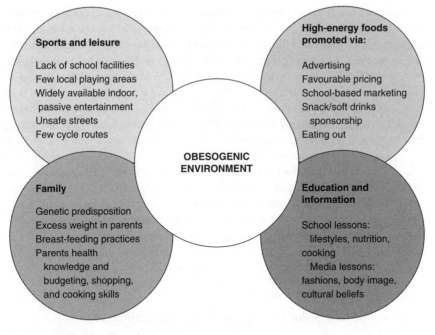

Sports and leisure

Lack of school facilities
Few local playing areas
Widely available indoor,
 passive entertainment
Unsafe streets
Few cycle routes

**High-energy foods
promoted via:**

Advertising
Favourable pricing
School-based marketing
Snack/soft drinks
 sponsorship
Eating out

**OBESOGENIC
ENVIRONMENT**

Family

Genetic predisposition
Excess weight in parents
Breast-feeding practices
Parents health
 knowledge and
 budgeting, shopping,
 and cooking skills

**Education and
information**

School lessons:
 lifestyles, nutrition,
cooking
 Media lessons:
fashions, body image,
cultural beliefs

Fig. 8.7 An obesogenic environment.
Source: Reproduced from International Obesity Task Force, and European Association for
the Study of Obesity (2002). Obesity in Europe: the case for action, IOTF & EASO,
London, with permission.

studied but the programme is certainly raising awareness amongst parents and schools
and providing data for close monitoring of the epidemic.

The evidence base in relation to the prevention of obesity is incomplete, but the
extent and severity of the epidemic makes it important to take a pragmatic approach
to changing the obesogenic factors identified above.

Individual approaches to obesity reduction depend on good motivation on the part
of the child and family. Whilst many families accept the potential harm of junk foods
and are critical of the heavy advertising of such foods in the media, many (particularly
young people) enjoy these foods and resist restrictions imposed on individual choice.
Targeted research has indentified some programmes which enable children to reduce
modifiable risk factors resulting in modest reductions in overweight and obesity. The
changes they bring about, although useful at a population level, are small from a
clinical point of view. There are two main individual level approaches: family programmes and health promoting school approaches.

Because of the limited success of individual programmes, population-based
approaches are critical. As the IOTF 'Obesity in Europe' paper stated some time ago,
Ministries of Health need to move away from the current ineffective approaches based
on opting for 'health education'. Instead, a more structured approach to identifying
the various forces and processes underlying the current 'toxic environment' is needed.
This will require cross-sector collaboration with other ministries.

Foods are a much harder target than tobacco for legislation because of the unending arguments about what is and what is not healthy. Companies who profit from food consumption have clouded the picture in order to avoid any restriction of their activities; suggestions for example that sugar might damage health leads to heavy lobbying by the sugar industry to prove the opposite. The length of time it has taken to restrict tobacco advertising, despite very good evidence against it, suggests that it could take even longer to do the same thing with food. In our profit-oriented society, the measures which are put in place are often those which do not challenge the 'for profit' sector, but there are also examples of co-operative action between major food retailers and producers to reduce obesogenic factors.

Declining levels of exercise in children are related to the growth of motor traffic (the convenience of which has made it very important to a large section of the population) and to television watching, electronic communication in the form of email, chat-rooms, personal blogs, and computer games. As parents themselves become less active, they are less inclined to participate in exercise with their children.

Policies which are generally accepted to have the greatest chance of success in preventing obesity at population level are listed below.

At local level (e.g. community/school)

- ◆ Whole-school approaches to improve nutrition and exercise including;
  - Provision and marketing of healthy options in school canteens
  - Breakfast clubs
  - Provision of free water
  - Provision of free fruit
  - Removal of vending machines selling sweet fizzy drinks and energy dense foods; this measure can be unpopular because vending machines create profit for schools
  - Food preparation and cooking classes for children and young people
  - Inclusion of parents; provision of nutritional information, recipes and cooking clubs and information on the effects of long hours watching television and using computers.
  - Increase in physical activity in the school curriculum and increase in information on the benefits of information
  - Development of Safer Routes to School programmes, which encourage walking or cycling to school
- ◆ Provision of family programmes (eg MEND, Families for Health) offering:
  - Motivation, empowerment, and support for change
  - Development of parents' relationship and behaviour management skills
  - Knowledge and skill in healthy eating: food habits, healthy and unhealthy foods, food labelling, portion sizes, meal preparation cooking
  - Encouragement and support for physical activity
- ◆ Provision of better sports facilities in schools and in the community

- Development of local cycle routes and facilities and promotion of walking and cycling
- Support of farmers' markets and other means to increase availability and reduce costs of healthy foods, especially fruit and vegetables
- Improving street safety for families

At national level

- The development of nutritional standards for school meals
- Co-operative action between the Food Standards Agency and major food manufacturer and retailers to reduce sugar, salt, and saturated and hydrogenated fats in processed foods.
- Changes in agricultural subsidies to encourage farmers to produce leaner meat and lower fat dairy products.
- Better labelling of nutritional content of food
- Food pricing policies
- More funding of sports facilities and support for sport and physical activity in schools
- Legislation to restrict marketing of unhealthy foods aimed at children, both in the media and in schools
- Road traffic reduction measures
- Funding for public transport and cycling, and environmental policies to support walking and cycling
- Support for Safer Routes to School programmes
- Promotion of breast-feeding

Who are the stakeholders?

There are many groups in society with the potential to influence the development of obesity, including farmers, the food industry, the physical activity industry (e.g. leisure companies), local and national governments, child health professionals, educationalists, NGOs – particularly those with an interest in sustainability and the transport sector. There are real political issues arising from the influence on government of food marketing corporations who invest large sums of money in persuading parents and children to purchase their products. The position of the government in maintaining a 'level playing field' is crucial, but most political parties tend to favour the interests of corporations over the public. The press also has a part to play and may attack government approaches which seem to restrict adults' ability to make their own choices about how much they drive their cars, what they eat, and what they feed their children: this is described as the 'nanny state', but is in fact making healthy choices easier to make.

An approach

Julie decides to establish a working party which includes members of the medical Royal Colleges, voluntary organizations, Department of Health, Department for Children Schools and Families, Department for Transport, the Food Standards

Agency, ministries concerned with farming and food, representatives from the food industry, local government and Primary Care Trusts. She established what has already been achieved over the last five years:

- Monitoring of childhood obesity in English schools and sending of information back to parents.
- Nutritional standards for schools developed and being implemented in Scotland and Wales
- Healthy vending machines, fruit tuck shops, free water, and breakfast clubs shown to be practical and implemented in 'beacon' schools
- Accessible information on healthy eating, e.g. the 'eatwell plate' developed to support teaching about food to children and parents
- Food labelling standards under negotiation with the food industry
- Sport England given additional funding for coaching facilities
- Food Standards Agency in discussion with the food industry about fat and sugar content of convenience foods. Some small successes achieved.

The working party takes stock of these achievements together with recent evidence providing some support for the belief that trends may be levelling out. It notes that more has been achieved with regard to nutrition than physical activity. They suggest that:

- Through the network of healthy schools, one in ten schools undertake an audit of physical activity and food each year relating to children and parents
- OFSTED includes breakfast clubs, vending machines, fruit and water provision, canteen options as well as curriculum content relating to food and activity in their school inspections
- Ring fenced funding is to be provided to local authorities to increase play and activity space in schools; to be eligible, schools need to have developed and be monitoring a comprehensive policy to increase children's activity levels at school.
- Primary Care Trusts to be monitored on activity to reduce childhood obesity including provision of family-based programmes.
- Food Standards Agency to press for further improvements in food content and labelling with consideration of legislative action in the next parliament if notable progress not achieved by voluntary means.
- Members of the European Parliament to work with civil servants in UK and Brussels to propose changes to agricultural subsidies that support farmers concerned with raising the nutritional standards in food
- Local Authorities to be encouraged to support Safe Route to Schools Scheme and develop 'play' streets.
- Consideration to be given to national legislation to prevent building on green spaces and develop their recreational potential.

Julie regards these recommendations as an important step forward. Whilst falling short of all that could be achieved, many will be challenging to implement and if successful would be very likely to make a difference.

Needless to say the report is met with considerable opposition from the tabloid press, who resent further advice to the public on food issues on the grounds that 'people know what's good for them'. Head teachers create an outcry about being given further responsibility to solve a problem that society has created and which does not effect educational outcomes. The voluntary sector criticizes the report for having no teeth and for failing to curb the marketing policies of the food industry and, in particular, the marketing of convenience foods on children's TV.

Much to her surprise Julie is able to remain as Minister of Public Health long enough to see some of these changes implemented. However the influence of the corporate sector on government is considerable and it remains to be seen whether the regulation of food companies is strong enough to reduce the impact of the obesogenic environment.

Further reading

Campbell, K., Waters, E., O'Meara, S., Kelly, S., and Summerbell, C. (2002) Interventions for preventing obesity in children (Cochrane review). *The Cochrane Library*; Issue **4**: Update Software, Oxford.

Ebbeling, C.B., Pawlak, D.B., and Ludwig, D.S. (2002) Childhood obesity: public health crisis, common sense cure. *Lancet*; **360**: 473–82.

Edmunds, L., Waters, E., and Elliott, E. (2001) Evidence-based management of childhood obesity. *BMJ*; **323**: 913–19.

Boonen, A., de Vries, N., de Ruiter, S., Bowker, S., and Buifjs, G. (2009) HEPS Guidelines on promoting healthy eating and physical activity in schools. www.hepseurope.eu

International Obesity Task Force and European Association for the Study of Obesity (2002) *Obesity in Europe: the case for action*. EASO, London.

Jago, R. et al (2005). BMI from 3–6 yrs of age is predicted by TV viewing and physical activity. *Internal Journal of Obesity*; **29**: 557–564.

Kipping, R., Jago, R., and Lawlor, D. (2008) Obesity in children. Part 1 Epidemiology, measurement, risk factors and screening. *BMJ*; **337**: 922–927.

Kipping, R., Jago, R., and Lawlor, D. (2008) Obesity in children. Part 2 Prevention and management. *BMJ*; **337**: a1848.

NHS Centre for Reviews and Dissemination. (1997) The prevention and treatment of obesity. *Effective Health Care Bulletin*; **3**(2).

O'Connor, T. and Jago, R. (2009) Engaging parents to increase youth physical activity: A systematic review. *American Journal of Preventive Medicine*; **37**(2): 87–172.

Robertson, W., Friede, T., Blissett, J., Rudolf, M., Wallis, M., and Stewart-Brown, S. (2008) Pilot of Families for Health: community-based family intervention for obesity. *Archives of Disease in Childhood*; **93**: 921–928. doi:10.1136/adc.2008.139162.

Robinson, T.N. (1999) Reducing children's television viewing to prevent obesity: a randomised trial. *Journal of the American Medical Association*; **282**: 1561–7.

Stamatakis, E., Primatesta, P., Chinn, S. Rona, R. and Falascheti, E (2005) Overweight and obesity trends from 1974 to 2003 in English children: what is the role of socioeconomic factors? *Archives of Disease in Childhood*. **90**: 999–1004.

Stewart-Brown, S. (2006) What is the evidence on school health promotion in improving health or preventing disease and, specifically what is the effectiveness of the health promoting schools approach? Copenhagen, WHO Regional Office for Europe's Health Evidence Network (HEN). http://www.euro.who.int/document/e88185.pdf accessed March 2006.

Wang, Y., and Lobstein, T. (2006) Worldwide trends in childhood overweight and obesity, *International Journal of Pediatric Obesity*; 1: 11–25.

World Health Organisation (2008). *Childhood overweight and obesity.* www.who.int/ dietphysicalactivity/chilhood/en/index.html

Scenario J: Tackling child malnutrition, a country approach

Case Study

Happiness Nzuma is the newly appointed Minister of Health in Zambezi, entering office after the first fair election in the country. This followed the death from a stroke of President Bugama, still in office at the age of 90. The country is beginning to recover (following five years of a unity government) from the ravages of corruption and mal-administration and an inflation rate which reached 10 sextillion percent. Large quantities of aid are coming into the country and trained Zambezians are returning from exile in South Africa and Europe. A new hope is felt but the problems are immense, not least the collapse of the agricultural system over the past 15 years. Child malnutrition is at an all-time high, affecting 50% of under-fives. The new President is putting child health at the top of his priority list and has given Mrs Nzuma (a former children's nurse and epidemiologist) carte blanche to work with other areas of government to eradicate malnutrition within ten years.

Nzuma's first action is to study successful examples of nutritional support in other poor countries globally, and the second to tour the country to establish exactly what the problems are from the people themselves, as well as exploring available data sources. The government is committed to take a new approach to its relationships with the outside world and to rigorously ensure that the poor come first and that self-sufficiency is put before the importing of high-tech equipment and large hospitals.

Background

Nzuma takes a systematic approach to the epidemiology of malnutrition. Data sources are inadequate owing to the collapse of the public health system in Zambezi in recent years. Accurate up to date survey data are not available but Nzuma requests her staff to provide answers, as far as is feasible, to the following questions:

What is the current prevalence of malnutrition in infancy, under fives, and older children?

The Fig. 8.8 below shows figures for stunting and wasting in Africa from data collected in 2005.

What is the rate of breast feeding at birth and at one year of age?

Though accurate local data are not available, it is clear that high rates of child malnutrition are present in all East and Central African countries and Nzuma decides that a common approach should be taken within the region. There are, though, specific factors in Zambezi to be addressed owing to the poor agriculture and loss of a local health service. Nzuma also recognizes that there are likely to be several nutritional components of malnutrition: protein, calorie, and micronutrient including iron, zinc and Vitamin A. Over-nutrition is not currently seen in Zambezi though is likely to emerge in the future with increasing prosperity.

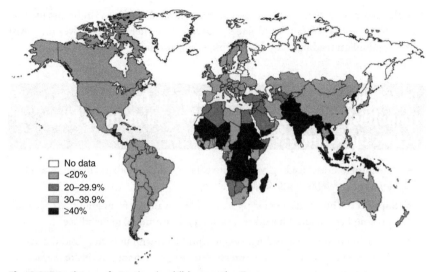

Fig. 8.8 Prevalence of stunting in children under 5.
Source: Reprinted from The Lancet, Vol 371, no. 9608, Black et al., Maternal and child undernutrition: global and regional exposures and health consequences, 243–60, Copyright (2008), with permission from Elsevier.

What is the incidence of associated diseases, specifically measles and diarrhoeal disease?

Once again local data are not available though it is known that there has been a resurgence of measles as vaccination clinics have not been held and the previously over 90% immunization rate has dropped dramatically. Also children were badly affected in the recent outbreak of cholera, which was eased dramatically when Zambezi accepted a major infusion of assistance from Cuba with a contingent of 200 doctors and public health experts.

The conditions with the strongest associations with malnutrition are diarrhoeal disease and measles. Malaria in pregnancy has an association with intra-uterine growth restriction.

Nzuma decides that any measures to combat malnutrition must also reduce the incidence of infectious disease and diarrhoea, through placing an emphasis on the maintenance of high immunization rates and the ready availability of oral rehydration solution.

What is the rate of breast feeding at birth and one year of age?

Once again it has not been possible to obtain up to date figures on breast feeding which was previously 80% at birth and 70% still exclusively breast feeding at 5 months (2000 survey data). It is likely that this figure has dropped significantly owing to maternal malnutrition, HIV infection and the decision of the Bugama government to import infant formula in place of Coca Cola, following a profitable deal with an infant formula manufacturer. However Nzuma suspects that the mothers most at risk will not have used infant formula since a week's supply cost 1 billion Zambezi dollars, a month's earnings for those able to remain in work.

In the absence of data, Nazuma has to rely on local opinions on breast feeding status. Fortuitously, Oxfam conducted a survey of mother's perspectives on breast feeding and infant feeding using focus groups. The results of this are in the Box.

Qualitative survey on breast feeding: Oxfam (unpublished) 20 focus groups of 8–10 mothers from across the country

- **Attitudes** to breast feeding: very positive, but working mothers (if work is available) would prefer to bottle feed

- **Support** for breast feeding: support is widely available from grandparents and other mothers and health workers are not normally turned to for advice

- **Maintenance** of breast feeding: very few problems with initiation, and the overwhelming majority use exclusive breast feeding up to 6 months owing to the lack of food available. However there is quite widespread use of bush teas and herbal drinks in the first 6 months.

- **Duration** of breast feeding: most mothers continue breast feeding until the second year and use breast feeding as a contraceptive, in the absence of readily available contraceptives. However pregnancy frequently intervenes and many mothers say that they prefer to stop when pregnant. They would use contraceptives if they could get them easily, and their husbands would accept this.

- HIV and breast feeding: mothers were not asked their HIV status but this issue did come up in the focus groups and they were aware that it is not necessary to stop breast feeding if the mother is HIV positive. However they did complain about the lack of availability of retroviral drugs during the recent emergency years, a problem being addressed urgently by the Department of Health together with the Gates Foundation (now under the aegis of WHO and newly enriched by additional funding from a UN tax on credit transfers following the recession of 2008-2010).

What is known about the nutritional causes of malnutrition in Zambezi?

Food shortages have been widely reported since 2000 when the production rate from rural farms began to plummet. Turning to international data, the causes of malnutrition can be grouped as shown in the Fig. 8.9.

What works

A governmental inter-departmental committee has been set up which will examine trade issues with the neighbouring Southern African Development Community (SADC – www.sadc.int) countries. This will place sustainability and a low carbon economy at the top of its priorities and will work with the newly established Fair Trade

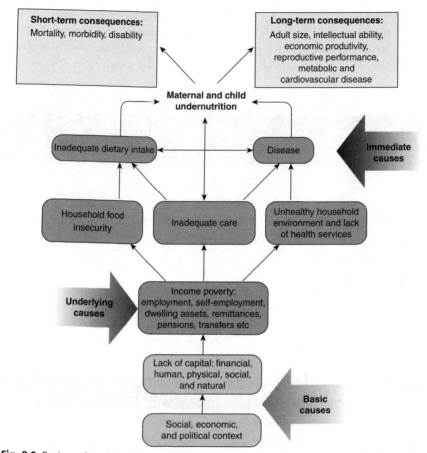

Fig. 8.9 Basic and underlying causes (distal and proximal determinants) of malnutrition. Source: Reprinted from The Lancet, Vol 371, no. 9608, Black et al, Maternal and child undernutrition: global and regional exposures and health consequences, 243–60, Copyright (2008), with permission from Elsevier.

Organization www.wfto.com which has replaced the notoriously rich-world centred World Trade Organization countries will trade locally wherever possible and will sell agricultural products only with fair trade and organic credentials. It has been decided to replace Zambezi's extensive and profitable tobacco farms with maize and wheat, since the world market for tobacco has dropped dramatically following China's institution of a public smoking ban. Part of the land will be used for a Public Cooperative Bank (successor to the World Bank) funded scheme for solar panels to source energy for all the SADC countries, which are expected to be self sufficient in energy within ten years.

It is recognized by the government that women's education is crucial to the success of family planning and child health programmes and there will be a major emphasis on this through public education, improved support for girls in school, and the use of role models – the new government is unique in Africa in having 40% of women ministers.

There will be an emphasis on primary health care, which recent research has shown to be effective in bringing health benefits which a vertical programme (see Box) is unable to do. (see Lancet 13th Sept 2008). Elements that will be included in primary health care, which is now strongly supported by WHO, are shown in the Box.

Primary health care in Zambezi as planned for the future (adapted from Lancet, 13th Sept 2008)

* Training of traditional birth attendants
* Provision of comprehensive family planning in rural clinics
* Curative and preventive care provided in the same clinic
* Use of integrated management of childhood disease (IMCI see Box below)
* Rational drug programme
* Community health workers

Vertical and Horizontal programmes

Vertical

* Programmes initiated centrally (eg at the level of region or country capital) which have a very specific aim eg
* Immunization
* Diarrhoeal Disease control
* HIV prevention
* Breast feeding support
* These programmes are delivered by a central organization without integration at district level. Whilst beneficial, they do not empower the local population and do not facilitate working together.

Horizontal

* A programme which is delivered in an integrated way at district level and includes cure, prevention, and rehabilitation. Primary health care (PHC) as described in the Alma Ata declaration is the prototype horizontal programme,

Elements of both types of programme may be beneficial, but in recent years WHO and UNICEF have favoured the vertical approach and there has been a relative decline in PHC.

Reduction of malnutrition

Experience of means of prevention of malnutrition was summarized in 2008 (see Bhutto).

- Effective interventions are available to reduce stunting, micronutrient deficiencies, and child deaths. If implemented at sufficient scale, they would reduce DALYs Disability Adjusted Life Years (see Chapter 7 for definition) by about a quarter in the short term

- Of available interventions, counselling about breastfeeding, and fortification or supplementation with vitamin A and zinc have the greatest potential to reduce the burden of child morbidity and mortality

- Improvement of complementary feeding through strategies such as counselling about nutrition for food-secure populations and nutrition counselling, food supplements, conditional cash transfers, or a combination of these, in food-insecure populations could substantially reduce stunting and related burden of disease

- Interventions for maternal nutrition (supplements of iron folate, multiple micronutrients, calcium, and balanced energy and protein) can improve outcomes for maternal health and births, but few have been assessed at sufficient scale

- Although available interventions can make a clear difference in the short term, elimination of stunting will also require long-term investments to improve education, economic status, and empowerment of women

Who are the stakeholders?

A regional approach is desirable hence Nzuma requests that SADC countries set up a task force on child malnutrition. This was extended to include maternal nutrition owing to the close association.

Within the government, Nzuma will need to work closely with the external trade minister, education and rural development departments, and the economic secretary. Since the abolition of the Zambezi army (following the example of Costa Rica), defence has become a regional function and this has released considerable funds for human development.

Within the country, other important stakeholders are the voluntary organizations (NGOs) working for improved nutrition, Oxfam and other development charities, local mayors, the traditional healers' organization and women's groups.

An approach

Nzuma summarizes her approach in a paper written for the SADC meeting which will set a ten year programme for the eradication of malnutrition in the region.

1 **Primary health care** Local clinics will be staffed by newly trained medical practitioners who will be well paid to signify their high importance and there will be the adoption of IMCI principles (see Box) and integration of curative with preventive care, particularly breast feeding and immunization. There will be close links with hospitals, and all hospital doctors will be expected to visit the clinics monthly for

follow up and teaching purposes.All hospitals will be expected to implement the UNICEF Baby Friendly principles.

2 **Women's education** The experience of Kerala and Cuba will be studied to find means of increasing the number of girls entering secondary education and there will be incentives to ensure that all girls as well as boys complete primary education

3 **Women's involvement in agriculture** New credit schemes will provide incentives for poor rural women to enter the agricultural sector and business associated areas

4 **Community development** The early experience of training of traditional birth attendants (TBA) which was carried out shortly after independence in Zambezi will be reviewed since the importance of the TBA in child birth is still recognized. Other areas of community support, for example in breast feeding, will also be established.

5 **Self sufficiency in energy** The region will move to reduce its import of fossil fuels through a massive increase in use of solar energy for heating and lighting and a re-introduction of bicycles and electric buses. Individuals will not be expected to own cars and there will be a punitive tax on the import of motor vehicles of all types. Government staff will be allowed to use pooled electric vehicles, but there will be carbon rationing to ensure that these are used fairly and video conferencing will replace international meetings.

Integrated Management of Childhood Illness (IMCI)

Seven out of every ten deaths of children less than five years in the majority world are due to five conditions: acute respiratory infections, diarrhoeal disease, malaria, measles, or malnutrition. There is considerable overlap of these conditions and a single diagnosis is often inappropriate.

IMCI was developed by WHO and UNICEF to improve the management and prevention of illness in children from one week to five years by improving health worker skills, improving aspects of the health system, and improving family and community practices using evidence based guidelines. The interventions are shown in the Box below. The case management approach is as follows:

1 assess the child and check immunization status

2 classify the illness and decide on degree of urgency

3 identify specific treatments

4 give practical treatment instructions to the parent including signs of deterioration

5 assess feeding in children under 2yrs and those with feeding problems, and offer guidance

6 organize follow up

Interventions included in the IMCI strategy

Promotion of growth and prevention of disease	Response to sickness
Home:	
Community/home based interventions to improve nutrition	Early case management
	Appropriate care seeking
Insecticide impregnated bednets	Compliance with treatment
Health services:	
Vaccination	Case management of disease
Complementary feeding and breast	Iron treatment
feeding counselling	Antihelminthic treatment
Micronutrient supplementation	

WHO has carried out Multi-country evaluation (MCE) of IMCI and this has shown the following results:

- IMCI improves health worker performance and their quality of care;
- IMCI can reduce under-five mortality and improve nutritional status, if implemented well;
- IMCI is worth the investment as, correctly managed, it costs up to six times less per child than current care;
- child survival programmes require more attention to activities that improve family and community behaviour;
- the implementation of child survival interventions needs to be complemented by activities that strengthen system support;
- a significant reduction in under-five mortality will not be attained unless large-scale intervention coverage is achieved.

Conclusion

This chapter illustrates how problems may present in many different ways – a concern voiced by members of the local community or a professional, via the media describing a critical incident, or as a result of national policy or local funding opportunities.

Case studies in clinical practice are designed to help inform the practitioner on how best to manage another patient with a similar problem or to illustrate a particular principle which is more generalizable. We hope the examples in this chapter provide some ideas on how to manage a particular child public health issue and perhaps a few general principles which may be useful in dealing with other areas. The framework we have used for structuring the 'problems'– assessing the epidemiology of the issue and evidence base for intervention, identifying the stakeholders, and agreeing an action plan – is the starting point. The subsequent management and monitoring of progress which goes with it is akin to regular review in clinic and is just as important. Both processes have in common that professionals may facilitate and initially manage the process, but the patient or the wider community are ultimately responsible for making it happen and sustaining the desired outcomes.

Further reading

Bhutto, Z.A. et al. (2008) What works? Interventions for maternal and child under nutrition and survival. *Lancet*, **371**: 414–440.

Black, R.E. et al. (2008) Maternal and child under nutrition: global and regional exposures and health consequences. *Lancet*, **371**: 243–260.

Lancet Child survival series (2003). *Lancet*; **362**: 65–71.

Lancet Maternal and Child undernutrition series (2008). *Lancet*; **371**: 243–260.

Editorial: A renaissance in primary health care (2008). *The Lancet*; **372**: 863.

Global Health Studies Resource Guide. Available from www.medact.org/content/Global%20 Health%20Studies%20complete%20file.pdf

Global Health Watch (2008) NGO alternative health report published in 2008 http://www. ghwatch.org/ghw2/ghw2_report.php

Southall, D. et al. (2008) Child Advocacy International: Manual of International Child Health http://www.childadvocacyinternational.co.uk/publications/international_child_health.htm

Blouin, C., et al (2009) Trade and social determinants of health. *Lancet*; **373**: 502–507.

Integrated Management of Childhood Illness see http://www.who.int/child_adolescent_health/ topics/prevention_care/child/imci/en/index.html

Index